Clinical and Pathological Aspects of Skin Diseases in Endocrine, Metabolic, Nutritional and Deposition Disease

Franco Rongioletti · Bruce R. Smoller
Editors

Clinical and Pathological Aspects of Skin Diseases in Endocrine, Metabolic, Nutritional and Deposition Disease

Springer

Editors
Franco Rongioletti
Department of Endocrinological and Medical Sciences (DISEM)
Section of Dermatology and Department of Pathology
University of Genova
Genova, Italy
franco.rongioletti@unige.it

Bruce R. Smoller
Department of Pathology
University of Arkansas for Medical Sciences
Little Rock, AR
USA
smollerbrucer@uams.edu

ISBN 978-1-4939-5099-7 ISBN 978-1-60761-181-3 (eBook)
DOI 10.1007/978-1-60761-181-3
Springer New York Dordrecht Heidelberg London

Printed on acid-free paper

Springer is part of Springer Science+Business Media (www.springer.com)

Foreword I

It is a pleasure to introduce this new book, *Clinical and Pathological Aspects of Skin Diseases in Endocrine, Metabolic, Nutritional, and Deposition Disease*, edited by two of my friends and respected colleagues, Franco Rongioletti and Bruce R. Smoller. In fact, I was very enthusiastic when I learned that they were preparing this work. Although endocrine, metabolic, w, and deposition diseases are regularly included in general textbooks of dermatology and dermatopathology, one gains the general impression that these topics receive little emphasis and are mainly included for completeness. The prospect of having all of this information in one volume, lovingly described and detailed by experts in the field, should be of great interest not only to dermatologists, pathologists, and dermatopathologists but also to internists and endocrinologists, who may well gain a different perspective on these disorders. As a dermatopathologist, I am also pleased that this project has been organized and undertaken by two distinguished authorities in cutaneous pathology. This assures a close integration of histopathology and other laboratory techniques with the clinical aspects of these disorders, which will make it possible – perhaps for the first time – to view these conditions in a truly comprehensive way.

So I invite you, the reader, to open this volume and dig in; be prepared for an eye-catching, intellectually stimulating, and ultimately rewarding experience!

Charlottesville, VA

James W. Patterson

Foreword II

Dermatopathology is a bridge between Dermatology and Pathology. In fact, dermatopathologists are drawn equally from both specialties.

The core of dermatopathology is clinical pathological correlation. While some conditions can be diagnosed on histological grounds alone, this is not without peril. What appears to be a simple seborrheic keratosis under the microscope could represent an epidermal nevus if present in a 2-year-old child. A dermal mucinous deposit makes a mucinosis, but which one? Is it a single lesion or are there multiple lesions? Is there a specific distribution of lesions? Is there an associated condition? The clinical information would likely clinch the right diagnosis.

There are a variety of good textbooks of dermatopathology. However, given the complexity, morphologic variations, and sheer number of dermatological conditions, it is nearly impossible for these textbooks to cover all topics in detail.

Thus, the *Clinical and Pathological Aspects of Skin Diseases in Endocrine, Metabolic, Nutritional, and Deposition Disease* by Franco Rongioletti and Bruce R. Smoller fills the gap by detailing this heterogeous group of conditions, which are often covered scantily and found scattered in different sections of other dermatopathology textbooks.

In a compact yet comprehensive way, this text and atlas covers these dreaded disorders. The blend of tables and photographs provides a concise and user-friendly format.

The combined experience of the editors Drs. Rongioletti and Smoller and their coauthors gives this book a distinct advantage.

I congratulate the editors and the authors for a job well done.

St. Louis, MO Daniel J. Santa Cruz

Preface

We are pleased to present this book entitled "*Clinical and Pathological Aspects of Skin Diseases in Endocrine, Metabolic, Nutritional, and Deposition Disease*" as a labor of love. Dr. Rongioletti has been studying, diagnosing, treating, and researching cutaneous mucinoses and deposition disorders for years and this work represents his dream of consolidating his amassed experiences into a concise atlas and text for the practicing dermatologist, pathologist, dermatopathologist, endocrinologist, and internist. Dr. Smoller has also been actively interested in cutaneous pathology as a window for systemic diseases and has written extensively on this topic. These editors have assembled a distinguished group of scholars to share their collective expertise regarding these entities. It is the hope of the authors that each chapter will provide insights into the clinical appearance and course of the diseases presented, followed by a review of pathogenesis for each disease, and a close inspection of histopathologic changes and any accompanying special studies that might be required to establish a diagnosis. Subsequent discussions address therapeutic options. For each chapter, key points are highlighted with bullet points to summarize the major features. Clinical photographs and photomicrographs have been included as rapid references for the busy clinician or as study aids for the student of most of the discussed cutaneous diseases.

Although we have tried to minimize repetition, some duplication of some diseases is present among the various chapters and reflects the overlapping features of the endocrine and metabolic pathways, in addition to the different perspectives on a disease process. Sometimes, repetition is the mother of the studies (in Latin repetita iuvant).

Dr. Smoller would like to take this opportunity to thank each of the authors who have contributed so generously their time and efforts in completing this project. He would also like to thank profusely his many students and colleagues who provide him with the continued inspiration to continue with his writings. He would also like to extend a work of public thanks to his coeditor, Franco, whose generous offer and hard work made this project a reality. Mostly, he would like to thank his loving wife of 30 years, without whom none of this work would be worth doing.

Dr. Rongioletti would like to thank his coeditor, Bruce, for his dedication and efforts in making this project possible, all the contributors for their expertise, hard work, and commitment, all the colleagues and friends for their encouragement, Richard A. Hruska, Editor, Clinical Medicine at Springer for his support, and his loving ladies, his mother and his perpetual fiancée, for their patience and sweetness. If a doctor in any part of the world makes a correct diagnosis after looking at a picture or treats a single patient in a proper way after reading a chapter or just a few lines of this book, our efforts will not have been in vain.

Little Rock, AR — Bruce R. Smoller
Genova, Italy — Franco Rongioletti

Contents

Contributors

Maxime Battistella, M.D.
Cutaneous Pathology, Department of Pathology, APHP Hôpital Saint Louis, Paris, France

Jameel Ahmad Brown, M.D.
University of Arkansas for Medical Sciences, Little Rock, AR, USA
JABrown@uams.edu

Kenneth B. Calder, M.D.
Department of Pathology and Cell Biology, University of South Florida, Tampa, FL, USA
kbcalder@uams.edu

Bernard Cribier, M.D.
Clinique Dermatologique, Université de Strasbourg/Faculté de Médecine,
Hôpitaux Universitaires de Strasbourg, Strasbourg, France
bernard.cribier@chru-strasbourg.fr

Angelo Massimiliano, D'Erme, M.D.
Department of Dermatological Sciences, University of Florence, Florence, Italy

Giampiero Girolomoni, M.D.
Department of Medicine, Section of Dermatology and Venereology,
University of Verona, Verona, Italy
giampiero.girolomoni@univr.it

Paolo Gisondi, M.D.
Department of Biomedical and Surgical Science, Section of Dermatology and Venereology,
University of Verona, Verona, Italy

Yann Charli-Joseph, M.D.
Instituto Nacional de Ciencias Médicas y Nutrición "Salvador Zubirán", México City, México

Jaqueline M. Junkins-Hopkins, M.D.
Division of Dermatopathology and Oral Pathology, Department of Dermatology,
Johns Hopkins Hospital, Baltimore, MD, USA
jjunkin1@jhmi.edu

Terrence Katona and Bruce R. Smoller
Richfield Laboratory of Dermatopathology, 9844 Redhill Drive, Cincinnati, OH 45242, USA
katonter@gmail.com

Jessica Linder, M.D.
Department of Dermatology, Miller School of Medicine, University of Miami, Miami, FL, USA

Torello Lotti, and Angelo Massimiliano D' Erme
Department of Dermatological Sciences, University of Florence, Via Lorenzo il Magnifico,
104, 50129 Florence, Italy
torello.lotti@unifi.it

Maria Miteva, M.D.
Department of Dermatology, Miller School of Medicine, University of Miami,
Miami, FL, USA

Martina Montinari, M.D.
Section of Dermatology, University of Genoa, Genova, Italy
martimontinari@libero.it

Aurora Parodi, M.D.
Section of Dermatology, DISEM, University of Genoa, Genova, Italy
aurora.parodi@unige.it

Alfredo Rebora, M.D.
Section of Dermatology, University of Genoa, Genova, Italy
rebdermo@unige.it

Camillo Ricordi, M.D.
Miller School of Medicine, Diabetes Research Institute, University of Miami,
Miami, FL, USA

Paolo Romanelli, M.D.
Department of Dermatology, Miller School of Medicine, University of Miami,
Miami, FL, USA
promanelli@med.miami.edu

Franco Rongioletti, M.D.
Department of Endocrinological and Medical Sciences (DISEM),
Section of Dermatology and Department of Pathology,
University of Genova,
Genova, Italy
franco.rongioletti@unige.it

Marcela Saeb-Lima, M.D.
Pathology Department, Instituto Nacional de Ciencias Médicas y Nutrición "Salvador
Zubirán", México City, México
marcela.saeblima@gmail.com

Bruce R. Smoller, M.D.
Department of Pathology, University of Arkansas for Medical Sciences, Little Rock, AR, USA
smollerbrucer@uams.edu

Uma Sundram, M.D, Ph.D.
Stanford University School of Medicine, Stanford, CA, USA
sundram@stanford.edu

Amena Usmani, M.D.
Department of Dermatology, Miller School of Medicine, University of Miami, Miami, FL, USA

Part I
Cutaneous Endocrine Disease

Chapter 1
Adrenal Disease

Kenneth B. Calder and Bruce R. Smoller

Key Points

- The clinical signs and symptoms of Cushing syndrome and adrenal insufficiency include a constellation of findings that can involve most major organ systems of the body, including the skin.
- There are no specific clinical manifestations of Cushing syndrome or adrenal insufficiency which are pathognomonic for these conditions, thus making the diagnosis a challenge.
- Cutaneous manifestations of hypercortisolism include: facial redness (plethora), epidermal atrophy, acne, purpura, hirsutism, and striae distensae.
- Hyperpigmentation is a feature of adrenocorticotropic hormone (ACTH)-dependent Cushing disease, while it is not a feature of Cushing syndrome due to primary adrenal hypercortisolism.
- The most common skin manifestation of Addison disease is hyperpigmentation, presenting as scattered hyperpigmented macules, diffuse homogenous hyperpigmentation, or hyperpigmentation of the palmar creases and flexural areas.
- Pheochromocytomas can rarely present with Addison-like hyperpigmentation or Cushing disease-like hyperpigmentation because of an increase in ectopic ACTH production.

Keywords Cushing syndrome • Addison disease • Pheochromocytoma

1.1 Introduction

As a major part of the neuroendocrine system, the hypothalamic–pituitary–adrenal axis is responsible for numerous physiologic responses including adaptation to stress, glucose metabolism, blood pressure control, sexuality, mood and emotion, and immune response [1]. Corticotropin-releasing hormone (CRH) is produced in the paraventricular nucleus of the hypothalamus and signals the production of pro-opiomelanocortin (POMC) in the anterior pituitary, where it is further processed into smaller peptide hormones resulting in the secretion of adrenocorticotropic hormone (ACTH) [2].

The outer most layer of adrenal cortex, the zona glomerulosa, is responsible for the production of aldosterone which regulates blood pressure via renal sodium and potassium excretion/absorption. The secretion of aldosterone is influenced by angiotensin II, potassium concentrations, and to a lesser extent ACTH. In the second layer of the adrenal cortex, the zona fasciculata, ACTH stimulates the production of androgens, androstenedione, and dehydroepiandrosterone (DHEA) [1]. Adrenal androgens can account for a major component (greater than 50%) of circulating androgens in premenopausal women, whereas in males this number is much lower because of testicular androgen production [3]. Adrenal androgens influence axillary hair growth, libido, and apocrine gland secretion. Finally, the inner most layer of the adrenal cortex is the zona reticularis, which produces cortisol. Cortisol is a diurnal stress hormone with its peak secretion prior to awakening. The physiologic effects of cortisol are diverse and include modification of gene expression in various metabolic pathways, alteration in the response of immune cells, and can cause psychological disturbances [1].

1.2 Clinical and Pathological Aspects of Skin Manifestations

1.2.1 Cushing Syndrome

Cushing syndrome is the eponym used to describe the clinical findings and symptoms related to overexposure to glucocorticoids. Currently, the most common cause of Cushing syndrome is due to exogenous or iatrogenic hypercorticism [4]. The term Cushing syndrome also includes cases of hypercortisolism secondary to functional tumors of the adrenal cortex. To be distinguished from the latter, the designation Cushing disease

K.B. Calder (✉)
Department of Pathology and Cell Biology, University of South Florida, 12901 Bruce B. Downs Blvd, MDC Box 11, Tampa, FL 33612, USA
e-mail: kbcalder@uams.edu

F. Rongioletti and B.R. Smoller (eds.), *Clinical and Pathological Aspects of Skin Diseases in Endocrine, Metabolic, Nutritional and Deposition Disease*, DOI 10.1007/978-1-60761-181-3_1,

includes cases of hypercortisolism due to over production of ACTH as a result of either pituitary overproduction or ectopic ACTH production. Tumors associated with ectopic ACTH production most commonly occur in men and are seen in cases of small cell carcinoma of the lung, bronchial carcinoid, and medullary thyroid carcinoma (MTC) [5].

Patients with the loss of diurnal variation of ACTH and cortisol secretion have sustained increased levels of cortisol and present with the following symptoms: weight gain, psychological disturbances, decreased libido, hyperglycemia, hypertension, and a constellation of skin findings.

The clinical cutaneous manifestations of hypercortisolism include *facial redness (plethora)*, *epidermal atrophy*, *acne* (Fig. 1.1), *purpura*, *hirsutism* (Fig. 1.2), *and striae* (Fig. 1.3). Changes in body habitus are also characteristic of hypercortisolism including: *progressive central obesity (centripetal obesity)* (Fig. 1.4), *fat deposition over the clavicles* (Fig. 1.5) and *the posterior neck (buffalo hump)*, *subcutaneous fat loss of the extremities*, *fat deposition in the cheeks (moon face)* (Fig. 1.6) [6], and rare cases of retro-orbital fat deposition causing exopthalmos [7]. Of note, none of the physical findings associated with Cushing's disease are pathognomonic. The symptoms of hypercorticism in patients with pituitary tumors usually develop over years, whereas those with ectopic ACTH production tend to have a sudden onset of symptoms [8]. In cases with ectopic ACTH production, patients are less likely to

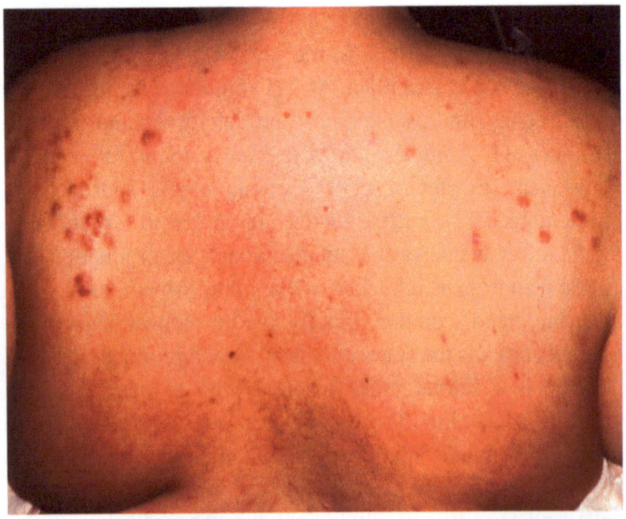

Fig. 1.1 Acne and central obesity in Cushing syndrome

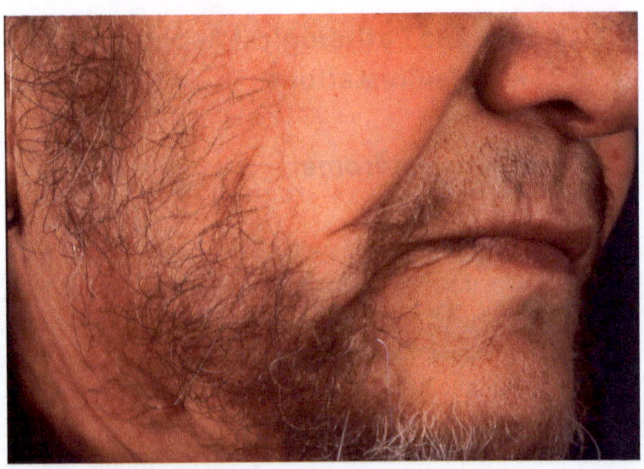

Fig. 1.2 Hirsutism in Cushing syndrome

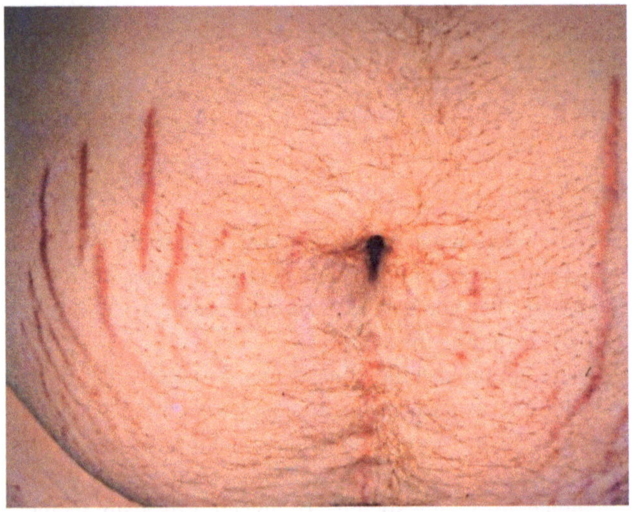

Fig. 1.3 Striae distensae in Cushing syndrome

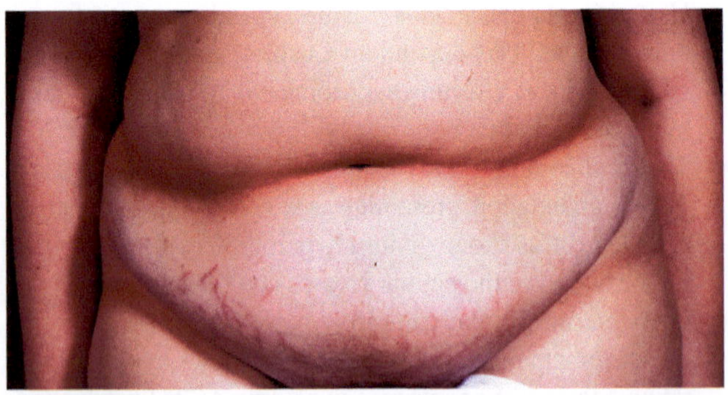

Fig. 1.4 Central obesity with striae in Cushing syndrome

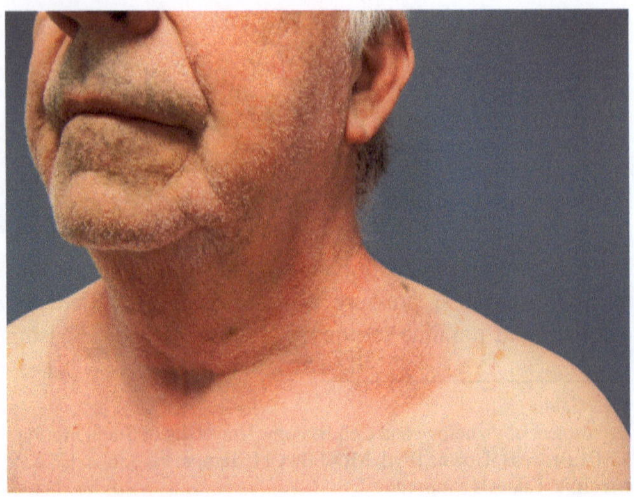

Fig. 1.5 Supraclavicular pad in Cushing syndrome

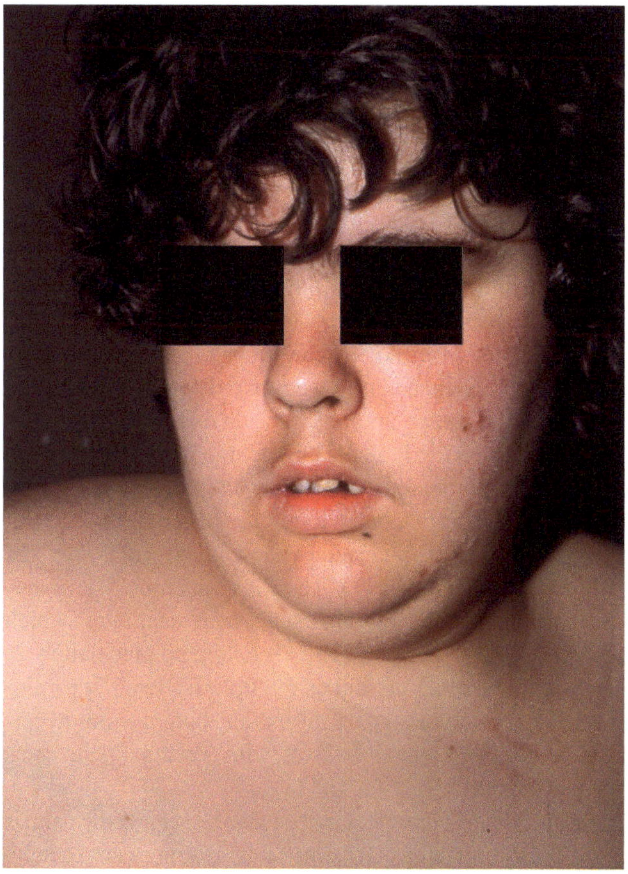

Fig. 1.6 Moon face in Cushing syndrome

be obese and more frequently present with complaints of muscle weakness and hypokalemia [9]. The findings of virilization are usually only seen in cases of adrenal carcinoma [8].

In patients with hypercorticism, the patient's skin can appear atrophic, paper-thin, and translucent. Histologically, there is thinning of the epidermis, loss of the normal rete dermoepidermal junction pattern, and loss of the ground substance between collagen and elastin in the dermis resulting in a disorganized appearance of the dermal fibers [10] (Fig. 1.7). These changes are secondary to glucocorticoid-related inhibition of type I and type III collagen synthesis and reduced hyaluronic acid content of the skin [11].

With the loss of dermal support and decreased elasticity, *ecchymoses or purpura* from minor trauma are more common in areas like the arms and legs. The plethoric appearance of skin is related to dilatation of weakened vessel walls in an already thin epidermis. *Cutis marmorata* and *purplish mottling of the lower extremities* (Fig. 1.8) can also be seen in the setting of hypercorticism because of decreased vascular tone [12]. Striae are characteristic in the setting of glucocorticoid excess, and are typically large, broad, and located on the trunk and extremities. In comparison to the usual striae seen in pregnancy and obesity, the striae in hypercorticism are deep, broad, and purple-colored because of dermal tearing and the translucency of the skin [13].

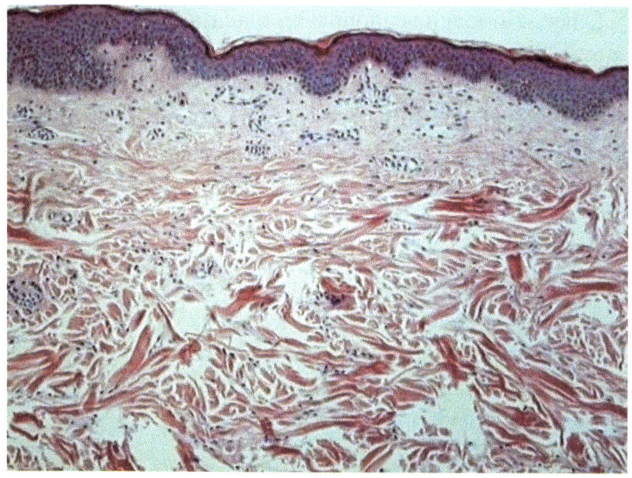

Fig. 1.7 Histopathology of atrophic skin in Cushing's syndrome (HE stain)

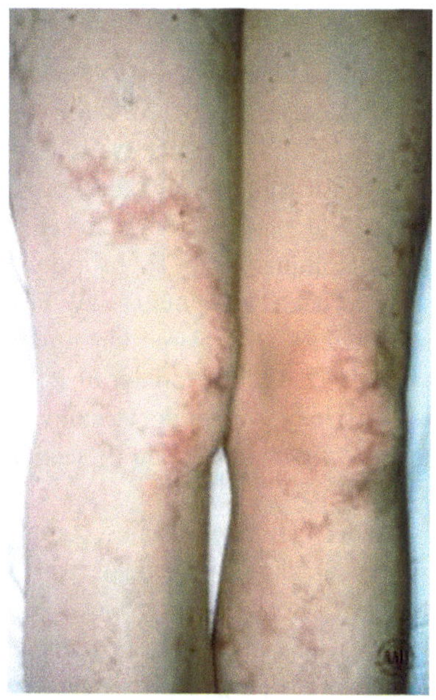

Fig. 1.8 Purplish mottling of the limbs

Hyperpigmentation is not a feature of Cushing syndrome due to primary adrenal hypercortisolism because the elevated levels of glucocorticoids inhibit the secretion of ACTH and MSH.

Other common skin findings associated with elevated glucocorticoids include *hypertrichosis*, *hirsutism*, and *acne*. The acne lesions associated with hypercorticism are typically uniform in appearance, and unlike acne vulgaris, comedones and cysts are rare. In general, acne and hirsutism tend to be more pronounced in cases of Cushing syndrome due to increased production of adrenal androgens which can also cause male-pattern baldness and clitoral hypertrophy. In Cushing disease, the features of increased androgen production are usually more mild and limited to hypertrichosis of the cheeks and upper lips with lanugo-like hair [13].

Other skin manifestations with important clinical implications include the *increased risk for infection* and *delayed wound healing*. The immunosuppressive effects of excess glucocorticoids make patients more susceptible to cutaneous staphylococcal, candidal, and dermatophyte infections. The classic hyper- or hypopigmented scaly macules of tinea versicolor can be seen over the chest and upper back, along with infections by such organisms as *Trichophyton rubrum* resulting in onychomycosis, tinea pedis, and/or tinea corporis [8]. In addition, there are reports of opportunistic infections involving deep fungal infections by aspergillus, zygomycosis, or phaeohyphomycosis in patients with hypercorticism [14].

1.2.2 Addison Disease

Addison disease is defined as primary adrenal gland insufficiency, which can be divided into three general categories: adrenal dysgenesis, impaired steroidogenesis, and adrenal destruction. In Addison disease, the ability of the adrenal cortex to produce glucocorticoids (cortisol) and mineralocorticoids (aldosterone) is compromised, resulting in increased levels of pituitary ACTH. In secondary adrenal insufficiency due to decreased pituitary ACTH production, glucocorticoid synthesis is impaired but mineralocorticoid production is not affected. Therefore, primary adrenal insufficiency is characterized by mineralocorticoid deficiency and hyperpigmentation, not characteristic of secondary adrenal insufficiency [1].

Historically, Addison disease was most common due to the destruction of adrenal glands in patients with tuberculosis. Autoimmune disease, autoantibodies to the adrenal cortex and/or 21 hydroxylase, is currently the most common cause of primary adrenal insufficiency [15]. Autoimmune Addison disease can also be seen as one of the major components of type 1 autoimmune polyglandular syndrome (APS) and type 2 APS. APS-1 and -2 are defined as multi-organ system autoimmune disorders. APS-1 is associated with an early onset (childhood or young adult) and is defined as having at least two of the triad including: chronic mucocutaneous candidiasis, acquired hypoparathyroidism, and autoimmune Addison disease. Other APS-1-associated conditions include chronic active hepatitis, malabsorption, alopecia universalis, vitiligo, and ectodermal dysplasias. The features of APS-2 include autoimmune Addison disease, autoimmune thyroid disease (Schmidt's syndrome), and/or immune-mediated type 1 diabetes (Carpenter's syndrome). The onset of APS-2 can occur at any age, but most commonly occurs in adults in their third decade [16].

The clinical presentation of Addison disease can be rather non-specific making it a challenging diagnosis. Patients can present with complaints of chronic fatigue and weakness, fasting hypoglycemia, behavioral changes, weight loss, salt craving, postural hypotension, nausea and vomiting, and skin hyperpigmentation [1]. The most common skin manifestation of Addison disease is *hyperpigmentation*, which occurs in 94% of cases [17]. The hyperpigmentation in Addison disease can present as multiple scattered hyperpigmented macules or as a more diffuse and homogenous hyperpigmentation throughout the body with accentuation in areas of sun exposure (Fig. 1.9a, b) [18].

Isolated hyperpigmentation can also be seen in the palmar creases, flexural areas, friction sites, recent scars, genital skin, areolae, and oral mucosa (Fig. 1.10) [19]. Darkening of pre-existing nevi and longitudinal pigmented bands on the nails has also been reported in patients presenting with Addison disease [20, 21]. The eruption of multiple new nevi has been reported as an early sign of Addison disease [22]. Of note, there are also reported cases of Addison disease which have been diagnosed in patients with no clinical evidence of hyperpigmentation [23]. Similar to Cushing disease, the *hyperpigmentation* of Addison disease is due to increased POMC production in response to the loss of cortisol-induced negative feedback on the pituitary. POMC synthesized in the pituitary is then cleaved to form MSH and

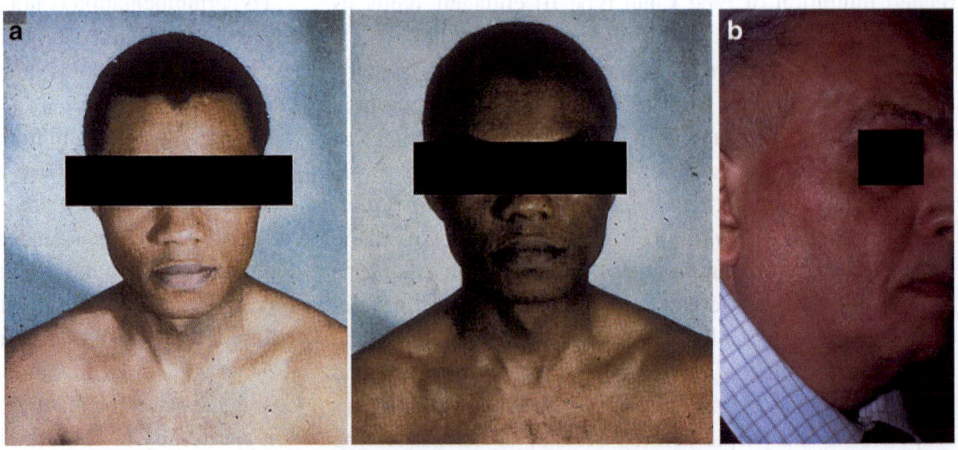

Fig. 1.9 Addison disease. (**a**) Progressive increasing darkening of the face. (**b**) Hyperpigmentation of the face

ACTH, both of which can stimulate melanocytes to increase pigmentation.

In Addison disease, melanin deposition is increased in both the epidermis and dermis with a normal number of melanocytes. In addition, no atrophy or inflammatory changes are present. Melanin granules can be seen throughout the epidermis, but are most concentrated in basal cells and in the tips of the rete ridges. Of note, the intracellular deposition of melanin granules in the basal cells can form a characteristic "cap" above the nucleus imparting a unique histological appearance. Melanin deposits in the dermis are present in melanophages. The proportion of melanin in the epidermis compared with the dermis can vary considerably, but pigment limited to the epidermis is unusual in this condition [24] (Fig. 1.11a, b).

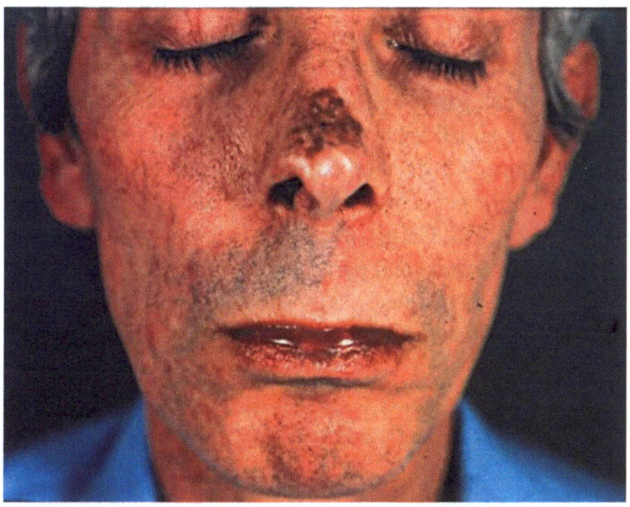

Fig. 1.10 Hyperpigmentation of the lips and nose in Addison disease

1.2.3 Pheochromocytoma

Pheochromocytomas are catecholamine-producing tumors derived from the chromaffin cells of the adrenal medulla. Similar tumors that arise from extra-adrenal tissue (i.e., sympathetic ganglia) are referred to as paragangliomas [25]. Catecholamine-secreting tumors are rare, with an annual incidence of two to eight cases per million [26]. Clinically, pheochromocytomas do not demonstrate a sex predilection, and are usually sporadic, benign, and unilateral neoplasms presenting in middle-aged patients. Patients can present with complaints associated with excess catecholamines, including sustained hypertension (approximately 50% of patients), episodic hypertension (30% of patients), anxiety, diaphoresis, headache, palpitations, angina, tremor, syncope, and nausea/vomiting [1]. Catecholamine-producing tumors have also been associated with ectopic hormone secretion including: ACTH, CRH, growth hormone-releasing hormone (GHRH), parathyroid hormone-related peptide (PTH-RP), and vasoactive intestinal polypeptide (VIP) [27–29].

There are rare reports of Cushing disease-like *cutaneous hyperpigmentation* associated with pheochromocytomas [29]. Skin findings in patients with pheochromocytomas and elevated ACTH include slate-like gray pigmentation of the face, helices of the ear, dorsum of the hands, with more pronounced pigmentation over the knuckles, knees, and elbows. Hyperpigmentation of old scars and of the oral mucosa have also been reported [30]. Cases of pheochromocytomas with associated Cushing syndrome have also been reported. The latter cases may present with features of Cushing's (i.e., centripetal fat deposition, moon facies, hirsutism, proximal muscle weakness, and hyperpigmentation) in addition to anorexia, anxiety, hypertension, headache, palpitations, and diaphoresis [31]. There have also been cases of

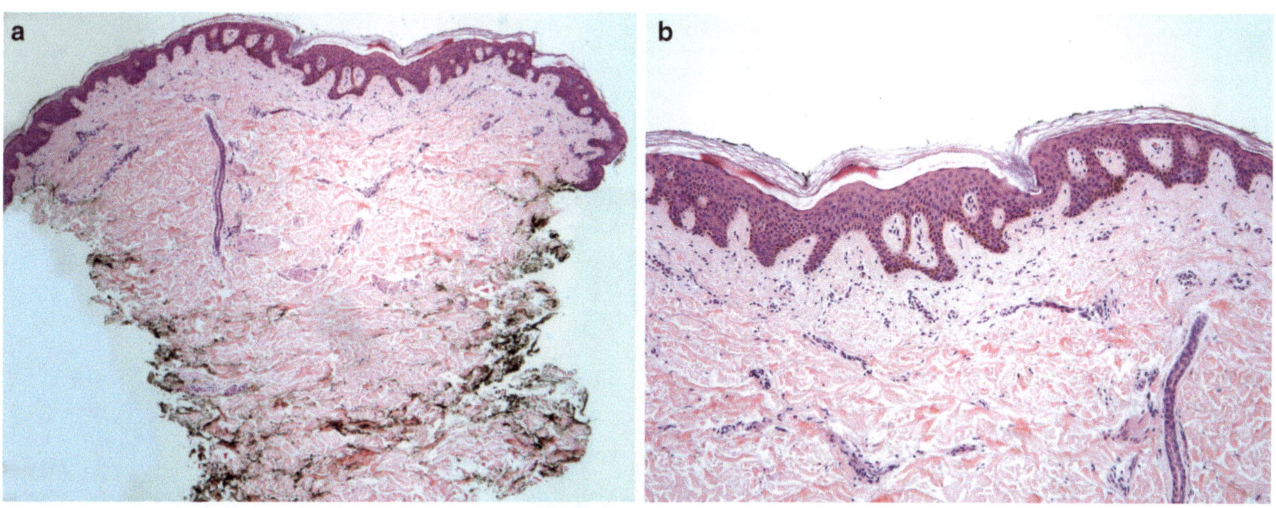

Fig. 1.11 Histopathology of Addison disease. (**a**) Epidermal hyperplasia and basal hyperpigmentation. (**b**) Hyperpigmentation because of melanin deposition is increased in both the epidermis and dermis, with a normal number of melanocytes (HE stain)

patients presenting with findings of Cushing syndrome, increased catecholamines, and hyperaldosteronism [32].

Many of the genetic and syndromic presentations of pheochromocytomas are also associated with characteristic skin and mucosal findings. In multiple endocrine neoplasia, type 2B (MEN-2B) patients can present with a marfanoid body habitus, *mucosal neuromas* (Fig. 1.12), pheochromocytomas (usually bilateral), and medullary thyroid carcinoma. In MEN-2A (Sipple's syndrome), which includes pheochromocytomas, medullary thyroid carcinoma, and hyperparathyroidism, lichen amyloidosus may develop (see Chap. 17). Skin manifestations of MEN-1 include angiofibromas (previously considered pathognomonic for tuberous sclerosis), collagenomas, lipomas, in addition to pituitary adenomas, primary hyperparathyroidism, pancreatic islet cell tumors, and rarely adrenal pheochromocytomas [33]. Angiofibromas are skin-colored, pink or light brown papules located on the central part of the face, histologically characterized by dermal fibrosis, ecstatic capillaries, and stellate cells in the upper dermis (Fig. 1.13a, b). Collagenomas are skin-colored-to-slightly hypopigmented firm papules located on the trunk and neck (Fig. 1.14a). Histopathology shows thickened dermis because of increased amount of collagen and normal or reduced numbers of elastic fibers (Fig. 1.14b–d).

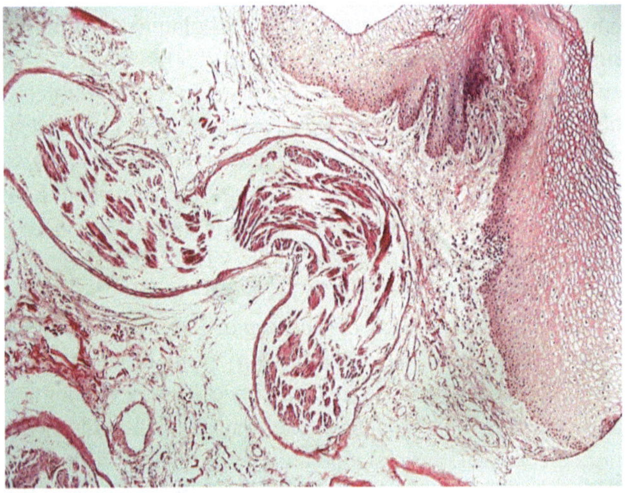

Fig. 1.12 Mucosal neuroma in MEN syndrome type 2B

Other conditions like neurofibromatosis type 1 (NF1) are also associated with pheochromocytomas in approximately 2% of cases [34]. In NF patients, pheochromocytomas can present as a solitary mass, bilateral pheochromocytomas, or as an abdominal paraganglioma. Skin manifestations of NF1 include café au lait spots, axillary and inguinal freckling, and neurofibromas. Other neurocutaneous syndromes which can present with a pheochromocytoma are ataxia-telangiectasia, tuberous sclerosis, Carney triad (gastric leiomyosarcoma, pulmonary chondroma, and paraganglioma), and Sturge–Weber syndrome. In the Carney triad, patients can also present with adrenal cortical adenomas leading to hypercorticism [35].

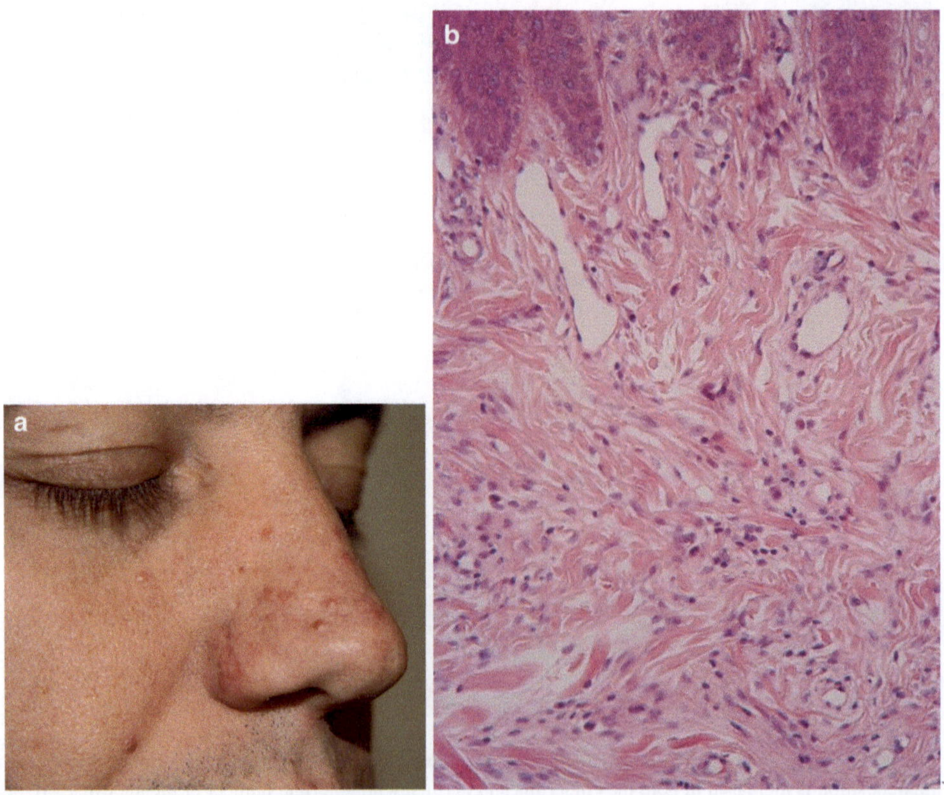

Fig. 1.13 (**a**) Angiofibromas on the face in MEN1. (**b**) Angiofibromas characterized by dermal fibrosis, dilated capillaries, and stellate cells in the upper dermis (HE stain) (Courtesy of B. Cribier, Strasbourg, France)

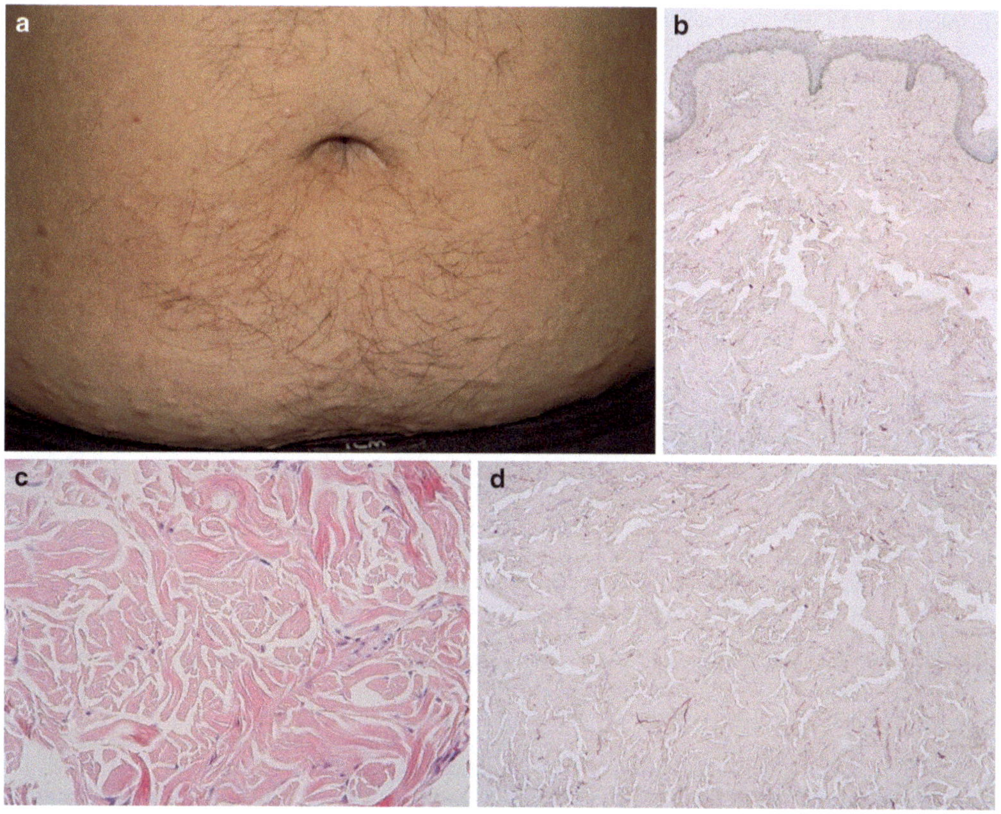

Fig. 1.14 (**a**) Multiple collagenomas in MEN1. (**b**) Histopathology of collagenoma showing thickened dermis because of increased amount of collagen. (**c**) Thickened collagen bundles in collagenoma. (**d**) Reduction to absence of elastic fibers in collagenoma (Courtesy of B. Cribier, Strasbourg, France)

1.3 Treatment and Prognosis

In Cushing disease, the severity of the manifestations does not always correlate with the biochemical indices of the disease. With the exception of striae distensae, cutaneous effects of endogenous hypercortisolism completely heal or improve within the first year after surgical cure of the disease, especially in children [36].

The hyperpigmentation of Addison disease is very responsive to treatment with physiologic levels of glucocorticosteroids, and is one of the more sensitive indices to monitor the maintenance therapy doses of replacement glucocorticoids [37]. In cases of hyperpigmentation secondary to ectopic ACTH production associated with pheochromocytoma, the hyperpigmentation rapidly resolved after the removal of tumor [30].

References

1. Stewart PM (2008) The adrenal cortex. In: Kronenberg HM, Melmed S, Polonsky KS, Larsen PR (eds) Kronenberg: Williams textbook of endocrinology, 11th edn. Saunders Elsevier, Philadelphia, pp 445–522
2. Smith AI, Funder JW (1988) Proopiomelanocortin processing in the pituitary, central nervous system, and peripheral tissues. Endocr Rev 9:159–179
3. Longcope C (1986) Adrenal and gonadal secretion in normal females. Clin Endocrinol Metab 15:213–228
4. Cizza G, Nieman LK, Doppman JL et al (1996) Factitious Cushing syndrome. J Clin Endocrinol Metab 81:3573–3577
5. Carpenter PC (1988) Diagnostic evaluation of Cushing's syndrome. Endocrinol Metab Clin North Am 17:445–472
6. Freinkel RK (1993) Cutaneous manifestations of endocrine diseases. In: Fitzpatrick TB, Eisen AZ, Wolf K et al (eds) Dermatology in general medicine, 4th edn. McGraw-Hill, New York, pp 2113–2131
7. Panzer SW, Patrinely JR, Wilson HK (1994) Exophthalmos and iatrogenic Cushing's syndrome. Ophthal Plast Reconstr Surg 10:278–282
8. Shibli-Rahhal A, Van Beek M, Schlechte JA (2006) Cushing's syndrome. Clin Dermatol 24:260–265
9. Ferrando AA, Stuart CA, Sheffield-Moore M et al (1999) Inactivity amplifies the catabolic response of skeletal muscle to cortisol. J Clin Endocrinol Metab 84:3515–3521
10. Lehmann P, Zheng P, Lavker RM et al (1983) Corticosteroid atrophy in human skin. A study by light, scanning and transmission electron microscopy. J Invest Dermatol 81:169–176
11. Oikerinen A, Autio P (1991) New aspects of the mechanism of corticosteroid-induced dermal atrophy. Clin Exp Dermatol 16:416–419
12. Davidovici BB, Orion E, Wolf R (2008) Cutaneous manifestations of pituitary gland diseases. Clin Dermatol 26:288–295
13. Yanovski JA, Cutler GB (1994) Glucocorticoid action and the clinical features of Cushing's syndrome. Endocrinol Metab Clin North Am 23:487–509
14. Callen J (2003) Dermatologic signs of systemic disease. In: Bolognia JL, Jorizzo JL, Rapini RP (eds) Dermatology. Mosby, New York, pp 718–719
15. Ten S, New M, Maclaren N (2001) Addison's disease. J Clin Endocrinol Metab 86:2909–2922
16. Neufeld M, Mclaren NK, Bilzzard RM (1981) Two types of autoimmune Addison's disease associated with different polyglandular autoimmune (PGA) syndromes. Medicine (Baltimore) 60:355–362

17. Thiboutot DM (1995) Dermatologic manifestations of endocrine disorders. J Clin Endocrinol Metab 80:3082–3087
18. Simpson SL (1950) Addison's disease. BMJ 4689:1164–1166
19. Nieman LK, Chanco Turner ML (2006) Addison's disease. Clin Dermatol 24:276–280
20. Feingold K, Elias P (1987) Endocrine–skin interactions. J Am Acad Dermatol 17:921–940
21. Erickson QL, Faleski EJ, Koops MK et al (2000) Addison's disease: the potentially life-threatening tan. Cutis 66:72–74
22. Ibsen HH, Clemmensen O (1990) Eruptive nevi in Addison's disease. Arch Dermatol 126:1239–1240
23. Kendereski A, Micic D, Sumarac M et al (1999) White Addison's disease: what is the possible cause? J Endocrinol Invest 22:395–400
24. Montgomery H, O'Leary PA (1930) Pigmentation of the skin in Addison's disease, acanthosis nigricans, and hemochromatosis. Arch Dermatol Syph 21:970–984
25. Lloyd RV, Tischer AS, Kimura N et al (2004) Adrenal tumors: introduction. In: DeLellis RA, Lloyd RV, Heitz PU et al (eds) World Health Organization classification of tumours: pathology and genetics of tumours of endocrine organs. IARC Press, Lyon, pp 136–138
26. Stenstrom G, Svardsudd K (1986) Phaechromocytoma in Sweden, 1958–81. An analysis of the National Cancer Registry Data. Acta Med Scand 220:225–232
27. Onozawa M, Fukuhara T, Minoguchi M et al (2005) Hypokalemic rhabdomyolysis due to WDHA syndrome caused by VIP-producing composite pheochromocytoma: a case in neurofibromatosis type 1. Jpn J Clin Oncol 35:559–563
28. Mune T, Katakami H, Kato Y et al (1993) Production and secretion of parathyroid hormone-related protein in pheochromocytoma: participation of an alpha-adrenergic mechanism. J Clin Endocrinol Metab 76:757–762
29. White A, Ray DW, Talbot A et al (2000) Cushing's syndrome due to pheochromocytoma secreting the precursors of adrenocorticotropin. J Clin Endocrinol Metab 85:4771–4775
30. Zawar VP, Walvekar R (2004) A pheochromocytoma presenting as generalized pigmentation. Int J Dermatol 43:140–142
31. Forman BH, Marban E, Kayne RD et al (1979) Ectopic ACTH syndrome due to pheochromocytoma: case report and review of the literature. Yale J Biol Med 52:181–189
32. Bourgoignie J, Dupont JCL, Noiret R (1964) Association d'un pheochromocytome et d'un hypercorticisme du type Cushing avec hyperaldosteronurie. Ann Endocrinol (Paris) 25:269
33. Schussheim DH, Skarulis MC, Agarwal SK et al (2001) Multiple endocrine neoplasia type 1: new clinical and basic findings. Trends Endocrinol Metab 12:173–178
34. Walther MM, Herring J, Enquist E et al (1999) von Recklinghausen's disease and pheochromocytomas. J Urol 162:1582–1586
35. Carney JA (1999) Gastric stromal sarcoma, pulmonary chondroma, and extra-adrenal paraganglioma (Carney triad): natural history, adrenocortical component, and possible familial occurrence. Mayo Clin Proc 74:543–552
36. Stratakis CA, Mastorakos G, Mitsiades NS, Mitsiades CS, Chrousos GP (1998) Skin manifestations of Cushing disease in children and adolescents before and after the resolution of hypercortisolemia. Pediatr Dermatol 15:253–258
37. Burk CJ, Ciocca G, Heath CR et al (2008) Addison's disease, diffuse skin, and mucosal hyperpigmentation with subtle "Flu-like" symptoms – a report of two cases. Pediatr Dermatol 25:215–218

Chapter 2
Pancreas Disease and Diabetes Mellitus

Franco Rongioletti

Key Points

- The main disease concerning the endocrine function of the pancreas is diabetes mellitus.
- Cutaneous manifestations are common in diabetes mellitus, with approximately 30% of patients experiencing some cutaneous involvement during the course of their illness.
- They can be classified as (1) non-infectious, including diseases with strong and weak associations with diabetes; (2) infectious; (3) related to complications because of vasculopathy and neuropathy; (4) related to complications of diabetes treatment.
- Skin manifestations generally appear during the course of diabetes but they may be first presenting sign or even precede the diagnosis of diabetes by many years.
- Patients with type 2 diabetes are more prone to develop skin infections, whereas those with type 1 more often have autoimmune-related diseases.

Keywords Diabetic skin conditions • Non-infectious • Infectious • Diabetic vasculopathy • Neuropathy • Iatrogenic

2.1 Introduction

Diabetes is a common metabolic disease characterized by high serum glucose levels and disturbances of carbohydrate and lipid metabolism that is estimated to affect 151 million people. Famous diabetic sufferers include actresses Sharon Stone and Elizabeth Taylor who went on to lead highly successful lives, despite being diagnosed diabetes at an early stage. Clinically, diabetes mellitus can be classified as type 1 and type 2. Type 1 diabetes mellitus, characterized by a specific autoimmune destruction of the insulin-secreting β-cells in the pancreatic islets, comprises 5–10% of all diabetes. Type 2 diabetes mellitus, which accounts for 80–90% of all cases, affects older and overweight patients and is characterized by a resistance to the action of insulin and inadequate insulin secretion from the pancreas. Other rare forms of diabetes include maturity onset diabetes of the youth characterized by familial incidence of hyperglycemia with monogenic autosomal dominant inheritance, gestational diabetes, drug-induced or chemically induced diabetes mellitus such as steroid diabetes. Hyperglycemia is common to all types of diabetes and leads to complex metabolic and immunologic dysfunctions that induce various patterns of pathology. Of particular importance to the development of clinical symptoms are microangiopathy, macroangiopathy, polyneuropathy, and changes to connective tissue texture [1].

Dermatologic problems are common in diabetes (Table 2.1), with approximately 30% of patients experiencing some cutaneous involvement during the course of their illness [2, 3]. Autoimmune skin lesions are more common in type 1 diabetics, whereas infectious involvement of the skin is more prevalent in type 2 diabetes mellitus [4]. Skin manifestations generally appear during the course of the disease in patients known to have diabetes, but they may also be the first presenting sign of diabetes or even precede the diagnosis by many years.

2.2 Clinical and Pathological Aspects of Skin Manifestations

Cutaneous manifestations in the setting of diabetes can be classified as following: (1) *non-infectious,* (2) *infectious,* (3) *related to complications because of vasculopathy and neuropathy, and* (4) *related to complications of diabetes treatment.*

F. Rongioletti (✉)
Department of Endocrinological and Medical Sciences (DISEM)
Section of Dermatology and Department of Pathology
University of Genova, Genova, Italy
e-mail: franco.rongioletti@unige.it

F. Rongioletti and B.R. Smoller (eds.), *Clinical and Pathological Aspects of Skin Diseases in Endocrine, Metabolic, Nutritional and Deposition Disease*, DOI 10.1007/978-1-60761-181-3_2, © Springer Science+Business Media, LLC 2010

Table 2.1 Skin manifestations associated with diabetes

Estimated prevalence (%)	Disease	Diabetes type	Comment
7–70	Diabetic dermopathy	Type 1 and type 2	Most common manifestation Sign of retinopathy, neuropathy, and nephropathy
20–30	Diabetic hand syndrome	Type 1 and type 2	Increase with age and limits joint mobility
50	Acquired perforating dermatosis	Type 2 > type 1	Patients with kidney failure
2.5–14	Sclerederma	Type 2	Permanent condition in long-standing diabetes
0.3–1.6	Necrobiosis lipoidica	Type 1 and type 2	Weak association in diabetics but 75% of affected patients have diabetes
0.5	Bullosis diabeticorum	Type 1 and type 2	Weak association. Long-standing diabetes with neuropathy
0.3	Granuloma annulare	Type 1 > type 2	Controversial association Weak link between disseminated form and type 1 diabetes
0.1	Eruptive xanthomas	Type 1 and type 2	Associated with high triglyceride-rich lipoproteins
1–7	Vitiligo	Type 1 > type 2	Sign of autoimmune syndrome
4.6–9	Psoriasis	Type 1 and type 2	Metabolic syndrome
0.3 (skin)40 (nail)	Yellow skin and nails	Type 2 > type 1	Palms, soles, and hallux nails
0.8–59	Rubeosis faciei	Type 2 > type 1	Functional microangiopathy
2.5–22	Xerosis	Type 1 and type 2	Sometimes, acquired ichthyosis-like pattern
1.3–3	Skin tags	Type 1 and type 2	Controversial association
20–40	Prurigo/pruritus	Type 1 and type 2	Controversial association; lack of evidence-based studies
1–37	Lichen planus	Type 1 and type 2	Controversial association, some evidence for oral lichen planus
90	Acanthosis nigricans	Type 2	Strong association in selected patients (obese young women of Afro-American and Hispanic ancestry)
49	Periungual telangiectasia	Type 1 and type 2	Common, functional microangiopathy
Unknown	Erysipela-like erythema (acral erythema)	Type 2 > type 1	Microcirculatory compromise mimicking erysipela
4.1	Palmar (plantar) erythema	Type 1 and type 2	Functional microangiopathy

2.2.1 Non-infectious Skin Manifestations

2.2.1.1 Necrobiosis Lipoidica

Necrobiosis lipoidica (*NL*) is a chronic granulomatous condition that occurs in all races and at any age, but it usually appears in the third and fourth decades and is three times more common in women. Although NL occurs in only 0.3–1.6% of diabetics, it precedes the onset of diabetes mellitus in 15% of patients [5], and 75% of patients with NL have or will develop diabetes mellitus [6]. Patients with type 1 diabetes develop NL at an earlier mean age than those with type 2 and those without diabetes. Familial cases of NL not associated with diabetes have been reported [7, 8]. The lesion starts as an asymptomatic, red-brownish papule that evolves into a non-scaling plaque with a yellow atrophic center, surface telangiectases, and an erythematous or violaceous border that may be elevated (Fig. 2.1). In most cases, the lesions are multiple, bilateral, and confined to the shins, but involvement of the face, scalp, trunk, upper extremities, penis, and abdomen at insulin injection sites has been reported. Ulceration occurs in up to 35% of cases, resulting in pain. Rarely, squamous cell carcinoma has been reported in older, ulcerated lesions. The Koebner phenomenon has been unusually associated. Sensory loss because of nerve damage, hypohidrosis, and alopecia has been reported [9]. Laboratory findings are not helpful in the diagnosis of NL, as it relies on histopathology. Histologically, NL is characterized by an interstitial and palisaded, necrobiotic granulomatous inflammation with histiocytes and a variable numbers of Langhans and foreign body giant cells in the lower two-thirds of the reticular dermis, extending into the septa of subcutaneous tissue (Fig. 2.2a). Aggregates of lymphoid cells with numerous plasma cells are typically present around the deeper vessels (Fig. 2.2b). Vasculopathy with thickening of the blood vessel walls and proliferation of the endothelial cells are found, especially in patients with diabetic microangiopathy (Fig. 2.2c) NL may also present with a collection of more typical epithelioid granulomas and less degenerated collagen and vasculopathy. This form seems to have a weaker association with diabetes than the classic one. Direct immunofluorescence studies show

IgM, IgA, C3, and fibrinogen in the blood vessels and at the dermoepidermal junction.

The main differential diagnosis is with necrobiotic xanthogranuloma, which is characterized by yellowish, indurated, often periorbital plaques and the presence of a monoclonal gammopathy, and histologically with granuloma annulare (GA) in which patchy, superficial, discrete foci of granulomatous inflammation with mucin deposition are observed.

The exact cause is unknown. NL diabeticorum has been considered as an antibody-mediated vasculitis with secondary collagen degeneration. Other factors implicated in the pathogenesis of NL include diabetic microangiopathy, impaired neutrophil migration, hyperlipidemia, venous reflux, and borrelia infection [10]. The findings of Glut-1 (human erythrocyte glucose transporter) expression in the areas of sclerotic collagen suggest that these abnormalities in glucose transport by fibroblast may have a role.

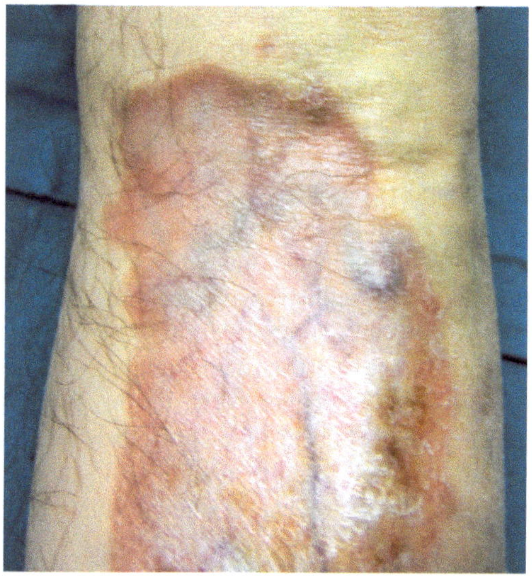

Fig. 2.1 Necrobiosis lipoidica on the shin

2.2.1.2 Diabetic Dermopathy

Diabetic dermopathy (DD) (i.e., *shin spots* and *pigmented pretibial papules)* is the most common cutaneous manifestation of diabetes occurring in 7–70% of all diabetic patients. It occurs twice as frequently in men compared with women, and the mean age is 50 years [4]. DD is commonly seen in diabetics with other end-organ damage such as retinopathy, neuropathy, and nephropathy. Coronary artery disease is present in 53% of patients with DD. Rarely, DD may precede abnormal glucose metabolism. Lesions consist of asymptomatic, bilateral, asymmetrical, well-demarcated, annular or irregular atrophic, brownish macules of 4–12 mm in diameter on the shins (Fig. 2.3). Involvement of the thighs and abdomen has been reported. The lesions do occur in patients without diabetes, but four or more lesions with typical features of DD are considered characteristic of diabetes mellitus [11]. Histopathology is not specific, especially in early lesions, and the diagnosis is a clinical one. Well-developed, atrophic macules exhibit epidermal atrophy, angioplasia of the superficial capillary plexus with hyaline microangiopathy, hemosiderin deposition, and a slight perivascular infiltrate of lymphocytes with plasma cells [12]. DD requires differentiation primarily from purpura pigmentosa chronica and stasis

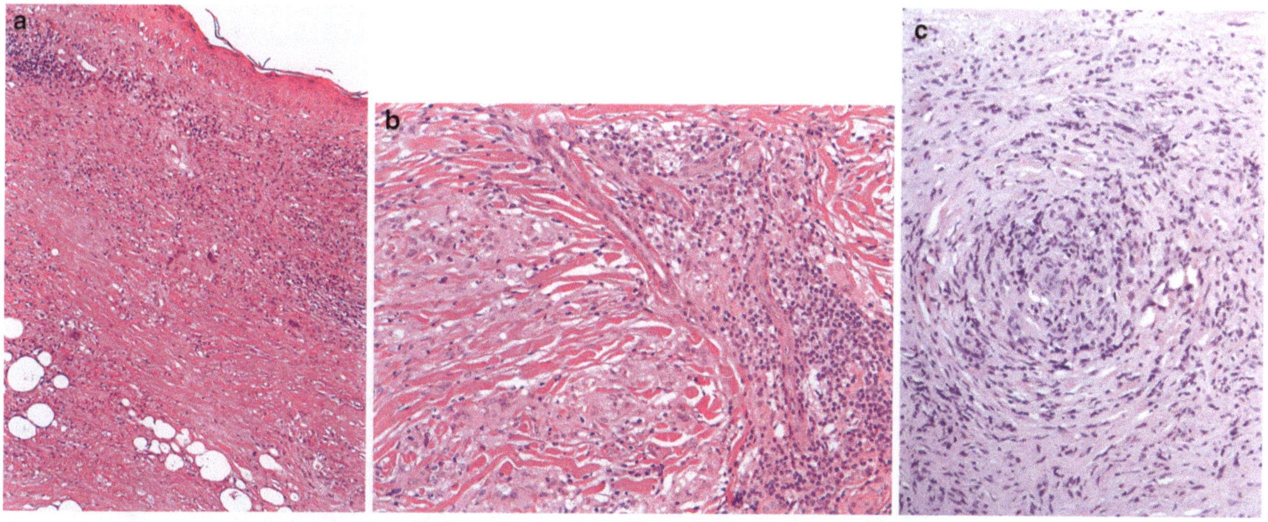

Fig. 2.2 Necrobiosis lipoidica. (**a**) Interstitial and palisaded, necrobiotic granulomatous inflammation with histiocytes and giant cells in the lower reticular dermis, extending into the subcutis. (**b**) Infiltrate with plasma cells and granulomatous features. (**c**) Microangiopathy in deep dermis (HE stain)

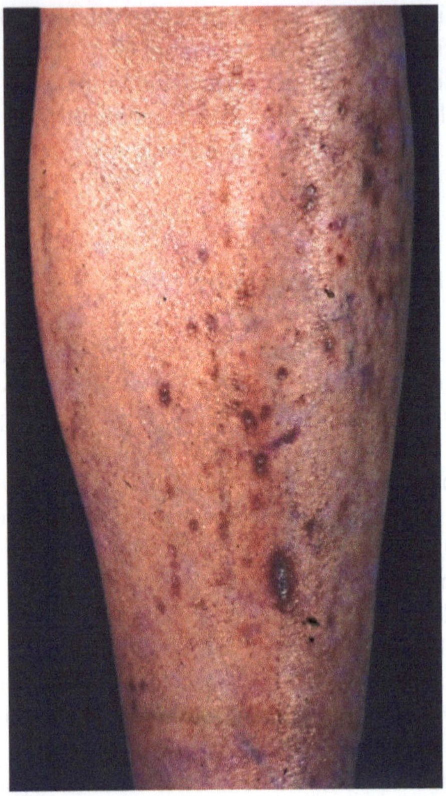

Fig. 2.3 Diabetic dermopathy

dermatitis. Atrophy and involvement of the shins in addition to diabetes are helpful. The cause is obscure but alterations in skin blood flow as part of diabetic microangiopathy and unnoticed trauma have been implicated.

2.2.1.3 Granuloma Annulare

Granuloma annulare (GA) is a benign self-limited, granulomatous inflammatory disease. When discussing skin conditions in the setting of diabetes, GA is always mentioned but the link between the two conditions has been debated. Recent studies have failed to show conclusively any link between GA and type 2 diabetes [13], although a weak link with type 1 diabetes has been demonstrated. This correlation seems to be more likely with the disseminated form than with localized variants [14]. GA has also been associated with autoimmune diseases like SLE, thyroid disease, HIV infection, giant cell arteritis, lymphoproliferative conditions, and solid tumors [15].

GA is typically a papular disease which can be divided into a localized, disseminated (more than ten lesions involving trunk and limbs), or linear type. The most common presentation is the localized, papular form (80% of cases) that occurs before the age of 30, most commonly in children and it is twice as often in females. The lesions typically are located on the dorsa of the hands and feet and are characterized by multiple, small, skin-colored or erythematous papules that coalesce into an arcuate or annular pattern (Fig. 2.4).

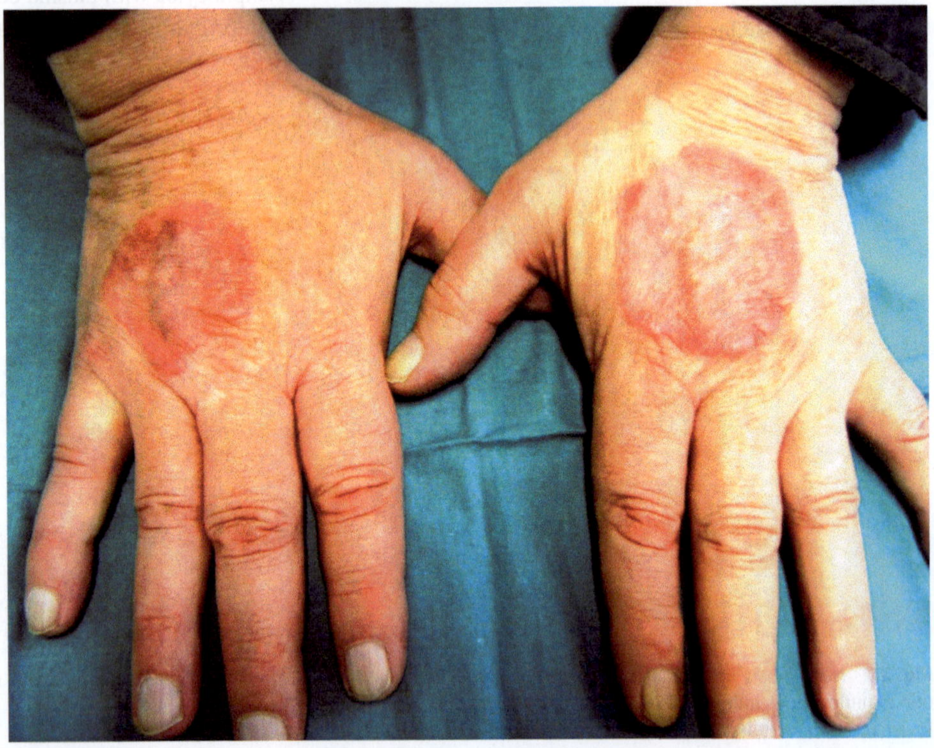

Fig. 2.4 Granuloma annulare

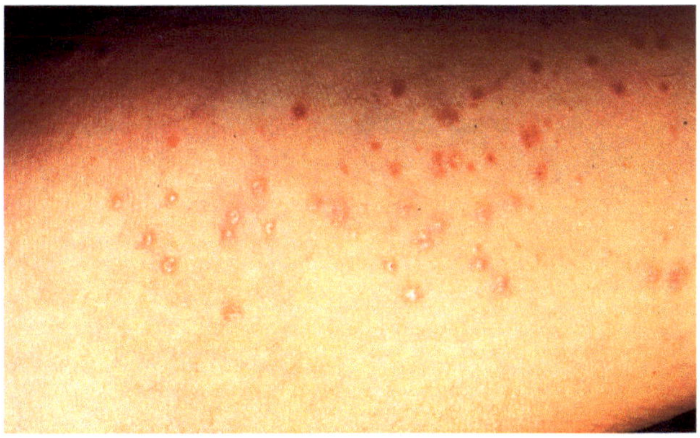

Fig. 2.5 Granuloma annulare papular type

The pure (micro) papular form without annular pattern is less frequent (Fig. 2.5). Disseminated, papular GA occurs in 15% of cases, prevailing in middle-aged and elderly patients. It is characterized by hundreds to thousands of small, skin-colored-to-erythematous papules that are distributed symmetrically on the extremities and trunk. Disseminated GA is the most common clinical pattern in HIV infection. Other main clinical variants include: perforating type with central umbilication or crusts, subcutaneous (deep) type (also known as pseudo-rheumatoid nodule) most commonly observed in children, and patch type characterized by red-brown patches without evident papular component or scale that may or may not have an annular configuration on the trunk and extremities (Fig. 2.6). GA is usually asymptomatic but an acute-onset, painful acral form has been described. Any atypical form of GA should alert to the possibility of a paraneoplastic link [16]. Follicular pustular cases have been rarely described as well as atypical site of involvement such as the face, the palms, and penis. Systemic involvement such as anterior uveitis is an exceptional event [17].

Three histological patterns are typically recognized: necrobiotic granuloma (classic) pattern, interstitial or "incomplete" form, and the sarcoidal or tuberculoid type.

The classic (necrobiotic granuloma pattern) consists of areas of degenerated collagen filled with mucin surrounded by histiocytes and a variable numbers of multinucleate giant cells in a peripheral rim, forming a palisaded pattern (Fig. 2.7). Occasionally, neutrophils or nuclear fragments are seen inside the granuloma. Vessel involvement with fibrinoid deposition and endothelial swelling and true vasculitis are rarely found and are said to be predictive of associated systemic disease [18]. A perivascular infiltrate of lymphocytes with some eosinophils may also be seen. In subcutaneous GA, areas of necrobiosis are often larger than in the superficial type and are located into deep dermis and/or subacutis. Eosinophils are said to be more common in this variant. In perforating GA, a central epidermal perforation communicates with underlying necrobiotic granuloma. The interstitial or "incomplete" form is the most common pattern, in which lymphocytes and histiocytes infiltrate between collagen fibers in the absence of areas of degenerated collagen with interstitial mucin (Fig. 2.8). The non-necrobiotic sarcoidal or tuberculoid type of GA is the least common pattern. Immunohistochemistry reveals a broad, intense expression of CD68/PGM1 in the histiocytic population [19].

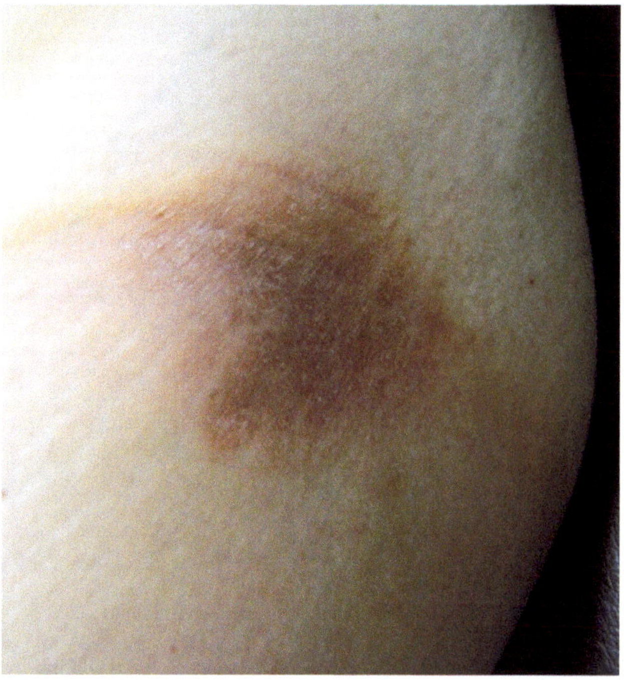

Fig. 2.6 Granuloma annulare patch type

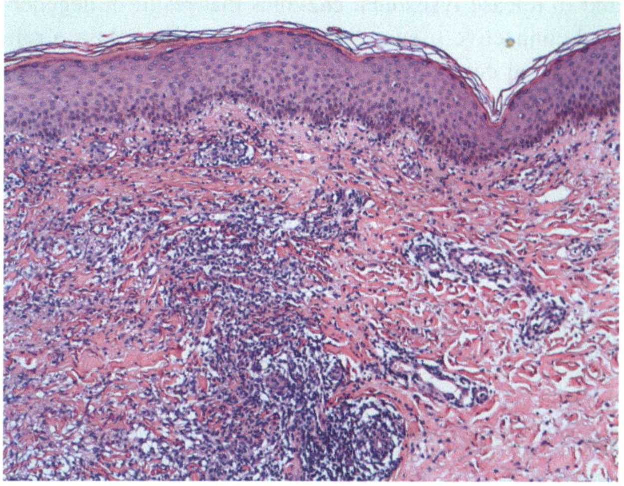

Fig. 2.7 Granuloma annular, necrobiotic pattern (HE stain)

GA is diagnosed based on clinical and pathological correlation and no laboratory tests are helpful. Although the pathogenesis of GA remains uncertain, GA is considered

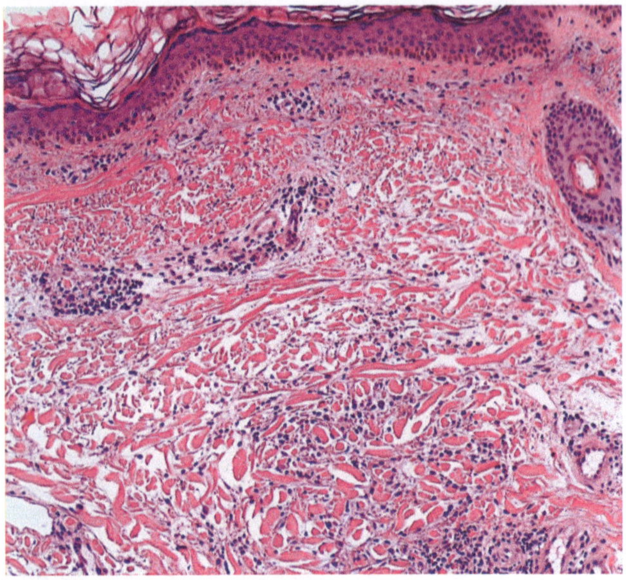

Fig. 2.8 Interstitial type of granuloma annulare (HE stain)

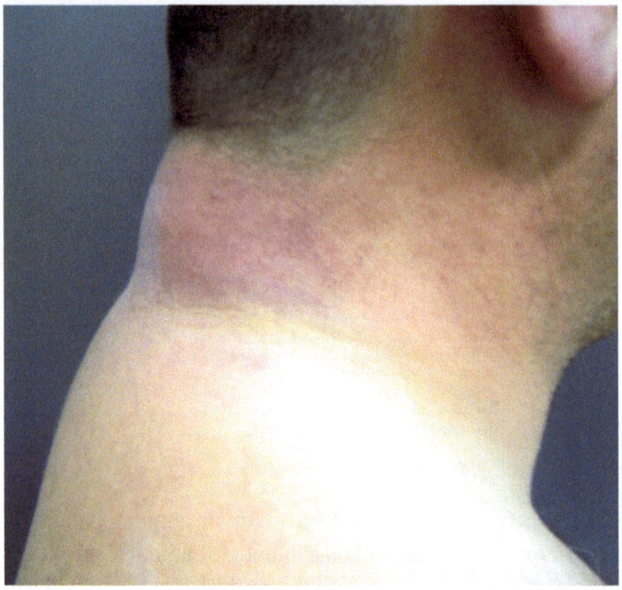

Fig. 2.9 Scleredema diabeticorum

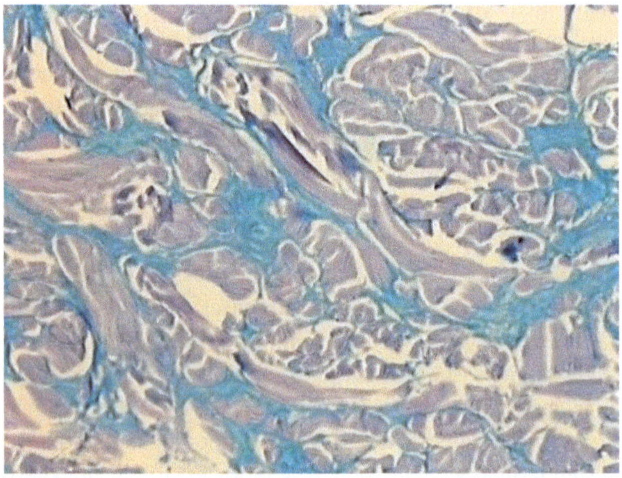

Fig. 2.10 Scleredema with large collagen bundles separated from one another by clear spaces filled with mucin (Alcian blue stain)

a Th1 inflammatory-delayed reaction with the release of cytokines, including macrophage inhibitor factor, which cause histiocytes to accumulate in the necrobiotic areas and to release lysosomal enzymes that result in degenerated connective tissue. A genetic component plays a role as familial cases have been reported and the generalized form has been significantly associated with HLA-BW35. An immunoglobulin-mediated vasculitis also has been proposed. Triggering pathogenetic associations include insect bites, Bartonella and Borrelia infection [20], HIV, Epstein-Barr virus, herpes zoster, hepatitis C virus, trauma, intralesional skin tests, erythema multiforme, exposure to ultraviolet light, and scars secondary to herpes zoster.

2.2.1.4 Diabetic Thick Skin

Diabetic thick skin is seen both in type 1 and type 2 diabetic patients. Diabetic patients with neurological disorders have a significant increase in skin thickness versus diabetic patients without neuropathy. Two forms are described: *scleredema* and *diabetic hand syndrome*, which share a common histopathology characterized by thickened dermis and deposition of mucin. As for pathogenesis, an irreversible glycosylation of collagen and resistance to degradation by collagenase could lead to an accumulation of collagen. Alternatively, excess stimulation by insulin, microvascular damage, and hypoxia could increase the synthesis of collagen and mucin.

Scleredema diabeticorum occurs in 2.5–14% of patients with obesity and long-standing, poorly controlled diabetes, with micro and macroangiopathies (see also Chap. 18). The clinical findings are characterized by symmetric non-pitting induration of the posterolateral aspects of the neck and upper back (Fig. 2.9), occasionally extending to the deltoid and lumbar regions. A *peau d'orange* appearance of the skin can occur, often with decreased sensitivity to pain and touch. The onset is subtle and the involvement persistent. Systemic manifestations may include serositis, dysarthria, dysphagia, myositis, parotitis, and ocular and cardiac abnormalities. Histopathology discloses thickening of the reticular dermis, with large collagen bundles separated from one another by clear spaces filled with mucin, resulting in fenestration of the dermis (Fig. 2.10). Direct immunofluorescence is usually negative, but IgG and C3 have been found at the dermal–epidermal junction. Mucin also accumulates in skeletal

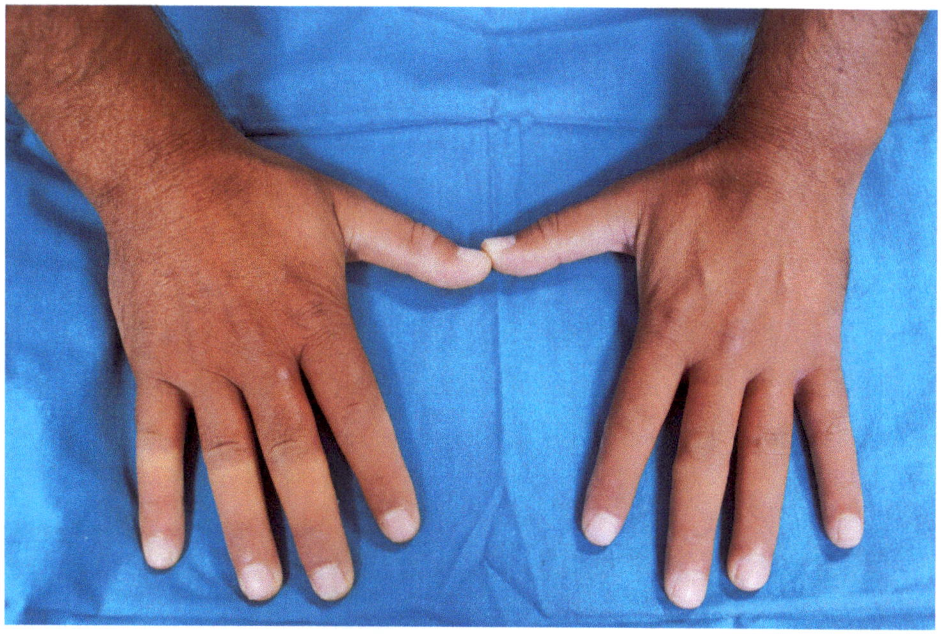

Fig. 2.11 Diabetic thick skin of the hand (pebble hands)

muscle and the heart. Diabetic scleredema does not undergo spontaneous resolution.

Thickening of the skin on the dorsum of the hands, also known as *diabetic hand syndrome* or *diabetic sclerodactyly*, occurs in 20–30% of both diabetic type 1 and diabetic type 2 patients [21]. Clinical presentations range from pebbled knuckles (or Huntley papules) that are multiple minute papules, grouped on the extensor side of the fingers, on the knuckles, or on the periungual surface that progress to stiffness of the metacarpophalangeal and proximal interphalangeal joints, limiting joint mobility (Fig. 2.11). Cheiroarthropathy, known as the prayer sign, is the inability to appose the palmar surfaces when pressing the hands together and is considered an indicator of limited joint mobility. Dupuytren contracture (or palmar fascial thickening) may further complicate diabetic hand syndrome. The thickening is measurable by ultrasonography and tends to increase with age. The histopathologic findings of diabetic sclerodactyly show a thick dermis, increased cross-linked collagen in the reticular dermis, and small amounts of mucin. It is important to distinguish between diabetic thick skin and scleroderma.

2.2.1.5 Bullosis Diabeticorum

Bullosis diabeticorum or diabetic bullae or bullous disease of diabetes is a non-inflammatory blistering condition occurring in 0.16–0.5% of patients with type 2 diabetes. The bullae are seen more frequently in adult men with long-standing diabetes and neuropathy but they may also be the first presentation of diabetes [22]. Diabetic bullae most often present as painless, tense, superficial bullae that occur in an acral distribution, mostly on the legs and feet (Fig. 2.12). Complications such as secondary bacterial infection, hemorrhage, or osteomyelitis may occur. Diabetic bullae have a heterogeneous histologic presentation as the blister may appear in a subcorneal, intraepidermal, or subepidermal location (Fig. 2.13). Dermal changes such as capillary wall thickening and dermal sclerosis reflect the patient's underlying diabetes mellitus. Caterpillar bodies typical of porphyria have been rarely reported. Direct immunofluorescence studies are negative. Trauma, diabetic neuropathy, and microangiopathy all could play a role. The differential diagnosis

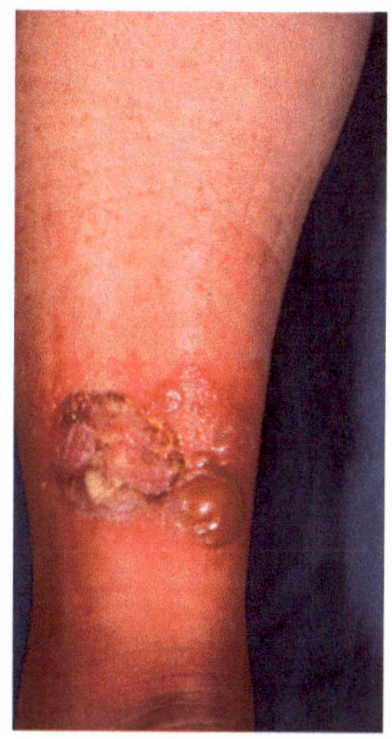

Fig. 2.12 Bullosis diabeticorum

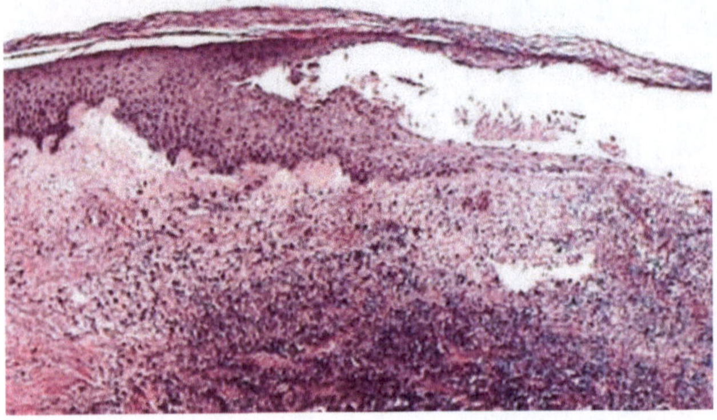

Fig. 2.13 Subepidermal and intraepidermal bulla of bullosis diabeticorum (HE stain)

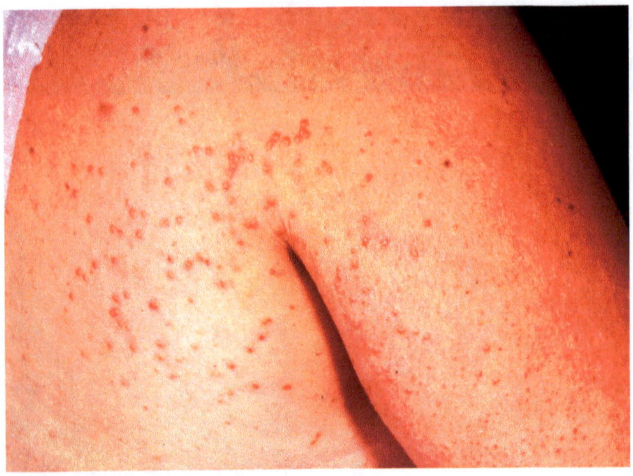

Fig. 2.14 Eruptive xanthomas

includes autoimmune bullous disorders, porphyria, and pseudo-porphyria

2.2.1.6 Eruptive Xanthomas

Eruptive xanthomas occur in the setting of chylomicronemia and hypertriglyceridemia caused by genetic abnormalities. Diabetes mellitus is a common cause of hypertriglyceridemia (diabetic lipemia), and the resultant eruptive xanthomas may be the first sign of an underlying untreated diabetes, usually of type 2 [23]. The incidence of eruptive xanthomas in diabetics is estimated at 0.1%. Eruptive xanthomas may also appear following alcohol abuse or ingestion of drugs such as estrogens or retinoids, or in the setting of hypothyroidism. Eruptive xanthomatosis manifests itself with the sudden appearance of yellowish-orange-to-red-brown, firm papules surrounded by a 1–4 mm wide erythematous halo (Fig. 2.14). They appear in crops on the buttocks, extensor surfaces of the extremities, and flexural creases. Pruritus and Koebner reaction may be present. Histologically, foamy macrophages with extravascular lipid deposits are present in the papillary and upper reticular dermis with an admixed inflammatory infiltrate of lymphocytes and neutrophils (Fig. 2.15). Touton type giant cells are usually absent.

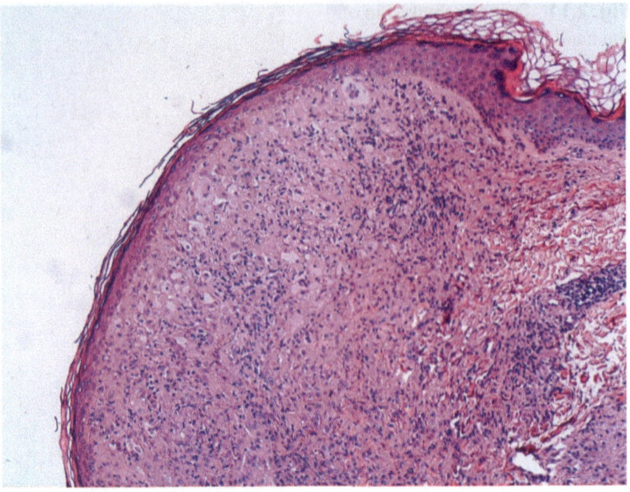

Fig. 2.15 Histopathology of eruptive xanthoma (HE stain)

2.2.1.7 Acquired Perforating Dermatosis

Acquired perforating dermatosis is a rare disorder seen in adult patients, especially those presenting with type 2 and type 1 diabetes mellitus (50%) and with chronic renal failure (73%) [24]. Most of the patients with diabetes mellitus (90.9%) had chronic renal failure because of diabetic nephropathy. It is characterized clinically by itching, hyperkeratotic, sometimes umbilicated or follicular papules and nodules with a central core, situated primarily on the extensor surfaces of the lower (Fig. 2.16a) and upper extremities, often in a linear fashion (Fig. 2.16b). Koebner phenomenon is seen in 32% of patients. The histological features are not uniform, and may resemble any of the four classic perforating disorders: *elastosis perforans serpiginosa, reactive perforating collagenosis, perforating folliculitis, or Kyrle's disease*. This classification is based primarily on the nature of the eliminated material and the type of epidermal disruption. In general, epidermal invagination filled with a keratotic plug admixed with basophilic cellular debris and neutrophils are the key features. If Masson trichrome and elastic van Gieson stains are negative in the epidermis and in the crater at the base of the lesion, the overall histological appearance is consistent with Kyrle's disease (Fig. 2.17). If vertically orientated collagen bundles are seen at the base of the cup-shaped invagination with transepidermal elimination, the overall histological appearance is consistent with reactive perforating collagenosis (Fig. 2.18a, b). If histochemical staining shows transepidermal elimination of degenerated elastic fibers, the overall histological appearance

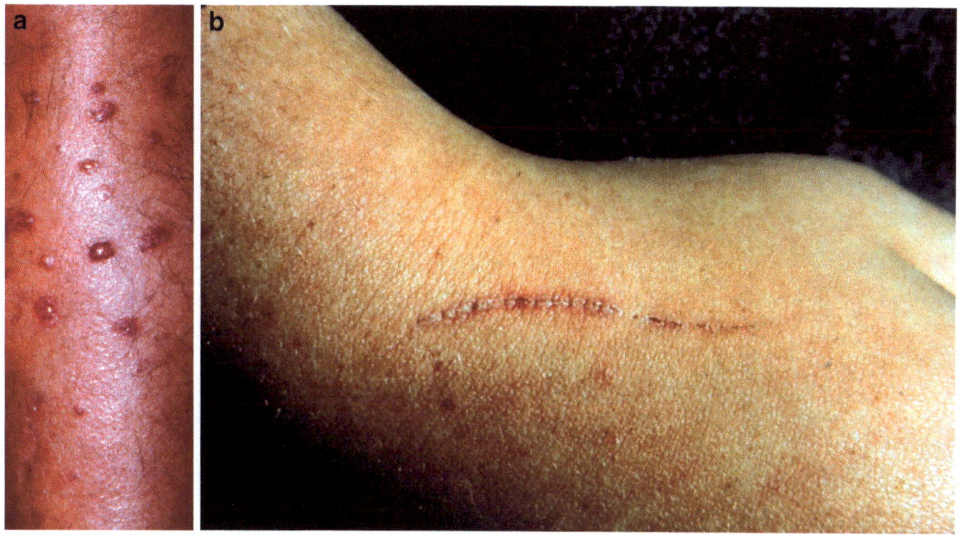

Fig. 2.16 Acquired perforating dermatoses in diabetic. (**a**) Kyrle's disease. (**b**) Reactive perforating collagenosis showing a linear arrangement due to Koebner phenomenon (Courtesy of James W. Patterson, Charlottesville, VA, USA)

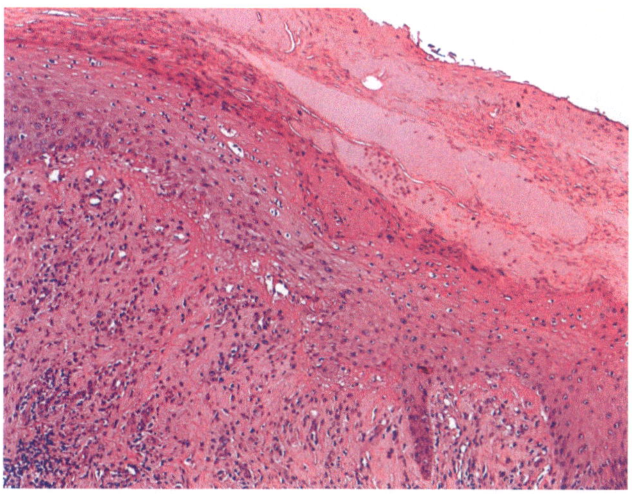

Fig. 2.17 Early lesion of Kyrle's disease with a central cup-like keratotic plug within an epidermal invagination (HE stain)

is consistent with elastosis perforans serpiginosa. When transepidermal elimination of collagen and elastic fibers occurs in many follicles, the features are consistent with perforating folliculitis (Fig. 2.19a, b). In diabetic patients, PAS staining may reveal thickening of the vessel walls in the upper dermis. The cause of APD is unknown, but it has been related to intense pruritus and subsequent scratching, to diabetic microangiopathy and hypoperfusion of dermal structures with an increase in matrix metalloproteinases, epidermal, or dermal change related to metabolic derangements, and to deposition of substances that cannot be removed with dialysis.

2.2.1.8 Acanthosis Nigricans

Acanthosis nigricans is a cutaneous manifestation of insulin-resistant diabetic patient and may indicate increased risk of type 2 diabetes mellitus [25]. Insulin resistance is the most common association of acanthosis nigricans in the younger age population. However, it can occur as a sign of malignancy (particularly stomach cancer), as an adverse effect of certain drugs (i.e., nicotinic acid and corticosteroids), in various endocrinopathies (i.e., acromegaly, Cushing syndrome, and leprechaunism), and associated with obesity (see also Chap. 9). Acanthosis nigricans presents as hyperpigmented, velvety plaques involving typical areas such as the posterior neck, the axilla, and flexural surfaces (Fig. 2.20). Although the lesions are generally asymptomatic, they can be painful, malodorous, or macerated. Acrochordons (skin tags) are often found in and around the affected areas. Histologic examination reveals hyperkeratosis, papillomatosis, and slight irregular acanthosis with minimal or no hyperpigmentation (Fig. 2.21). The dermal papillae project upward as finger-like projections, with occasional thinning of the adjacent epidermis. Clinical hyperpigmentation is secondary to the hyperkeratosis and not to increased melanocytes or increased melanin deposition. The pathogenesis is most likely related to high levels of circulating insulin, which binds to insulin-like growth factor receptors to stimulate the growth of keratinocytes and dermal fibroblasts.

2.2.1.9 Miscellanea

"Yellow nails and skin" is a benign condition associated with diabetes whose significance is unknown. The tinctoral change may be due to either high levels of carotene or non-enzymatic glycosylation of dermal collagen. The yellow color is best appreciated at the distal hallux of the nails, palms, and soles (Fig. 2.22).

The association between diabetes and lichen planus is controversial. Some studies have showed a significantly

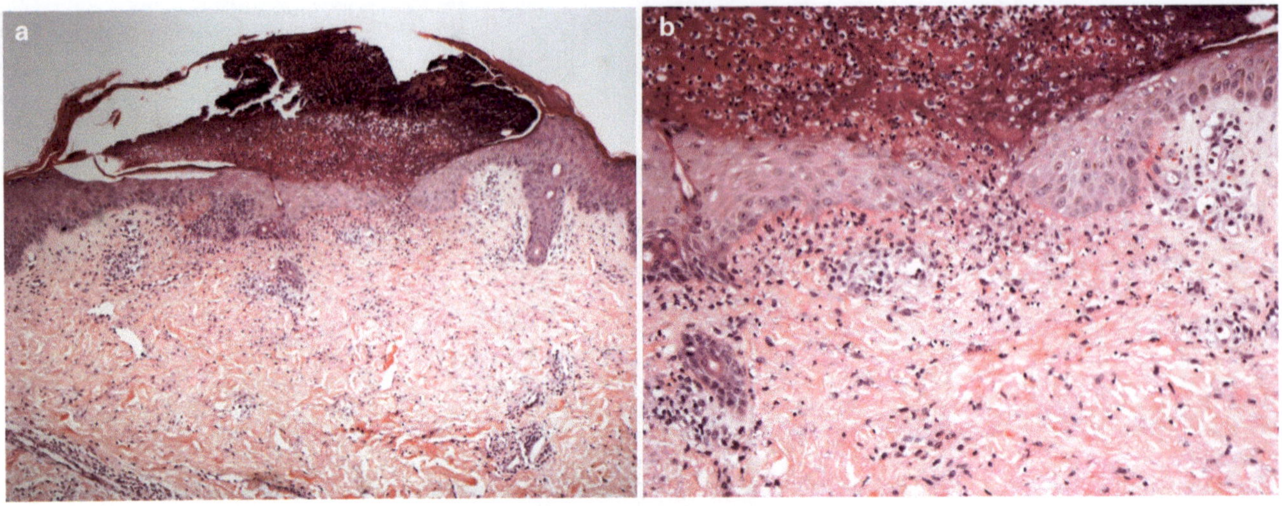

Fig. 2.18 Reactive perforating collagenosis. (**a**) Epidermal invagination filled with a keratotic plug admixed with basophilic cellular debris (HE stain) (Courtesy of James W. Patterson, Charlottesville, VA, USA). (**b**) Transepidermal elimination of collagen fibers (Courtesy of James W. Patterson, Charlottesville, VA, USA)

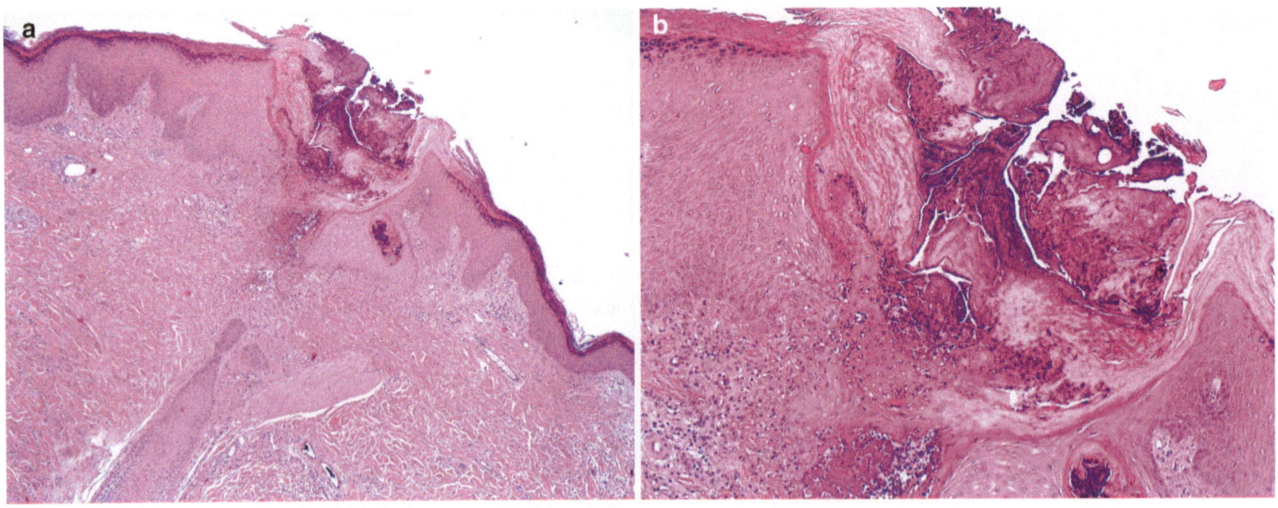

Fig. 2.19 Perforating folliculitis. (**a**) Transepidermal elimination of basophilic cellular debris and neutrophils throughout the follicle. (**b**) Close-up of follicular transepidermal elimination (HE stain)

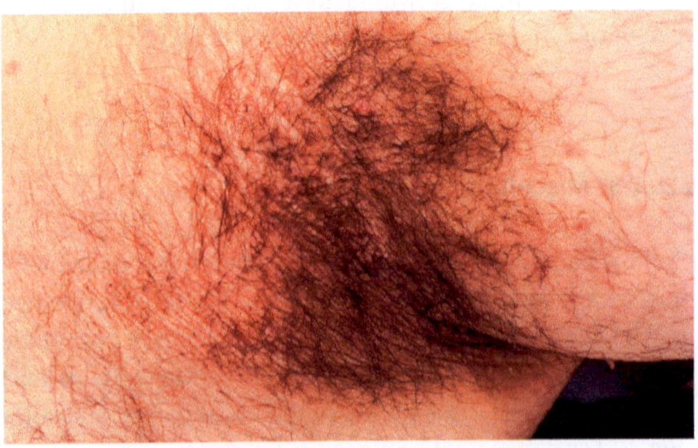

Fig. 2.20 Acanthosis nigricans with skin tags on the axilla

higher prevalence of lichen planus, especially oral lichen planus, in type 1 diabetic patients [26].

Vitiligo occurs with increased frequency in type 1 diabetic patients. From 1 to 7% of all diabetic patients have vitiligo versus 0.2 to 1% of the general population [4]. The association is based on autoimmune mechanisms and is a warning sign for polyglandular autoimmune syndrome.

Although skin tags are common lesions, over 25% of patients with acrochordons had diabetes and 8% had impaired glucose tolerance in a controlled study [4]. Acquired ichthyosis, especially in type 1 diabetic patients [27], is commonly described, while pruritus associated with diabetes mellitus, although commonly reported, is a controversial association. The described pruritus is often localized to the vulva or anus and usually is due to candidal infection. Cutaneous signs of diabetic microangiopathy are periungual telangiectasia, palmar (plantar) erythema, rubeosis faciei, and erysipelas-like erythema, which is a well-demarcated erythema on the lower leg or dorsum of the foot that correlates with radiological evidence of underlying bone destruction, and incipient gangrene.

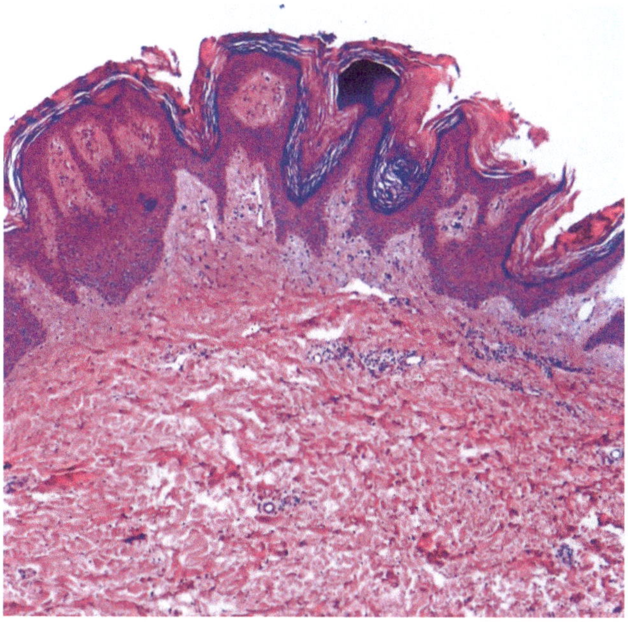

Fig. 2.21 Histopathology of acanthosis nigricans (HE stain)

2.2.2 Cutaneous Infections

Skin infections occur in 20–50% of diabetic patients (more often in those with type 2 diabetes) and are often associated with poor glycemic control.

2.2.2.1 Bacterial Infections

Pyodermic infections such as folliculitis, furuncolosis, impetigo, erysipelas, and cellulitis are more severe and widespread in diabetics and are caused by *Staphylococcus aureus* or hemolytic streptococci. Staphylococcal sepsis can complicate even the smallest wound. Necrotizing fasciitis is a life-threatening condition that may occurs in diabetics (Fig. 2.23). This infection is typically polymicrobial, involving group A streptococci, enterococci, *S. aureus*, enterobacteriaceae, and various anaerobes.

Non-clostridial gas gangrene occurs in 17% of diabetics admitted to the hospital for gangrene or ulceration.

Erythrasma is a brown-red dyscoloration of the intertriginous areas of the skin due to *Corynebacterium minutissimum*. It is seen with increased frequency in obese diabetics.

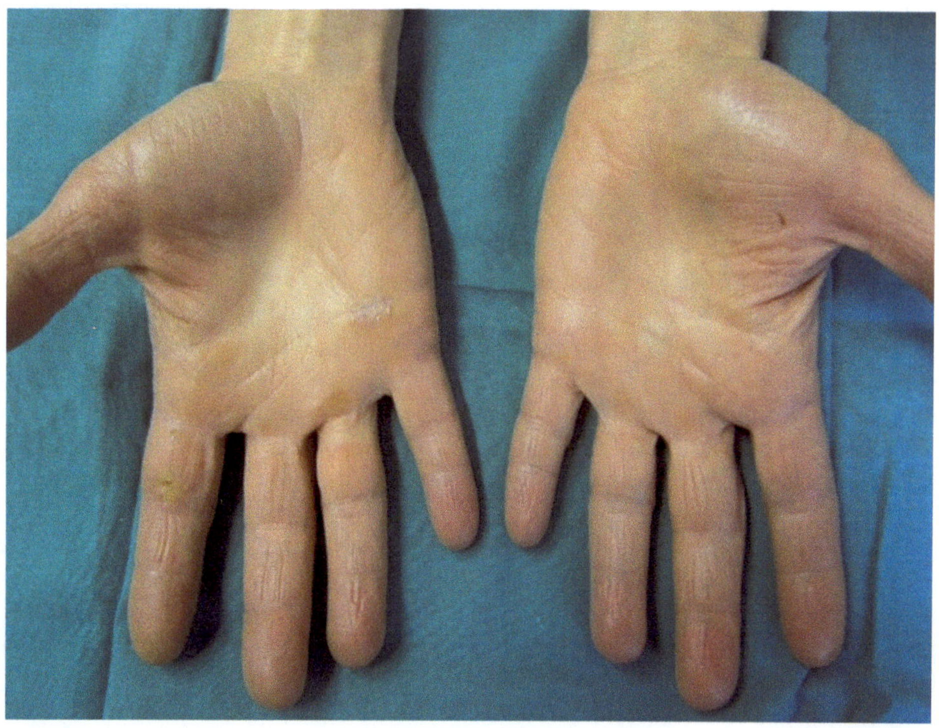

Fig. 2.22 Yellow palms in a diabetic type 2

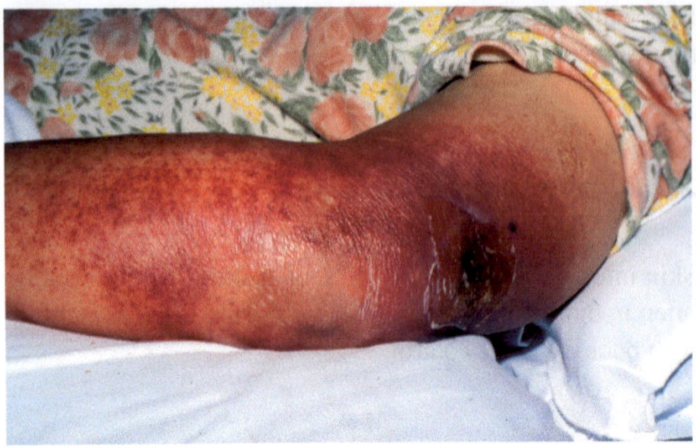

Fig. 2.23 Necrotizing fasciitis in a diabetic with poor glycemic control

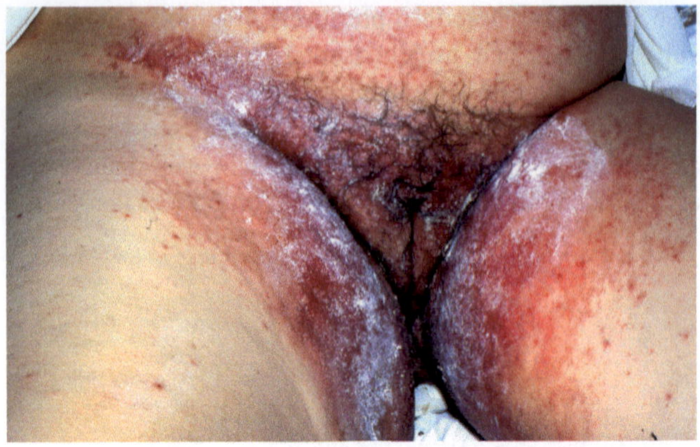

Fig. 2.24 Intertrigo and vulvovaginitis in a diabetic woman

2.2.2.2 Candida Infections

Candida infections may be an early sign of undiagnosed diabetes and commonly develop in patients with poorly controlled disease. They include candidal angular stomatitis (perleche), median rhomboid glossitis, paronychia, erosion interdigitale blastomycetica characteristically involving the web space between the middle and fourth finger, vulvovaginitis with intertrigo (Fig. 2.24), balanitis, and phimosis.

2.2.2.3 Dermatophyte Infections

Although dermatophyte infections are not more frequent in diabetics compared with controls, tinea pedis and onychomycosis because of *Trychophyton rubrum* and *Trychophyton mentagraphytes* can result in significant morbidity as they can act as a portal of entry for bacterial infection.

2.2.2.4 Rare Infections

A few infections, such as malignant otitis externa, and rhinocerebral mucormycosis occur almost exclusively in patients with diabetes. Malignant otitis externa involves middle-aged, diabetic patients and is usually due to *Pseudomonas aeruginosa*. Infection starts with severe ear pain and otorrhea in the external auditory canal and spreads to adjacent soft tissue, cartilage, and bone.

Mucormycosis is caused by various ubiquitous molds (Phycomycetes). Invasive disease occurs in patients with poorly controlled diabetes and ketoacidosis. Fungi colonize the nose and paranasal sinuses with periorbital or perinasal pain, swelling, and induration, spreading to adjacent tissues by invading blood vessels and causing soft tissue necrosis, bony erosion, and cerebral abscesses (Fig. 2.25).

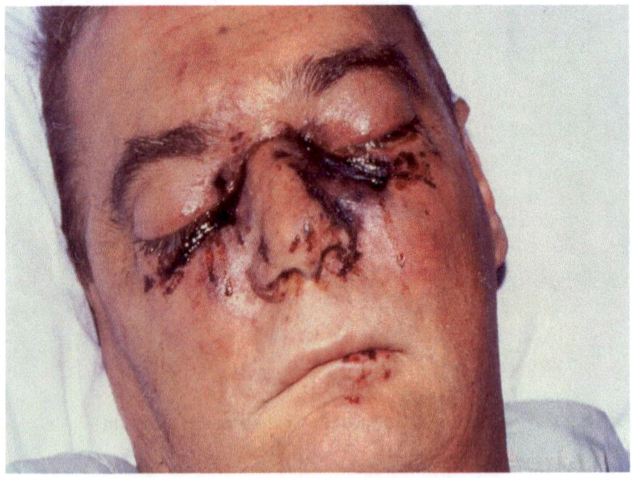

Fig. 2.25 Rhinocerebral mucormycosis in a diabetic

2.2.3 Complications Due to Diabetic Neuropathy and Vasculopathy

Diabetic foot ulcers are common complications that occur in 15% of diabetic patients at some time during their lifetime. A total of 12–24% of individuals with a foot ulcer requires amputation (Fig. 2.26). Indeed, diabetes is the leading cause of non-traumatic lower extremity amputations. Foot complications occur in both forms of diabetes (type 1 and type 2) and are related more to the period of time that the illness has been present than to the age of onset. A number of factors are involved in the development and maintenance of a diabetic foot ulcer, including: sensorimotor and autonomic polyneuropathy, mechanical overload, peripheral arterial disease and infection. Diabetic peripheral neuropathy causes altered or complete loss of feeling in the foot and/or leg. There are two types of diabetic foot: (a) neuropathic foot that is warm, painless with palpable pulses, characterized by diminished sweating and dry skin prone to fissuring; (b) neuroischemic foot that is cool, painful, and pulseless characterized by thin, shiny skin. The typical perforating foot ulcer is a circular deep ulcer with a hyperkeratotic ring on areas most subjected to weight bearing, such as the heel, plantar metatarsal head areas (Fig. 2.27), the tips of the most prominent toes (usually the first or second), and the tips of hammer toes. Histologically, changes are related to the time of biopsy and are not specific. Hyperkeratosis is conspicuous, particularly at the edges of the lesion. The dermis is hypertrophic with a greater degree of fibrosis, frequently disrupting the normal structure of the extracellular matrix. An inflammatory infiltrate, mainly represented by leukocytes and macrophages, is present with variable granulation tissue [28].

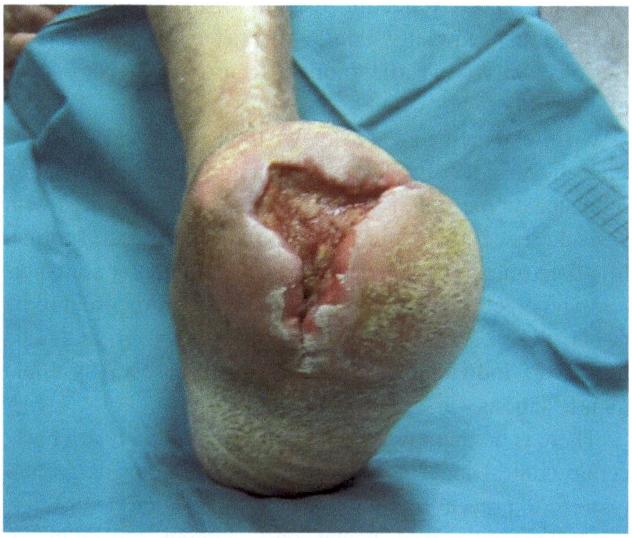

Fig. 2.26 Diabetic foot undergone to amputation for necrosis of toes

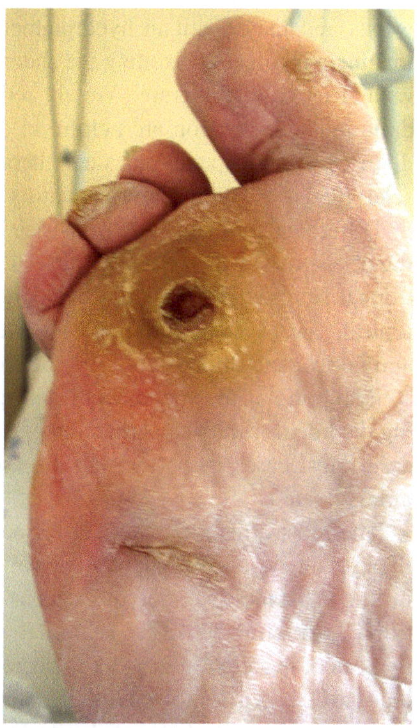

Fig. 2.27 Perforating foot ulcer

Calciphylaxis, also known as calcific uremic arteriolopathy, is a small-vessel vasculopathy accompanied by mural calcification with intimal proliferation, fibrosis, and thrombosis (see also Chaps. 5 and 21). Poor-healing, necrotizing skin ulcers with a livedo-like reticular pattern are seen. In renal failure patients, women, white, obese, or diabetic patients (especially those with type 2 diabetes) are considered at risk [29]. Penile necrosis has been described in patients with a long history of diabetes, who were on dialysis [30].

2.2.4 Complications Due to Diabetes Treatment

Maculopapular rash, generalized erythema, and urticarial reactions may be induced by first-generation sulfonylureas such as chlorpropamide and tolbutamide in the first month of therapy and may resolve spontaneously, even if therapy is not stopped. Second-generation sulfonylureas (glipizide and glimepiride) are less likely to cause skin reactions. Metformin, the first choice oral drug in type 2 diabetes, may cause leucocytoclastic vasculitis.

Allergic reactions due to insulin range from IgE-mediated local erythematous reactions to more generalized reactions with angioedema and urticaria, and to delayed reactions characterized by an itching nodule at the site of injection. Biphasic reactions, with immediate itching and burning at the injection site, followed by a more sustained induration and generalized reaction 4–8 h later may occur. Such reactions may result from the insulin itself or from impurities, preservatives, additives, or retarding agents such as zinc or protamine and occur within 1–4 weeks of starting treatment. The use of recombinant human insulin preparations has decreased the incidence of insulin reactions to a rate of 0.1–2.4%. Lipoatrophy characterized by depressed areas at injection sites is actually rare (Fig. 2.28) while lipohypertrophy clinically mimicking lipomas can still occur due to the lipogenic action of insulin. Keloids, hyperkeratotic papules, localized hyperpigmentation, and purpuric reactions have also been reported.

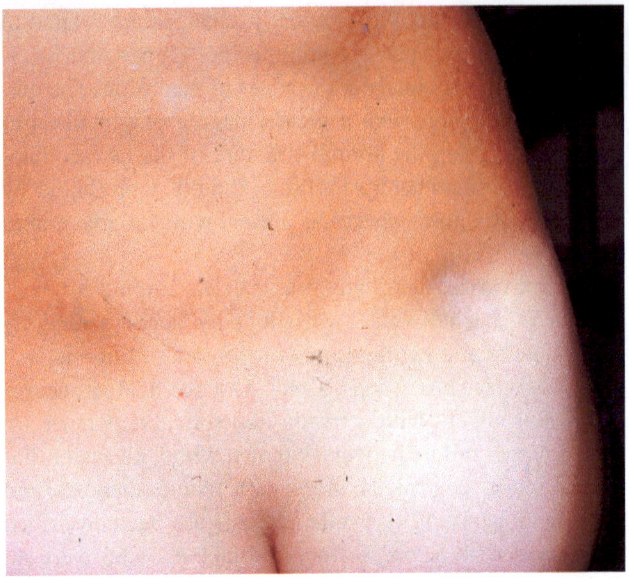

Fig. 2.28 Insulin lipoatrophy

2.3 Treatment and Prognosis

NL tends to chronicity. No robust studies have demonstrated any particularly effective therapy to date. Topical and intralesional corticosteroids are empirically considered as a first-line treatments lessening the inflammation of early active lesions and the active borders, but worsening the atrophy. Many recent therapies have been tried with variable success including topical tacrolimus, topically applied bovine collagen, mycophenolate mofetil, cyclosporin A, UVA1 therapy, photodynamic therapy, and pulse dye laser. Excision and grafting have been successful, but recurrence may occur. Anti-tumor necrosis factor alpha (TNF-α) agents such as etanercept and infliximab have been used for refractory, ulcerative NL [31]. Treatment of the hyperglycemic state does not change the cutaneous lesions, although improvement following pancreas transplantation has been reported [32]. Because localized trauma can cause NL to ulcerate, protection of the legs with elastic support stockings and leg rest is useful.

The evolution of DD is variable and does not appear to be affected by glycemic control. The lesions may persist or resolve spontaneously with scar formation and recur in crops. Treatment is not very effective. Particular attention should be placed on the detection and prevention of diabetic complications such as retinopathy, neuropathy, nephropathy, and coronary heart disease, as patients with DD are more inclined to develop microangiopathies.

No well-designed randomized controlled studies have demonstrated any particularly effective therapy for GA. Localized disease generally is self-limited and resolves within 2 months to 2 years, whereas disseminated disease may last 3–4 years or as long as 10 years. For localized disease, topical or intralesional glucocorticoids, tacrolimus and pimecrolimus, imiquimod, pulse dye laser, and cryotherapy have been used with variable success. Because localized GA is self-limited, a "wait and see approach" is also warranted. For disseminated disease, treatment modalities include retinoids, antibiotics, nicotinamide, dapsone, pentoxyfilline, cyclosporine, fumaric acid esters, antimalarials, photodynamic therapy, and ultraviolet therapy including UVA1 phototherapy [33]. Regarding TNF-α inhibitors, there are reports reflecting resolution of the disease with this treatment modality while others show no benefit [34]. Lesions may resolve after biopsy. Recurrences occur in 40% of cases.

No effective treatment is known for scleredema diabeticorum. Control of the hyperglycemia does not have any influence on the skin. Many treatments have been tried with variable success. Phototherapy such as UVA1, cyclosporine, low-dose methotrexate, intravenous immunoglobulin therapy, and electron-beam therapy have all been reported to be of benefit [35, 36]. Aggressive therapies, however, should be limited to individuals with disabling disease or systemic manifestations.

There is no therapy for diabetic hand, although strict glycemic control may be helpful. Physical therapy is recommended to prevent limitations in the range of motion [37].

Diabetic bullae heal spontaneously without scarring in 2–6 weeks, but they may be recurrent. Blisters may turn into chronic foot ulcers with complications [38]. Glycemic control does not appear to have a direct correlation with blister formation.

Eruptive xanthomas usually resolve spontaneously over weeks and may result in hyperpigmented scars. Adequate treatment involves controlling the underlying hyperlipidemia with strict dietary therapy. Weight reduction and carbohydrate intake restriction are helpful in cases associated with diabetes. Eruptive xanthomas may herald the risk of atherosclerotic disease and acute pancreatitis.

Different treatments have been tried for acquired perforating dermatosis with variable results, such as topical or intralesional steroids, phototherapy including narrowband UVB, topical, and systemic retinoids, systemic antihistamines, antibiotics, and allopurinol [39]. Although there have been some reports of the spontaneous disappearance of perforating disorders with the stabilization of diabetes and renal disease, most cases of perforating disease continue for years unless treated.

The most effective treatment for acanthosis nigricans is lifestyle alteration. Weight reduction and exercise can reduce insulin resistance. Keratolytics such as ointments containing salicylic or retinoic acid can be used to reduce thicker lesions in areas of maceration in order to decrease odor. Oral agents that have shown some benefits include etretinate, isotretinoin, metformin, and dietary fish oils. Dermabrasion and laser therapy may also be used to reduce the bulk of the lesion.

Foot ulcers in diabetes require multidisciplinary assessment, usually by diabetes specialists, dermatologists, and surgeons. Treatment consists of appropriate bandages, strict infection control, skin grafts, skin substitutes, debridement, and arterial revascularization [40]. Hyperbaric oxygen therapy reduce the risk of amputation and may improve the healing.

References

1. Ahmed I, Goldstein B (2006) Diabetes mellitus. Clin Dermatol 24:237–246
2. Schneider JB, Norman RA (2004) Cutaneous manifestations of endocrine-metabolic disease and nutritional deficiency in the elderly. Dermatol Clin 22:23–31
3. Oumeish OY (2008) Skin disorders in patients with diabetes. Clin Dermatol 26:235–242
4. Van Hattem S, Bootsma AH, Thio HB (2008) Skin manifestations of diabetes. Cleve Clin J Med 75:772–787
5. Paron NG, Lambert PW (2000) Cutaneous manifestations of diabetes mellitus. Prim Care 27:371–383
6. Peyrí J, Moreno A, Marcoval J (2007) Necrobiosis lipoidica. Semin Cutan Med Surg 26:87–89
7. Roche-Gamón E, Vilata-Corell JJ, Velasco-Pastor M (2007) Familial necrobiosis lipoidica not associated with diabetes. Dermatol Online J 13:26
8. Shimanovich I, Erdmann H, Grabbe J, Zillikens D, Rose C (2008) Necrobiosis lipoidica in monozygotic twins. Arch Dermatol 144:119–120
9. Fernandez-Flores A (2008) Necrobiosis lipoidica and cutaneous anaesthesia: immunohistochemical study of neural fibres. Folia Neuropathol 46:154–157
10. Eisendle K, Baltaci M, Kutzner H, Zelger B (2008) Detection of spirochaetal microorganisms by focus floating microscopy in necrobiosis lipoidica in patients from central Europe. Histopathology 52:877–884
11. Ngo BT, Hayes KD, DiMiao DJ, Srinivasan SK, Huerter CJ, Rendell MS (2005) Manifestations of cutaneous diabetic microangiopathy. Am J Clin Dermatol 6:225–237
12. Houck GM, Morgan MB (2004) A reappraisal of the histologic findings of pigmented pretibial patches of diabetes mellitus. J Cutan Pathol 31:141–144
13. Nebesio CL, Lewis C, Chuang TY (2002) Lack of an association between granuloma annulare and type 2 diabetes mellitus. Br J Dermatol 146:122–124
14. Erkek E, Karaduman A, Bukulmez G, Senturk N, Ozkaya O (2001) An unusual form of generalized granuloma annulare in a patient with insulin-dependent diabetes mellitus. Acta Derm Venereol (Stockh) 81:48–50
15. Yáñez S, Val-Bernal JF, Peña-Sagredo JL, Jiménez-Gómez I, Vazquez-Rodriguez TR, Gonzalez-Gay MA (2008) Generalized granuloma annulare and giant cell arteritis. Clin Exp Rheumatol 26:S108–S110
16. Rongioletti F, Cerroni L, Massone C et al (2004) Different histologic patterns of cutaneous granulomas in systemic lymphoma. J Am Acad Dermatol 51:600–605
17. Reddy HS, Khurana RN, Rao NA, Chopra V (2008) Granuloma annulare anterior uveitis. Ocul Immunol Inflamm 16:55–57
18. Magro CM, Crowson AN, Regauer S (1996) Granuloma annulare and necrobiosis lipoidica tissue reactions as a manifestation of systemic disease. Hum Pathol 27:50–56
19. Stefanaki K, Tsivitanidou-Kakourou T, Stefanaki C, Valari M, Argyrakos T, Konstantinidou CV, Karentzou O, Katsambas A (2007) Histological and immunohistochemical study of granuloma annulare and subcutaneous granuloma annulare in children. J Cutan Pathol 34:392–396
20. Ziemer M, Grabner T, Eisendle K, Baltaci M, Zelger B (2008) Granuloma annulare – a manifestation of infection with Borrelia? J Cutan Pathol 35:1050–1057
21. Yosipovitch G et al (2003) Medical pearl: scleroderma-like skin changes in patients with diabetes mellitus. J Am Acad Dermatol 48:109
22. Lopez PR, Leicht S, Sigmon JR, Stigall L (2009) Bullosis diabeticorum associated with a prediabetic state. South Med J 102:643–644
23. Nayak KR, Daly RG (2004) Images in clinical medicine. Eruptive xanthomas associated with hypertriglyceridemia and new-onset diabetes mellitus. N Engl J Med 350:1235
24. Saray Y, Seçkin D, Bilezikçi B (2006) Acquired perforating dermatosis: clinicopathological features in twenty-two cases. J Eur Acad Dermatol Venereol 20:679–688
25. Fagot-Campagna A, Pettitt DJ, Engelgau MM et al (2000) Type 2 diabetes among North American children and adolescents: an epidemiologic review and a public health perspective. J Pediatr 136:664–672
26. Seyhan M, Ozcan H, Sahin I, Bayram N, Karincaoğlu Y (2007) High prevalence of glucose metabolism disturbance in patients with lichen planus. Diabetes Res Clin Pract 77:198–202
27. Pavlović MD, Milenković T, Dinić M, Misović M, Daković D, Todorović S, Daković Z, Zecevi RD, Doder R (2007) The prevalence of cutaneous manifestations in young patients with type 1 diabetes. Diabetes Care 30:1964–1967
28. Piaggesi A, Viacava P, Rizzo L, Naccarato G, Baccetti F, Romanelli M, Zampa V, Del Prato S (2003) Semiquantitative analysis of the histopathological features of the neuropathic foot ulcer: effects of pressure relief. Diabetes Care 26:3123–3128
29. Wilmer WA, Magro CM (2002) Calciphylaxis: emerging concepts in prevention, diagnosis, and treatment. Semin Dial 15:172–186
30. Ohta A, Ohomori S, Mizukami T, Obi R, Tanaka Y (2007) Penile necrosis by calciphylaxis in a diabetic patient with chronic renal failure. Intern Med 46:985–990
31. Hu SW, Bevona C, Winterfield L, Qureshi AA, Li VW (2009) Treatment of refractory ulcerative necrobiosis lipoidica diabeticorum with infliximab: report of a case. Arch Dermatol 145:437–439
32. Souza AD, El-Azhary RA, Gibson LE (2009) Does pancreas transplant in diabetic patients affect the evolution of necrobiosis lipoidica? Int J Dermatol 48:964–970
33. Piaserico S, Zattra E, Linder D, Peserico A (2009) Generalized granuloma annulare treated with methylaminolevulinate photodynamic therapy. Dermatology 218:282–284
34. Rosmarin D, LaRaia A, Schlauder S, Gottlieb AB (2009) Successful treatment of disseminated granuloma annulare with adalimumab. J Drugs Dermatol 8:169–171
35. Kroft EB, de Jong EM (2008) Scleredema diabeticorum case series: successful treatment with UV-A1. Arch Dermatol 144:947–948
36. Barde C, Masouyé I, Saurat JH, Le Gal FA (2009) Scleroedema adultorum Buschke in a diabetic subject: intravenous immunoglobulin therapy. Ann Dermatol Vénéréol 136:360–363
37. Infante JR, Rosenbloom AL, Silverstein JH et al (2001) Changes in frequency and severity of limited joint mobility in children with type 1 diabetes mellitus between 1976-78 and 1998. J Pediatr 138:33–37
38. Larsen K, Jensen T, Karlsmark T, Holstein PE (2008) Incidence of bullosis diabeticorum – a controversial cause of chronic foot ulceration. Int Wound J 5:591–596
39. Hoque SR, Ameen M, Holden CA (2006) Acquired reactive perforating collagenosis: four patients with a giant variant treated with allopurinol. Br J Dermatol 154:759–762
40. Edmonds M (2006) Diabetic foot ulcers: practical treatment recommendations Drugs 66:913–929

Chapter 3
Thyroid Disease

Alfredo Rebora and Franco Rongioletti

Key Points

- Dermatological manifestations as a sign of thyroid disturbances occur either in thyreotoxic states or in the evolution of autoimmune diseases of the thyroid that is in apparent euthyroidism, or in overt hypothyroidism.
- Pretibial myxedema and thyroid acropachy are typical manifestations of hyperthyroidism, in particular of Graves' disease. Vitiligo, diffuse alopecia (both telogen effluvium and alopecia areata), and chronic urticaria can be associated with autoimmune disease of the thyroid.
- Generalized myxedema is the most common skin manifestation of hypothyroidism characterized by yellowish, cold, and dry skin filled with mucin, nonpitting edema of face and extremities, dry and brittle hairs, resulting in diffuse or partial alopecia.
- In generalized myxedema, skin symptoms subside with thyroxine administration, while treatment of pretibial myxedema and thyroid acropachy remains problematic.

Keywords Hyperthyroidism • Pretibial myxedema • Thyroid acropachy • Hypothyroidism • Generalized myxedema

3.1 Introduction

The thyroid gland is a highly vascular organ that synthesizes the hormones thyroxine (T3) and triiodothyronine (T_4). T_3 and T_4 are iodine-containing amino acids whose task is to regulate the body's metabolism. The thyroid functioning unit is the follicle, a cavity lined by epithelial cells and contains colloid, a proteinaceous material composed by the thyroid hormones and thyroglobulin. Thyroglobulin is used by the gland to produce the thyroid hormones. In addition, the parafollicular cells, which are scattered among follicles, produce calcitonin.

The follicular cells have three functions: to collect and transport iodine, to synthesize thyroglobulin, and to release T_3 and T_4 from the latter at the rate of 4 μg and 80 μg per day, respectively. The secretion is regulated by the pituitary thyroid-stimulating hormone (TSH), which, in turn, is stimulated by the thyrotropin-releasing hormone (TRH) secreted by the hypothalamus. TSH binds to a specific receptor (TSH-R) in the thyroid cell membrane.

When thyroid hormones enter cells, most of the T_4 is converted to T_3. T3 finds a specific receptor (in fact, there are two of them, hTR-α1 and hTR-β1, variously represented in the body) and increases the expression of specific genes that, in turn, are responsible for the many effects of thyroid hormones. In brief, thyroid hormones stimulate oxygen consumption, affect tissue growth and maturation, regulate lipid metabolism, and increase cardiac contractility and intestinal absorption of carbohydrates.

Five types of thyroid dysfunction can be encountered: *hyperthyroidism* (sometimes assimilated to thyrotoxicosis in which the levels of T_4, T_3, or both are elevated), including diseases that are a subset of thyrotoxicosis caused by an excess of thyroid hormone, and excluding exogenous thyroid hormone intake and subacute thyroiditis; *hypothyroidism* caused by a deficiency of thyroid hormones; *goiter* caused by an excess of TSH; *thyroid neoplasms and abnormal thyroid function tests in a clinically euthyroid subject.*

Thyroid diseases are frequently "diseases in progress," and most dermatological manifestations are indicative of thyroid disturbance in general, occurring either in thyrotoxic states or in the evolution of autoimmune diseases of the thyroid, that is, in apparent euthyroidism, or in overt hypothyroidism.

3.2 Clinical and Pathological Aspects of Skin Manifestations

3.2.1 *Hyperthyroidism*

Almost 60% of cases of thyrotoxicosis are represented by Graves' disease [1]. Graves' disease is an autoimmune

A. Rebora (✉)
Clinica Dermatologica, University of Genova,
Viale Benedetto XV, 7, Genova, Italy
e-mail: rebdermo@unige.it

F. Rongioletti and B.R. Smoller (eds.), *Clinical and Pathological Aspects of Skin Diseases in Endocrine, Metabolic, Nutritional and Deposition Disease*, DOI 10.1007/978-1-60761-181-3_3, © Springer Science+Business Media, LLC 2010

disorder with a variety of circulating antibodies including thyroid-stimulating immunoglobulin (TSI), which binds to TSH-R and activates the thyroid hormone synthesis and release, and induces the thyroid to grow. Extremely elevated levels of T3 and a diffusely enlarged thyroid are typical features. Periorbital and conjunctival edema, injection, and proptosis of the eyes are common. More rarely, there is a dermopathy over the lower extremities (see below). As in most autoimmune conditions, other cell-mediated autoimmune diseases (pernicious anemia, myasthenia gravis, vitiligo, adrenal insufficiency, alopecia areata, and type 1 diabetes mellitus) may be associated.

Subacute thyroiditis accounts for about 15–20% of cases of thyrotoxicosis. In the first phase of subacute thyroiditis, hormone levels can be extremely elevated as a result of destruction of the thyroid follicle and release of preformed thyroid hormone into the circulation. In the second phase, lasting up to 2 months, thyroid hormone is depleted, and the patient may become mildly hypothyroid. Eventually, almost all patients return to euthyroidism. Silent thyroiditis, painful or granulomatous thyroiditis, and postpartum thyroiditis are the most common causes. Toxic multinodular goiter (Plummer's disease) represents 15–20% of thyreotoxic patients, most commonly elderly with a long-standing goiter. Thyroid hormone levels are only mildly elevated but may increase after high iodine intake (namely, radiocontrast or amiodarone administration). Accordingly, symptoms are mild (apathetic hyperthyroidism). Diagnosis is made by means of nuclear scintigraphy. Toxic adenoma is rare and is caused by a benign monoclonal tumor. Again, diagnosis is based on nuclear scintigraphy.

In hyperthyroidism, the skin is smooth, soft, warm, and moist with increased pigmentation, especially on the palms and soles. There is a flushed face, increased sweating, and accelerated nail growth. Skin manifestations are more prominent in Graves' disease and are typically represented by the triad of *pretibial myxedema* (4%), *thyroid acropachy* (<1%), and *exophthalmos* (Fig. 3.1) in 30% of patients [2]. English actor Marty Feldman (who starred in several films such as Young Frankenstein) was notable for his bulging eyes, caused by Graves' disease. Gynecomastia may be observed in men [3].

Pretibial myxedema [4, 5] occurs up to 14 years after ophthalmopathy, but it has also been reported in patients with hypothyroidism (Hashimoto's thyroiditis, primary hypothyroidism) and euthyroidism, apparently unrelated to the levels of thyroid hormone (see also Chap. 18). Its incidence peaks in the fifth to sixth decades of life. Myxedema may also involve other skin areas, such as arms, head, neck, and elsewhere on the legs. There are four main clinical variants of pretibial myxedema: diffuse, nonpitting edema (43%); plaque (27%); nodular (18%); and elephantiasis (5%). The lesions can vary in color and may exhibit a characteristic *peau d'orange* (orange peel) appearance and texture owing to prominent hair follicles (Fig. 3.2). The pure nodular form is an uncommon presentation (Fig. 3.3). The elephantiasic form is the most symptomatic and debilitating, consisting of nodular, polypoid, or fungating lesions with marked lymphedema (Fig. 3.4). Histopathology reveals an abundant deposition of mucin (glycosaminoglycans) throughout the reticular dermis, particularly in the middle to the lower part, with separation of collagen fibers (Fig. 3.5a). The mucin stains with Alcian-blue at pH 2.5 and colloidal iron stains (Fig. 3.5b). The overlying epidermis shows acanthosis with hyperorthokeratosis, follicular plugging, and sometimes, papillomatosis (Fig. 3.6). Fibroblasts are normal in number, and stellate forms are often observed. Elastic fibers are reduced in number.

Pathogenesis is unclear, but it appears that pretibial fibroblasts are targets of the autoimmune attack. Trauma in the legs, which result in cytokine release from inflammatory cells, arterial or venous insufficiency, and smoking may be

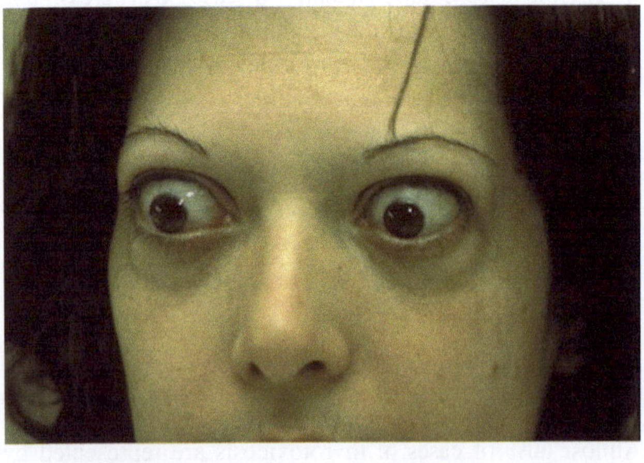

Fig. 3.1 Exophtalmos (Courtesy of C. Varotti, Bologna, Italy)

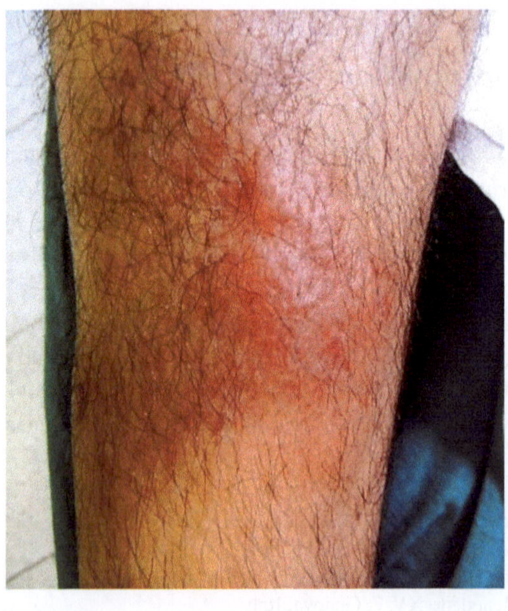

Fig. 3.2 Pretibial myxedema (plaque-type)

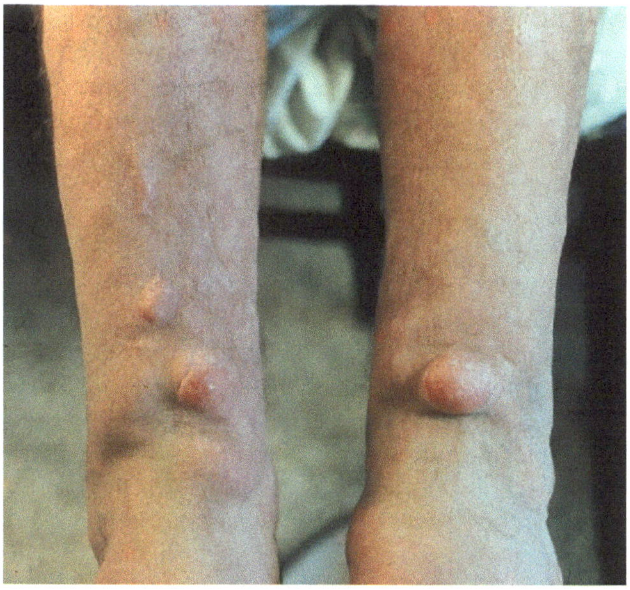

Fig. 3.3 Pretibial myxedema (nodular type)

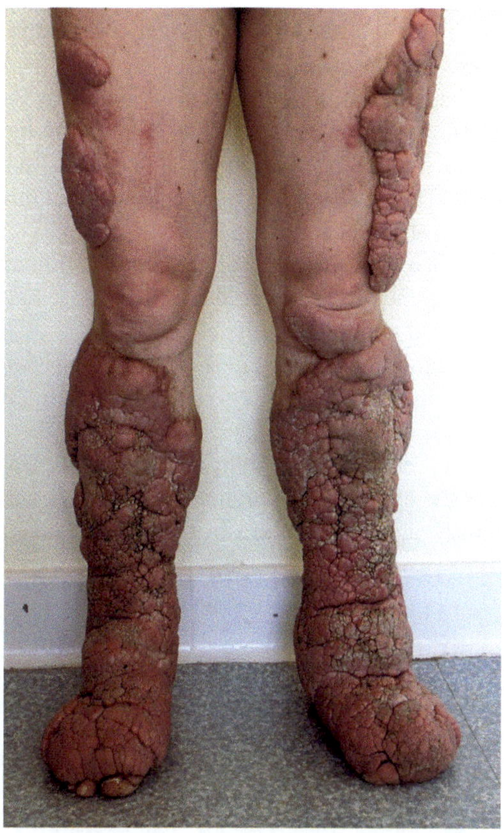

Fig. 3.4 Localized elephantiasic, fungating myxedema of hyperthyroidism (Courtesy of B. Cribier, Strasbourg, France)

favoring factors. Two hypotheses have been advanced to explain the excess hyaluronic acid production by fibroblasts. According to the first one, pretibial fibroblasts have TRH-R antibody binding sites or, alternatively, T cells react with

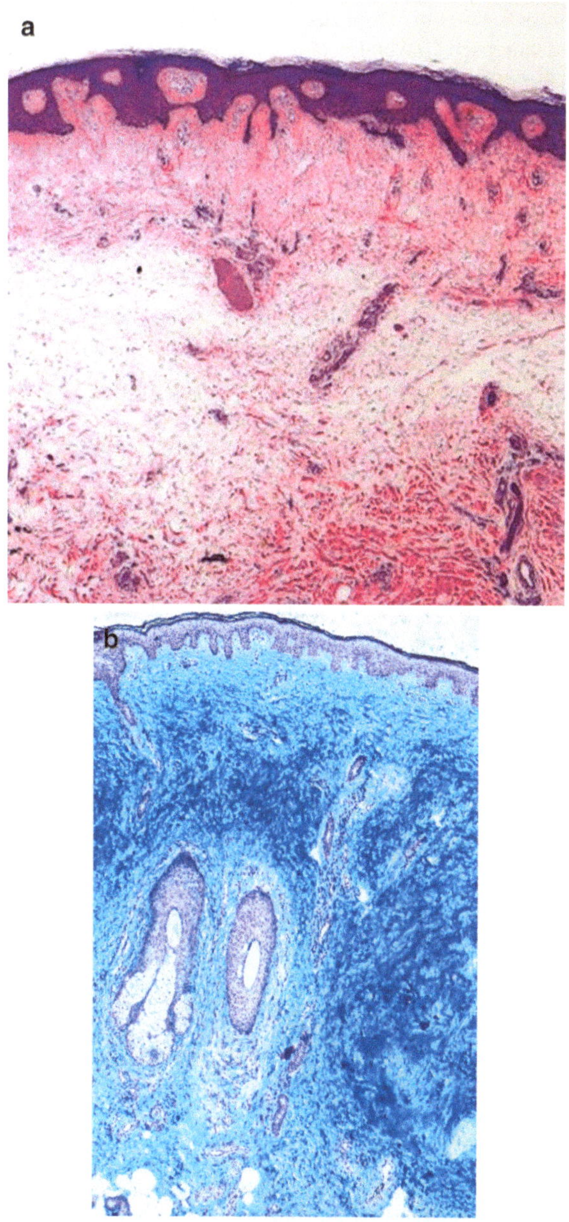

Fig. 3.5 (**a**) Pretibial myxedema (HE stain). (**b**) Pretibial myxedema (Colloidal iron stain)

TRH-R on pretibial fibroblasts causing fibroblast-stimulating cytokine release. In addition, germline mutations in TRH-R have been reported [5].

Thyroid acropachy [6] occurs up to 25 years after the onset of thyroid disease and often after hyperthyroidism has been treated. Women are affected four times as often as men. Acropachy has never been reported in the absence of exophthalmos. It consists in digital clubbing (Fig. 3.7a) and diaphysial proliferation, which on radiograph appears as irregular, lacy, bubbly new bone. Onycholysis, spoon nails, and Hippocratic nails may be observed (Fig. 3.7b). The soft tissues swell over the hypertrophic bones as a result of mucin deposition in between dense collagen bundles (Fig. 3.8).

In men with Graves' disease, *gynecomastia* may be related to the increased conversion of testosterone to estradiol. *Vitiligo* [7] (Fig. 3.9) and *diffuse alopecia* [8, 9] (Fig. 3.10) (mostly due to telogen effluvium) have been found to be more common in autoimmune hyperthyroidism. The association between thyroid autoimmunity and *chronic idiopathic urticaria* [10] has long been recognized, although prevalence rates differ from 12 to 29%. The significance of the association of alopecia areata (Fig. 3.11) with Hashimoto's thyroiditis and Graves' disease deserves further study, as does the association between Duhring's disease and autoimmune hyperthyroidism.

3.2.2 Hypothyroidism

Hypothyroidism may result from a primary insufficient hormone production by the gland or from a secondary failure of TSH pituitary secretion from the pituitary gland. It may even be tertiary when the failure involves TRH secretion from the hypothalamus [11]. Usually, the patient is asymptomatic for a long time or, rarely, undergoes coma (myxedema coma). Hashimoto's thyroiditis is the most common cause in the Western world. Hypothyroidism may also be congenital (cretinism), but this occurs much more rarely. As a consequence of the hormone deficiency, all metabolic processes are slowed down and mucin accumulates in the tissues. Cardiac enlargement and decreased cardiac output, achlorhydria and slow intestinal transit, delayed puberty and infertility, LDL hypercholesterolemia and insulin resistance are common findings.

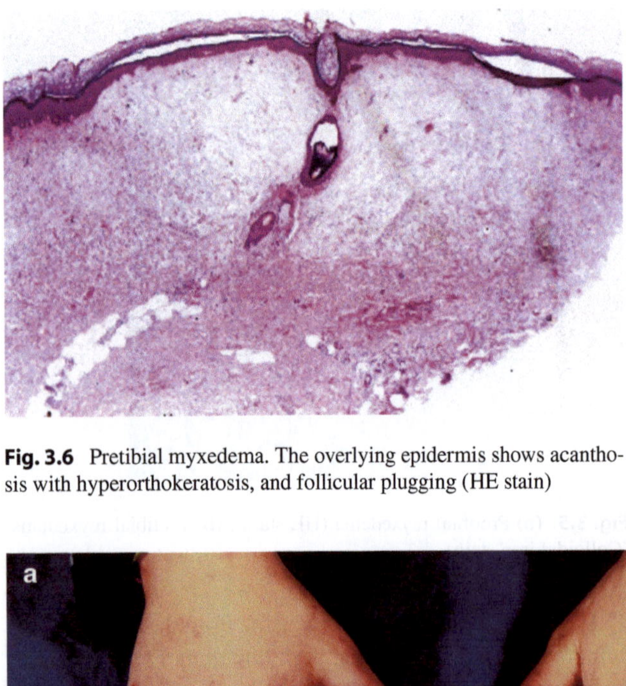

Fig. 3.6 Pretibial myxedema. The overlying epidermis shows acanthosis with hyperorthokeratosis, and follicular plugging (HE stain)

The etiology is multifarious. The most common cause is Hashimoto's thyroiditis, in which the progressive destruction of the gland results from a lymphocytic infiltration. Antiperoxidase antibodies are usually present and are of diagnostic importance. Of particular dermatological interest is postpartum thyroiditis that develops in 10% of women, 2–10 months after delivery. The condition, which can be preceded by a short thyrotoxic state (see above), is usually transient (2–4 months), but the risk for permanent hypothyroidism is not insignificant. Probably associated with postpartum thyroiditis is the telogen effluvium often observed in some women, 2–3 months after delivery.

Inflammatory conditions or viral syndromes may be associated with transient hyperthyroidism followed by transient hypothyroidism (de Quervain or painful thyroiditis, subacute thyroiditis). These are often associated with fever, malaise, and a painful and tender gland.

Amiodarone, interferon alpha, thalidomide, lithium, and radioactive iodine for treatment of Graves' disease have also been associated with primary hypothyroidism.

Thyroidectomy and external neck irradiation (for solid cancers or Hodgkin disease) may result in hypothyroidism as well.

Secondary or tertiary hypothyroidism results from the damage of the hypothalamic-pituitary axis. Many conditions like pituitary adenomas, tumors of the hypothalamus, brain

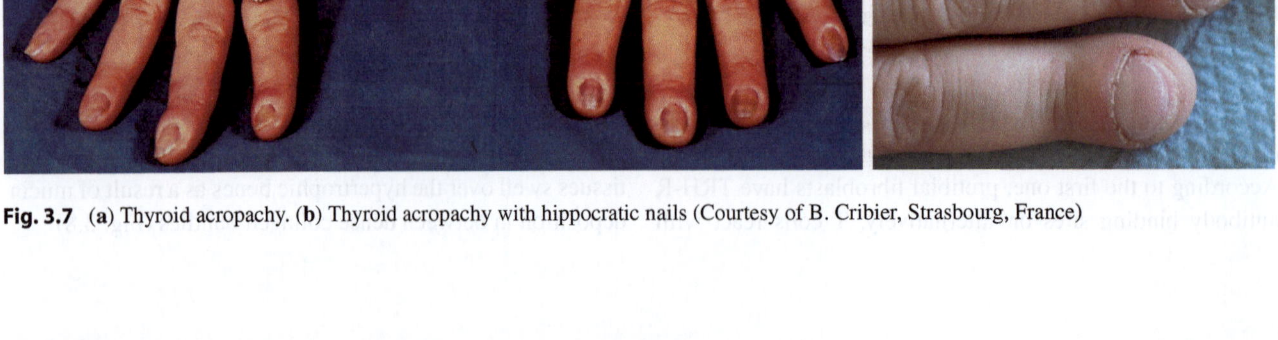

Fig. 3.7 (**a**) Thyroid acropachy. (**b**) Thyroid acropachy with hippocratic nails (Courtesy of B. Cribier, Strasbourg, France)

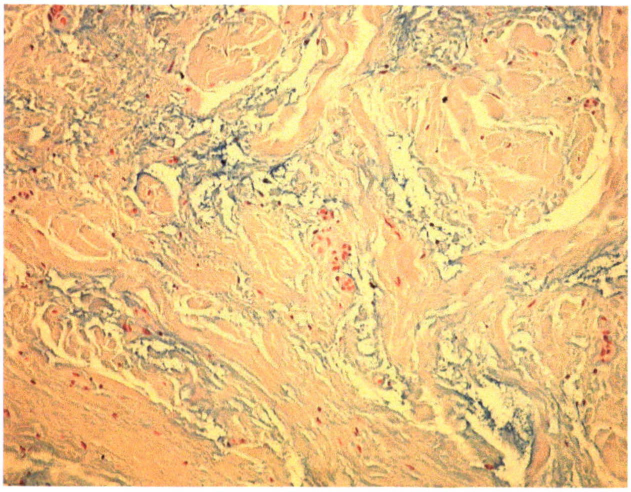

Fig. 3.8 Mucin deposition in between dense collagen bundles in thyroid acropachy (HE stain) (Courtesy of B. Cribier, Strasbourg, France)

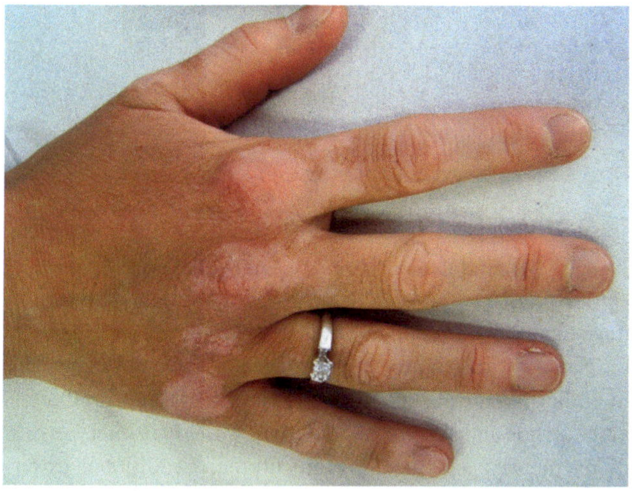

Fig. 3.9 Vitiligo in Graves' disease

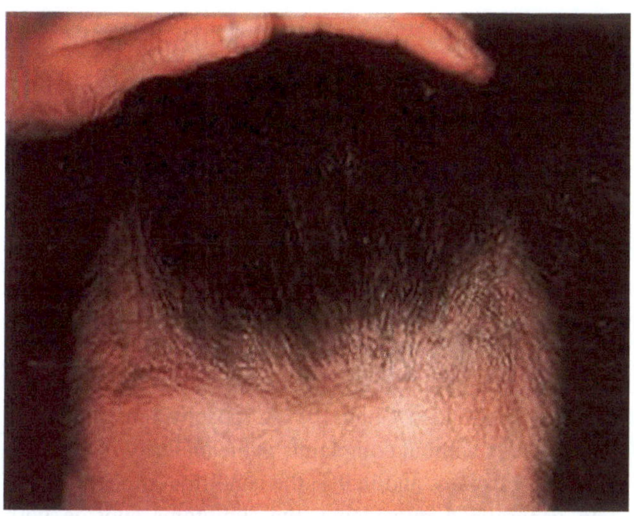

Fig. 3.10 Telogen effluvium in hyperthyroidism

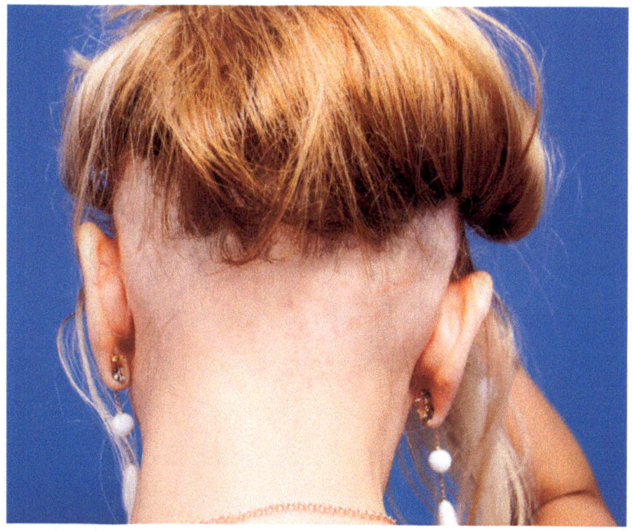

Fig. 3.11 Alopecia areata (ophiasis type) in Graves' disease

irradiation, and drugs such as dopamine and lithium may evolve into this result.

Primary generalized myxedema is the most common skin manifestation of hypothyroidism, resulting from the impaired secretion of thyroid hormone. It may be the end stage of a chronic inflammation of the gland (Hashimoto's thyroiditis) or Graves' disease, or may be due to the surgical or radiologic removal of the thyroid or due to the ingestion of substances or drugs.

There are three forms that are similar in their presentation, differing only in the age of onset, including cretinism in the early childhood, the juvenile form in childhood, and the most common adult form.

In cretinism, the patient appears as a retarded dwarf. Hypertelorism and thickened eyelids with confluent eyebrows are common. The hair changes are typical. Scalp hairs are coarse, dry, and dull, and brittle with reduced diameter, while axillary and pubic hairs fail to develop at puberty. An infrequent sign is hypertrichosis on the back, shoulders, and outer aspects of the arms and legs.

The juvenile form of myxedema is similar and is accompanied by retarded bone growth, but mental retardation is absent.

In the adult form, fatigue and weight gain, cold intolerance, hoarseness of voice, physical slowness, mental retardation, and constipation are common features. The face is round with periorbital edema (Fig. 3.12), enlarged and protruding lips, macroglossia, and a broad nose. There are episodes of malar flushing, and sweating is reduced or absent. Cold, nonpitting edema involves both the hands and feet. In hypothyroidism, the skin is usually thick, yellowish (due to carotenemia), cold, and dry with livedo on the extremities. Acquired ichthyosis and/or asteatotic eczema (Fig. 3.13) are often reported [12]. The thyroid hormone is well known to

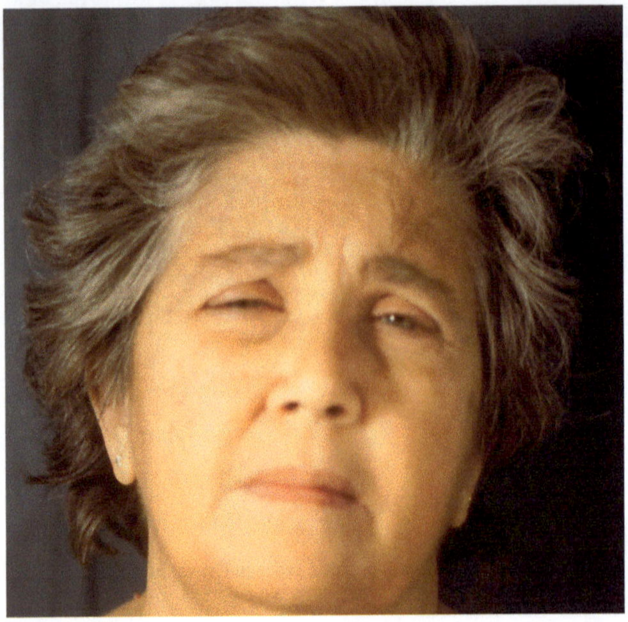

Fig. 3.12 Generalized myxedema. Typical facies

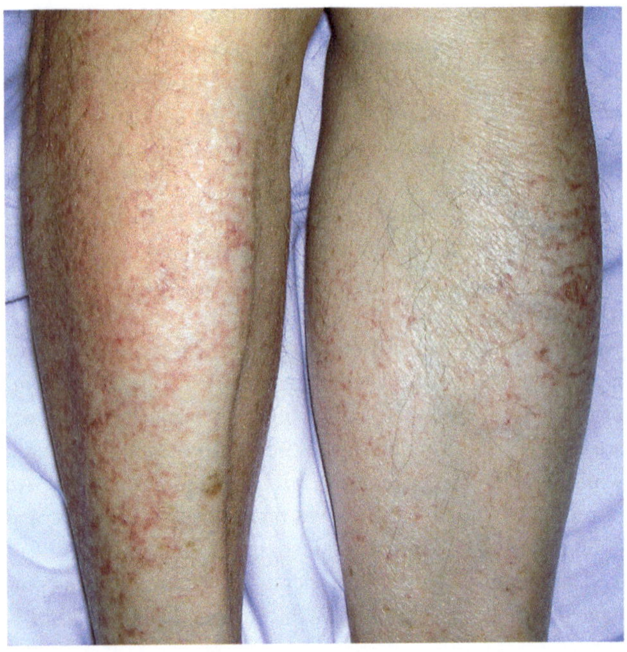

Fig. 3.13 Asteatotic eczema on the legs

regulate fatty acid metabolism and cholesterol biosynthesis. As a consequence, hypothyroidism can be associated with abnormalities in the epidermis and a disordered stratum corneum. Hairs are dry, coarse, and brittle, contributing to the diffuse or partial alopecia of the scalp (Fig. 3.14), groin, and even lateral eyebrows. The etiopathogenesis is unclear, although thyroid therapy may reverse the hair changes. Nails are brittle and thick and grow slowly. Bruising is easy with poor wound healing.

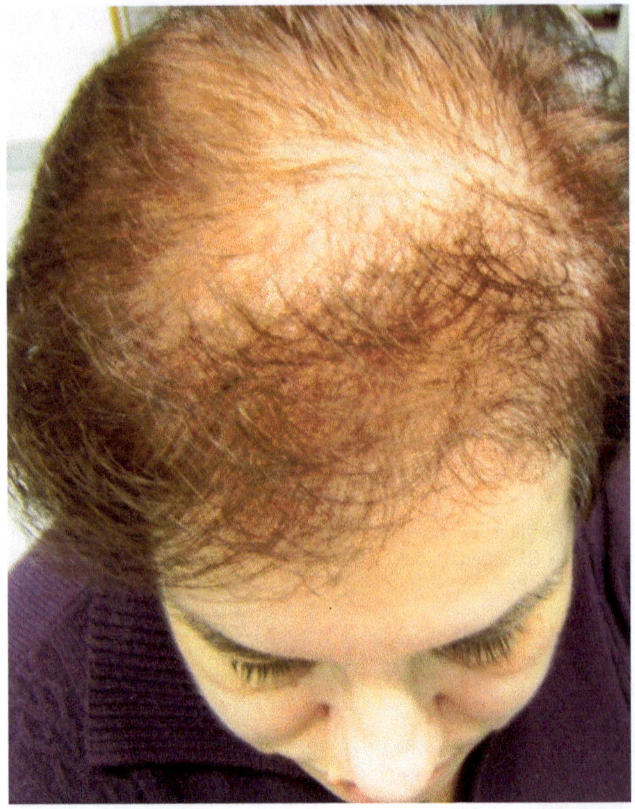

Fig. 3.14 Alopecia in hypothyroidism

Secondary myxedema depends on the failure of the pituitary gland to stimulate thyroid. The symptoms and signs are the same as in primary myxedema, but goiter, obesity, and hypothermia are absent. The voice is less coarse, and there is amenorrhea and absence of lactation, while in primary myxedema menses and lactation are normal. Additional differences are the normal levels of cholesterol and the decreased levels of serum TSH.

3.3 Treatment and Prognosis

Pretibial myxedema may benefit from corticosteroids either in occlusive medication or in intralesional injection [3]. Plasmapheresis, gradient pneumatic compression, and octreotide with and without surgical shave removal have been of some benefit. Therapy for the associated hyperthyroidism does not improve the cutaneous lesions, and often, localized myxedema develops after treatment. Localized myxedema may also clear spontaneously. Surgical intervention should be avoided (see also Chap. 18). Acropachy remains stable over the years without complaints in the majority of patients. In 14%, it resolves, and in 9%, the condition improves.

In generalized myxedema, the symptoms subside with thyroxine administration and recur if it is discontinued.

Overall, the most common problem in hypothyroidism is dryness of the skin. It is important to use a gentle cleansing soap with light abrasive properties and to moisturize the skin with petrolatum-based creams, urea (10–20%), or alpha-hydroxy acids.

Hair loss may be a diagnostic problem before becoming a therapeutic challenge. It is essential to distinguish hair problems due to insuffcient thyroid hormones (hair dull and brittle) from hair loss as a sign of a paralleling autoimmune attack. In the first instance, thyroid hormone administration is mandatory, while in the second a corticosteroid medication, possibly topical, may be beneficial in the long term (at least 4 months).

References

1. Nayak B, Hodak SP (2007). Hyperthyroidism. Endocrinol Metab Clin North Am 36:617–656
2. Anderson CK, Miller OF 3rd (2003) Triad of exophthalmos, pretibial myxedema, and acropachy in a patient with Graves' disease. J Am Acad Dermatol 48:970–972
3. Burman KD, McKinley-Grant L (2006) Dermatologic aspects of thyroid disease. Clin Dermatol 24:247–255
4. Georgala S, Katoulis AC, Georgala C, Katoulis EC, Hatziolou E, Stavrianes HG (2002). Pretibial myxedema as the initial manifestation of Graves' disease. J Eur Acad Dermatol Venereol 16:380–383
5. Fatourechi V (2005) Pretibial myxedema: pathophysiology and treatment options. Am J Clin Dermatol 6:295–309
6. Fatourechi V, Ahmed DD, Schwartz KM (2002) Thyroid acropachy: report of 40 patients treated at a single institution in a 26-year period. J Clin Endocrinol Metab 87:5435–5441
7. Alkhateeb A, Fain PR, Thody A, Bennett DC, Spritz RA (2003) Epidemiology of vitiligo and associated autoimmune diseases in Caucasian probands and their families. Pigment Cell Res 16: 208–214
8. Artantaş S, Gül U, Kiliç A, Güler S (2009) Skin findings in thyroid diseases. Eur J Intern Med 20:15–161
9. Niepomniszcze H, Amad RH (2001) Skin disorders and thyroid diseases. J Endocrinol Invest 24:628–638
10. Roberts CG, Ladenson PW (2004). Hypothyroidism. Lancet 363: 793–803
11. Dreskin SC, Andrews KY (2005) The thyroid and urticaria. Curr Opin Allergy Clin Immunol 5:408–412
12. Brazzelli V, Prestinari F, Barbagallo T, Bellani E, Calcaterra V, Larizza D, Lauriola MM, Borroni G (2005) Acquired ichthyosis and hypertrichosis due to autoimmune thyroiditis: therapeutic response to thyroxine replacement. Pediatr Dermatol 22: 447–449

Chapter 4
Pituitary Gland Diseases

Martina Montinari and Franco Rongioletti

Key Points

- Excessive secretion of pituitary hormones, as well as their deficiency, may cause a constellation of clinical and pathological manifestations involving major organ systems of the body, including the skin.
- There are no specific cutaneous signs or symptoms that are pathognomonic for the main manifestations of pituitary gland diseases such as acromegaly, hyperprolactinemia, Cushing's disease, or hypopituitarism.
- In addition to tissue hyperplasia, which is the hallmark of the disease, patients with acromegaly present with skin thickening, excessive sebaceous, eccrine and apocrine secretion, skin tags, and cutis verticis gyrata.
- In the setting of hyperprolactinemia, galactorrhea in women and gynecomastia or impotence in men are associated with acne vulgaris, seborrhea, androgenetic alopecia, and hirsutism.
- Rubeosis faciei, epidermal atrophy, acne, purpura, hirsutism, and striae distensae are the main features of ACTH-dependent Cushing's disease in association with hyperpigmentation.
- Skin manifestations, although not pathognomonic, may be the first sign of underlying pituitary gland disease and can allow early detection and intervention, reducing the adverse medical implications.

Keywords Acromegaly • Hyperprolactinemia • Cushing's disease • Panhypopituitarism

4.1 Introduction

The pituitary gland is also called the "master" gland of the endocrine system since it administers the functions of the other endocrine glands. It is a complex organ connected to the hypothalamus by the pituitary stalk. Sending signals to the thyroid gland, adrenal glands, ovaries, and testes, this gland modulates the production of a variety of hormones that have important effects on metabolism, blood pressure, sexuality, reproduction, growth, milk production, and other vital body functions [1]. The pituitary is a pea-sized gland that is housed within a bony structure (sella turcica) at the base of the brain and has two distinct parts: the anterior lobe (adenohypophysis) and the posterior (neurohypophysis) lobe, anatomical extension of the hypothalamus [1].

Under the influence of the hypothalamus, the adenohypophysis synthesizes and secretes important endocrine hormones, such as growth hormone (GH), thyrotropin (TSH), adrenocorticotropic hormone (ACTH), prolactin (PRL), endorphins, follicle stimulating hormone (FSH), luteinizing hormone (LH).

Hypothalamic hormones are secreted into the anterior lobe via a special capillary system, called the hypothalamic-hypophyseal portal system. The posterior pituitary gland stores and releases oxytocin (OT) and antidiuretic hormone (ADH, also known as vasopressin). Table 4.1 summarizes the main disorders involving the pituitary gland.

Excessive secretion of pituitary hormones, as well as hormone deficiencies, may cause characteristic cutaneous manifestations that sometimes may be the first sign of the underlying disease.

4.2 Clinical and Pathological Aspects of Skin Manifestations

4.2.1 *Acromegaly*

Acromegaly is the clinical syndrome that results from excessive secretion of the growth hormone. The diagnosis is based on an increase serum GH concentration unsuppressed after an oral glucose load and an increased insulin-like growth factor-1 (IGF-1). In more than 95% of cases, the primary cause is a secreting pituitary adenoma [2]. Rarely, familial syndromes such as McCune–Albright syndrome, MEN type 1, and Carney complex are associated with

M. Montinari (✉)
Clinica Dermatologica, University of Genova,
Viale Benedetto XV, 7, Genova, Italy
e:mail: martimontinari@libero.it

F. Rongioletti and B.R. Smoller (eds.), *Clinical and Pathological Aspects of Skin Diseases in Endocrine, Metabolic, Nutritional and Deposition Disease*, DOI 10.1007/978-1-60761-181-3_4, © Springer Science+Business Media, LLC 2010

Table 4.1 Disorders involving the pituitary gland

Hyperpituitarism	Anterior	Acromegaly, Hyperprolactinaemia, Pituitary ACTH hypersecretion
	Posterior	Syndrome of inappropriate secretion of antidiuretic hormone (SIADH)
	General	Nelson's syndrome (rapid enlargement of a pituitary adenoma that occurs after the removal of both adrenal glands)
Hypopituitarism	Anterior	Kallmann syndrome (hypothalamic hypogonadotropic hypogonadism) Growth hormone deficiency, ACTH deficiency
	Posterior	Neurogenic diabetes insipidus
	General	Empty sella syndrome, Pituitary apoplexy, Sheehan's syndrome, Lymphocytic hypophysitis

acromegaly. Extrapituitary causes for acromegaly are infrequent and include pancreatic islet cell tumors that secrete either GH or GH-releasing hormone.

Tissue hyperplasia is the hallmark of the syndrome and is a consequence of the stimulation of GH and IGF [1, 3], which promote sulfation of collagen and synthesis of RNA and DNA. In patients with acromegaly, the skin is thickened and has a doughy feel owing to dermal mucin accumulation and edema [4]. The main clinical features are broadened hands and feet with widened, thickened, and stubby fingers. The *facial aspect* is typical with coarse features including a widened nose, thick lips, frontal bossing, and deep facial lines (Fig. 4.1). Oily skin with widened skin pores and hypertrichosis are also frequent findings, while acne is a less common feature [5]. The skin is also wet with an offensive body odor due to excessive eccrine and apocrine hyperhidrosis leading to a heightened incidence of abscesses in the axillae and intergluteal cleft. However, eccrine and sebaceous gland morphology and number do not differ from healthy controls, proving that the excessive sebum and sweat production is due to an overactivity of the glands.

Numerous pigmented *skin tags* are found in up to 45% of patients (Fig. 4.2). As skin tags are associated with insulin resistance, diabetes mellitus, and dyslipidemia in the general population, it is not clear if skin tags are a direct consequence of acromegaly or the dysmetabolic syndrome which frequently coexists with acromegaly. In almost half of the patients, skin pigmentation is increased, a phenomenon that appears to be due to the effect of melanocyte-stimulating hormone (MSH). Occasionally, acanthosis nigricans is also a finding (Fig. 4.2) [6].

Cutis verticis gyrata, a scalp condition where there are convoluted folds and deep furrows that resemble the surface of the cerebral cortex can be another sign of acromegaly (Fig. 4.3). Scalp hair is usually coarse, but in late stages, it is often fine, silky, and sparse. A relationship between psoriasis and acromegaly has been reported [7], based upon an increase of serum GH in some psoriatic patients and an improvement of the dermatitis after surgical pituitary tumor excision [8] or after treatment with somatostatin or dopamine analogs [9–11]. However, these data have not been confirmed by other investigators [12, 13].

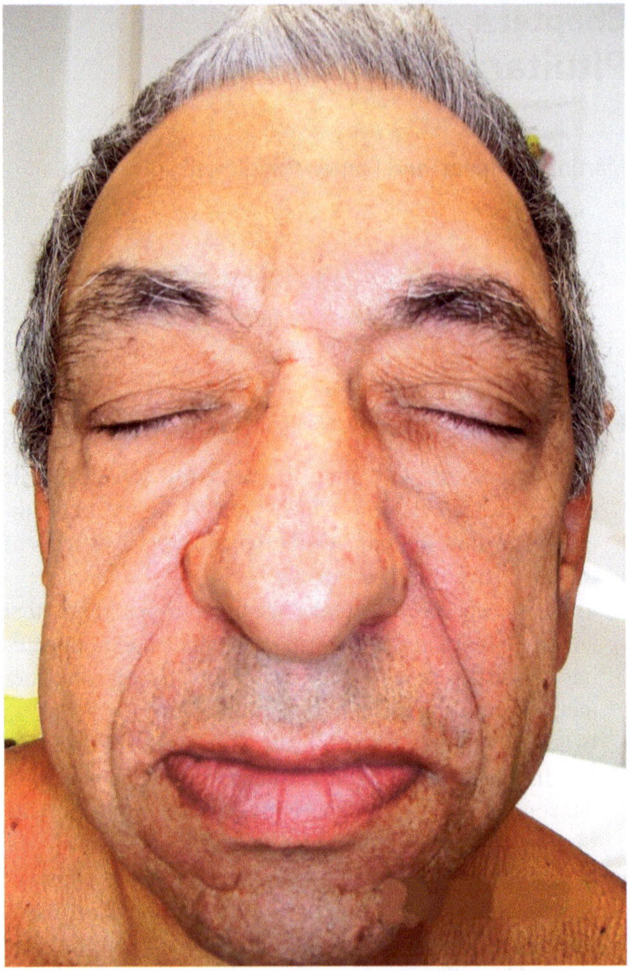

Fig. 4.1 Acromegaly. Patient with frontal bossing, prognathism, nasal bone hypertrophy, deep nasolabial folds, and enlarged pores

The disease also has rheumatologic, cardiovascular, respiratory, and metabolic consequences which determine its prognosis.

4.2.2 Hyperprolactinemia

Prolactin is a pituitary hormone that plays a fundamental role in a variety of reproductive functions. It is an essential factor for normal production of breast milk following childbirth. An excess of prolactin, or hyperprolactinemia, is a commonly encountered clinical condition due to a prolactin-secreting

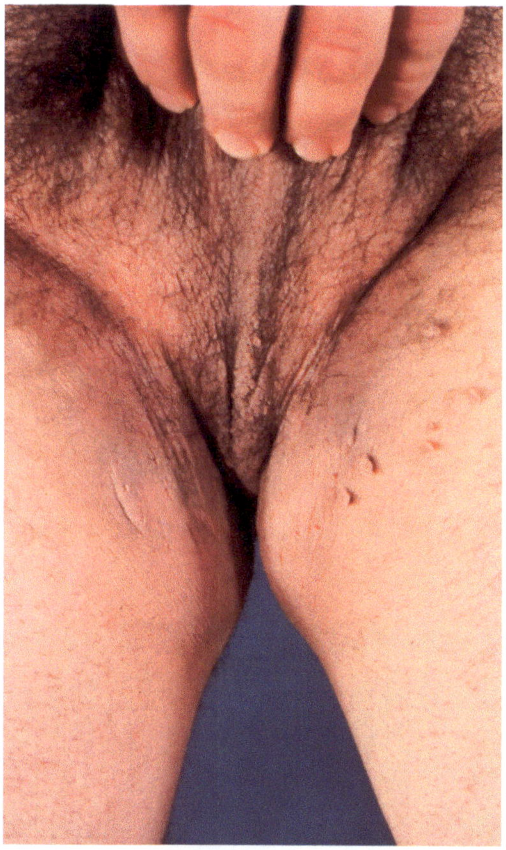

Fig. 4.2 Pigmented skin tags and acanthosis nigricans in acromegaly

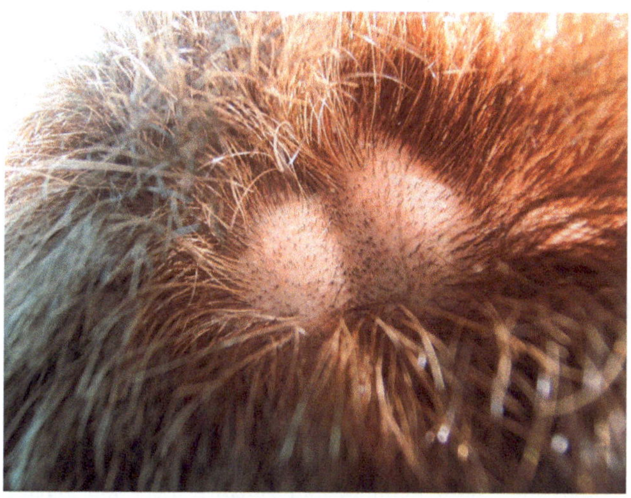

Fig. 4.3 Cutis verticis gyrata in acromegaly

adenoma (prolactinoma). Several drugs may result in a significant increase in prolactin serum concentration such as antipsychotic, antidepressant with serotoninergic activity, prokinetics, opiates, estrogens, antiandrogens, antihypertensive drugs, H2-receptor antagonists, anticonvulsivants, and cholinomimetics [14–16]. Other pathologic conditions inducing hyperprolactinemia are kidney failure, granulomatous diseases of the pituitary gland, and disorders that interfere with the hypothalamic inhibition of prolactin release, for example, in response to the hypothyroid state. Ectopic (nonpituitary) production of prolactin may also occur.

The most frequent symptoms are decreased libido, infertility, oligomenorrhea/amenorrhea, and galactorrhea in women and decreased libido, infertility, gynecomastia (Fig. 4.4), or impotence in men. The skin in hyperprolactinemia becomes thickened, coarse, and greasy, with enlarged pores. Acne vulgaris and seborrhea may develop; androgenetic alopecia may occur also in children and adolescents, where the straight hairline conforms to the adult configuration (calvities frontalis adolescentium). In fact, prolactin plays a role in the hair cycle, promoting the anagen phase [17]. Estrogen is a potent stimulator of prolactin release and prolongs the anagen phase of the hair cycle, explaining the increased frequency of hypertrichosis observed during pregnancy. Hyperprolactinemia is one recognized cause of *hypertrichosis or hirsutism* occurring on the extremities, the anterior chest, abdomen, lower back, and in the beard area (Fig. 4.5).

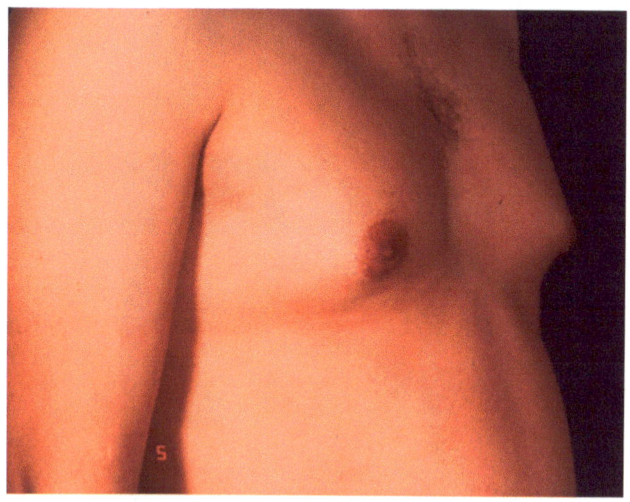

Fig. 4.4 Gynecomastia in a young man with hyperprolactinemia

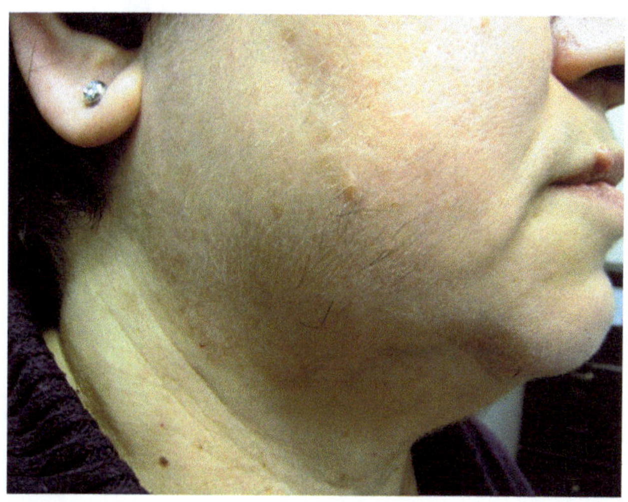

Fig. 4.5 Hypertrichosis in a woman with hyperprolactinemia

Acanthosis nigricans may occur, especially in women with hyperprolactinemia and polycystic ovary disease. An association between psoriasis and the level of prolactin has been suggested, and psoriasis has been linked to the development of a prolactinoma [18, 19].

4.2.3 Cushing's Disease

The term "Cushing's disease" is reserved for the pathological condition that is caused by excessive secretion of ACTH by a pituitary adenoma (usually microadenoma) with subsequent suprarenal hyperplasia. Roughly, two-thirds of the cases of endogenous Cushing's syndrome are caused by "Cushing's disease".

Clinical features associated with the metabolic consequences of excess cortisol include progressive central obesity (Fig. 4.6), hypertension, abnormal glucose metabolism, osteoporosis, excess protein breakdown with myopathy, psychiatric disturbances, and amenorrhea [1, 20].

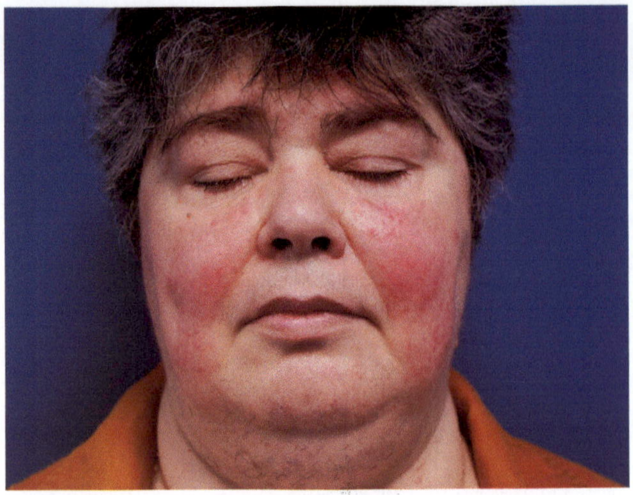

Fig. 4.7 Rubeosis, moon face, and acne in Cushing's disease

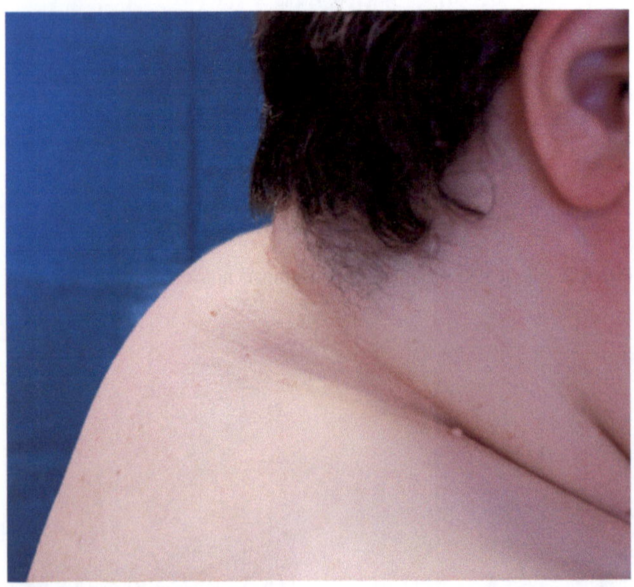

Fig. 4.8 Cushing's disease. "*Buffalo hump*"

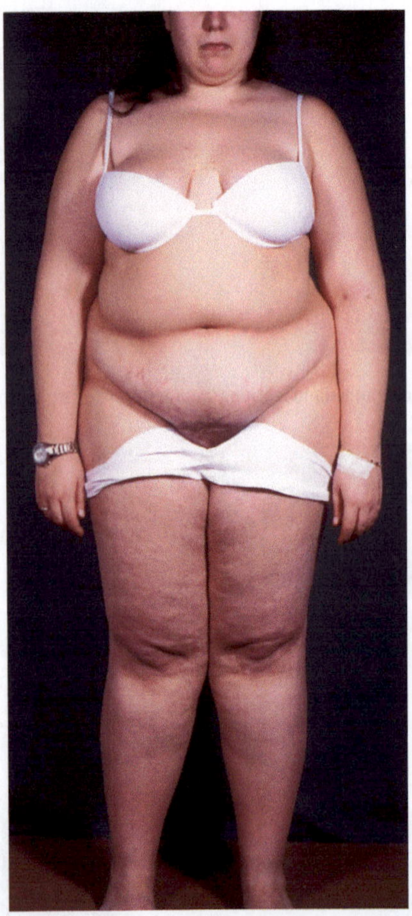

Fig. 4.6 Cushing's disease with central obesity in a young woman

The cutaneous manifestations of Cushing's disease include accumulation of fat tissue with a characteristic distribution (facial, truncal, and back of the neck) causing the "*moon face*" with plethora and *rubeosis* over the cheeks (Fig. 4.7) and "*buffalo hump*" (Fig. 4.8) [1, 20]. Corticosteroids, among other effects, inhibit epidermal cell division, impair synthesis of collagen and mucopolysaccharides, and increase catabolism of proteins. *Violaceous striae* extending greater than 1 cm in diameter on the abdomen and lower flanks are a pathognomonic sign (Fig. 4.9). The skin eventually becomes atrophic, fragile and may peel off with adhesive tape-like damp tissue paper (*Liddle's sign*). Atrophy results in easy bruising manifesting with *petechiae* and *ecchymoses* over the extremities. *Hyperpigmentation* is particularly expressed

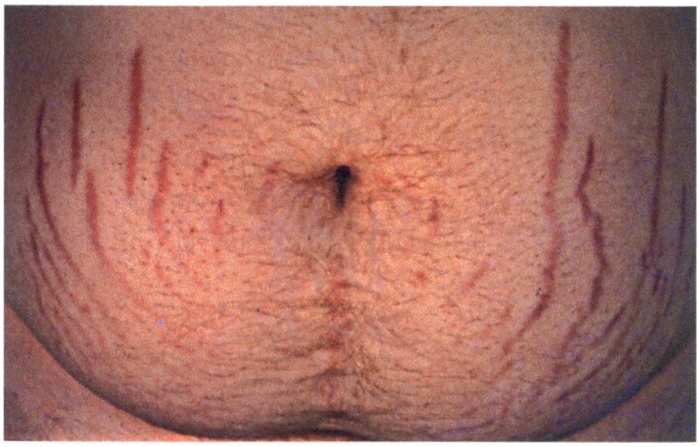

Fig. 4.9 Cushing striae

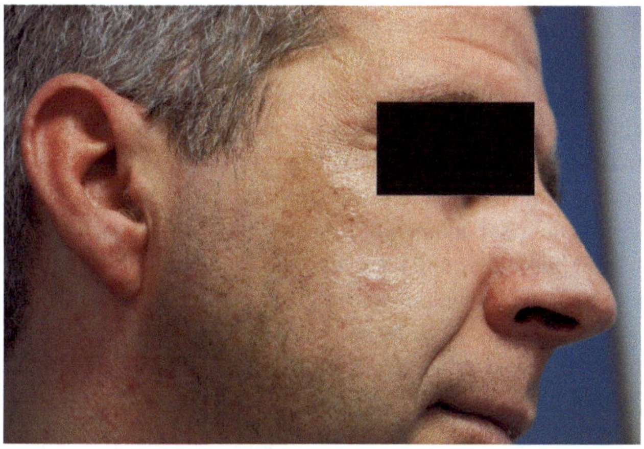

Fig. 4.10 Hyperpigmentation of sun-exposed area in Cushing's disease

with the ectopic ACTH syndrome, less frequently with Cushing's disease and almost absent with adrenal Cushing's syndrome. The hyperpigmentation is a result of the action of ACTH and MSH on melanocyte-stimulating receptors inducing melanogenesis. Clinically, the pigmentation is generalized but accentuated in sun-exposed areas (Fig. 4.10) and sites of friction or trauma. It has been reported that scars that occur during the period of elevated ACTH become hyperpigmented and remain discolored despite subsequent reduction in ACTH. On the other hand, scars that are present prior to an elevation in ACTH are not hyperpigmented. Hyperpigmentation can also occur on the inner mucosa of the lips and buccal mucosa along the line of dental occlusion. Acanthosis nigricans may be linked to hyperinsulinism and insulin resistance. *Hypertrichosis* is common, as well as *acne*, but differently from acne vulgaris, the lesions are monomorphic, without comedones and cysts. Associated features in women are clitoridomegaly and *androgenetica alopecia with male pattern* (Fig. 4.11) [21]. Poikiloderma-like changes with "cigarette paper" wrinkling on the back of the hands and elbows have been rarely reported. Patients are more prone to develop mycoses such as dermatophytosis and pityriasis versicolor. Minor wounds heal slowly and can be often infected secondarily.

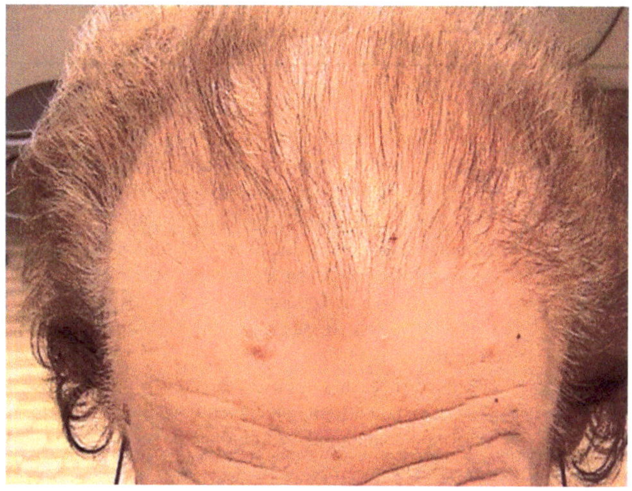

Fig. 4.11 Androgenetic alopecia with male pattern in Cushing's disease

4.2.4 Panhypopituitarism

Hypopituitarism is a condition in which there is diminished or absent secretion of one or more pituitary hormones, resulting either from a primary disorder of the secretory cells of the anterior pituitary gland or as a secondary consequence of reduced stimulation by the releasing hormones of the hypothalamus. When the deficiency of anterior pituitary hormones is generalized, the condition is referred to as panhypopituitarism.

The most common cause is a pituitary tumor (chromophobe adenoma, craniopharyngioma), but vascular abnormalities (ischemic necrosis), granulomatous inflammation (sarcoidosis), autoimmune disorders (autoimmune hypophysitis), trauma (stalk destruction), infections (syphilis, tuberculosis), Langerhans cell histiocytosis, congenital disorders (Rathke's cleft cyst), and iatrogenic damage (surgery, radiotherapy) also cause hypopituitarism. A particular well-described cause of acquired hypopituitarism is postpartum pituitary necrosis or Sheehan's syndrome [1, 22, 23]. Table 4.2 summarizes the extracutaneous manifestations of hypopituitarism.

Most of the dermatological signs and symptoms are similar to those that occur with a primary deficiency of that gland. TSH deficiency results in signs and symptoms of hypothyroidism (*see Chap. 3*) including pale and dry skin with a yellow tinge of the palms, soles, and nasolabial folds (carotenemia), although these changes are less frequent than in primary hypothyroidism (<10%). Puffiness of the face and dermal accumulation of acid glycosaminoglycans (myxedema) are striking features (Fig. 4.12a, b). *Mucin deposits,* mainly perivascular

Table 4.2 Extracutaneous manifestations in hypopituitarism

Hormone	Major clinical manifestations of deficiency
ACTH	Weakness, malaise, nausea, vomiting, and collapse hypoglycemia; hypothermia; loss of libido in women
TSH	Fatigue; constipation; weight gain; cold intolerance Severity of manifestations is generally less than that seen in primary hypothyroidism
GH	Impaired quality of life; altered musculoskeletal composition; impaired cardiac function; increased cardiovascular risk diminished vigor and decreased tolerance to exercise and social functioning
LH/FSH	Amenorrhea and atrophy of the breasts in women, testicular atrophy and erectile dysfunction in men, and diminished libido both sexes
PRL	Alactogenesis
ADH	Diabetes insipidus
OT	None

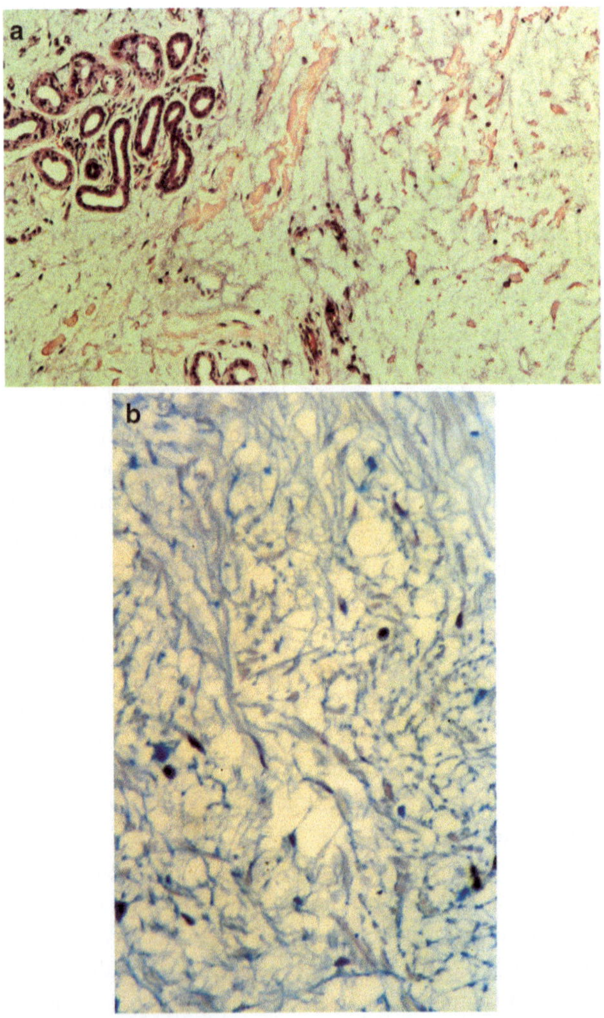

Fig. 4.12 Generalized myxedema. (**a**) Mucin deposition in the deep dermis around eccrine glands (HE stain). (**b**) Mucin stains positively with Alcian blue stain

and periadnexal, splay collagen bundles and may extend to the subcutaneous fat and nerves. Fibroblasts are not increased in number, but elastic fibers are reduced. Scalp hair becomes dull, coarse, and brittle with partial or diffuse alopecia due to a premature arrest of the anagen of the hair cycle [24]. Loss of hair from the lateral third of the eyebrow is characteristic [25]. Onycholysis, longitudinal ridging, and brownish discoloration of the nail plate may occur.

In addition to amenorrhea and erectile dysfunction, deficiency of gonadotropins such as luteinizing hormone (LH) and follicle-stimulating hormone (FSH) results in loss of body hair, which is observed in all patients early in the course. Men show a slowing of beard growth and uniformly decreased body hair, usually starting in the axillae. In women, most androgens are produced by the adrenal glands. The loss of LH-mediated ovarian androgens, therefore, does not have a significant impact on axillary or pubic hair, although prepubertal women may have loss of other secondary sexual characteristics. Scalp hair tends to be fine and dry, and there may be generalized thinning. The loss of androgen-mediated collagen synthesis and maturation causes a thinning of the dermis and subcutaneous tissues with the development of fine wrinkling around the eyes and mouth, giving the patient a premature aging appearance [26].

GH deficiency causes atrophic, dry, and pruritic skin that may be easily traumatized with a delayed time of wound healing.

ACTH deficiency gives rise to signs similar to those found in adrenal insufficiency (See also Chap. 1), except for the absence of hyperpigmentation.

The decreased MSH production also results in generalized hypopigmentation, especially in the sexual areas. The inability to tan may lead to severe sunburn after sunlight exposure [27].

Less commonly, deficiency in arginine vasopressin (AVP) results in diabetes insipidus in which anhidrosis has been described.

4.3 Treatment and Prognosis

Controlling GH and IGF-1 oversecretion improves most cutaneous manifestations of acromegaly, although a full regression is difficult to be attained, especially in patients with long-lasting disease. Facial features improve and puffiness decreases. Ring size decreases along with shoe size, and acanthosis nigricans, cutis verticis gyrata, and psoriasis also improve [28].

The cutaneous manifestations of hyperprolactinemia improve with systemic therapy. Medical treatment with dopamine agonist drugs (bromocriptine, 10–15 mg daily) is currently the gold standard approach for both microprolactinomas and macroprolactinomas. Bromocriptine as a treatment for prolactinoma has been associated with good therapeutic response of psoriatic lesions.

The treatment of Cushing's disease is directed at the source. Once the disease is under control, the cutaneous signs, except the violaceous striae, significantly improve; the color fades when the disease is arrested, but the atrophy, obviously, remains.

Concerning hypopituitarism, partial relief from skin dryness can be obtained with emollient creams, but the real treatment is the management of disease that consists of replacing the individual peripheral hormones through oral, transdermal, intramuscular, intranasal, or subcutaneous routes. It is essential that patients are aware about the importance of hormone supplementation and (in the case of cortisol) about the requirement for dosage modifications during acute illness or stress.

Restoration of euvolemia with desmopressin in anhidrosis induced by diabetes insipidus restores sympathetic nerve activity and sweating function [29, 30].

References

1. Davidovici BB, Orion E, Wolf R (2008) Cutaneous manifestations of pituitary gland diseases. Clin Dermatol 26:288–295
2. Melmed S, Kleinberg D (2003) Anterior pituitary. In: Larsen PR, Kronenberg HM, Melmed S, Polonsky KS (eds) Williams textbook of endocrinology, 10th edn. Saunders, Philadelphia, PA, pp 177–279
3. Ben-Shlomo A, Melmed S (2006) Skin manifestations in acromegaly. Clin Dermatol 24:256–259
4. Braham C, Betea D, Pierard-Franchimont C et al (2002) Skin tensile properties in patients treated for acromegaly. Dermatology 204:325–329
5. Centurion SA, Schwartz RA (2002) Cutaneous signs of acromegaly. Int J Dermatol 41:631–634
6. Stone OJ (1993) Acanthosis nigricans – decreased extracellular matrix viscosity: cancer, obesity, diabetes, corticosteroids, somatotrophin. Med Hypotheses 40:154–157
7. Weber G, Neidhardt M, Schmidt A (1981) Korrelation von Wachstumshormon und klinischem Bild der Psoriasis. Arch Dermatol Res 270:129–140
8. Todd DJ, Eedy DJ, McMillan JC (1991) Acromegaly and psoriasis. Clin Exp Dermatol 16:222–223
9. Weber G, Klughardt G, Neidhardt M (1981) Psoriasis and human growth hormone: aetiology and therapy. Arch Dermatol Res 270:361–365
10. Valentino A, Fimiani M, Bilenchi R et al (1984) Therapy with bromocriptine and behavior of various hormones in psoriasis patients. Boll Soc Ital Biol Sper 60:1841–1844
11. Guilhou JJ (1990) Growth hormone, somatostatin and psoriasis. Dermatologica 181:81–82
12. Mackie RM, Beastall GM, Thomson JA (1984) Growth hormone levels in psoriasis. Arch Dermatol Res 275:207–208
13. Vernier A, De Simone C, Forri L et al (1988) Treatment of severe psoriasis with somatostatin: four years of experience. Arch Dermatol Res 280(Suppl):51–54
14. La Torre D, Falorni A (2007) Pharmacological causes of hyperprolactinemia. Ther Clin Risk Manag 3:929–951
15. Peveler RC, Branford D, Citrome L et al (2008) Antipsychotics and hyperprolactinaemia: clinical recommendations. J Psychopharmacol 22(2 Suppl):98–103
16. Ghafoor S (2009) Drug-induced hyperprolactinaemia. Nurs Stand 24:59
17. Paus R (1991) Does prolactin play a role in skin biology and pathology? Med Hypotheses 36:33–42
18. Giasuddin ASM, El-Sherif AI, El-Ojali SI (1998) Prolactin: does it have a role in the pathogenesis of psoriasis. Dermatology 197:119–122
19. Regana S, Millet PU (2000) Psoriasis in association with prolactinoma: three cases. Br J Dermatol 143:864–867
20. Jabbour SA (2003) Cutaneous manifestations of endocrine disorders: a guide for dermatologists. Am J Clin Dermatol 4:315–331
21. Findling JW, Raff H (2001) Diagnosis and differential diagnosis of Cushing's syndrome. Endocrinol Metab Clin North Am 30:729–747
22. Geller JL, Braunstein GD (2006) Dermatologic manifestations in hypopituitarism. Clin Dermatol 24:266–275
23. Borlu M, Tanriverdi F, Koc CA et al (2006) The effects of severe growth hormone deficiency on the skin of patients with Sheehan's syndrome. J Eur Acad Dermatol Venereol 21:199–204
24. Leonhardt M, Heymann WR (2002) Thyroid disease and the skin. Dermatol Clin 20:473–481
25. Grando SA (1993) Physiology of endocrine skin interrelations. J Am Acad Dermatol 28:981–992
26. Freinkel RK (1993) Cutaneous manifestations of endocrine diseases. In: Fitzpatrick TB, Eisen AZ, Wolf K et al (eds) Dermatology in general medicine, 4th edn. McGraw-Hill, New York, pp 2113–2131
27. Jabbour SA, Miller JL (2000) Endocrinopathies and the skin. Int J Dermatol 39:88–99
28. Maison P, Demolis P, Young J et al (2000) Vascular reactivity in acromegalic patients: preliminary evidence for regional endothelial dysfunction and increased sympathetic vasoconstriction. Clin Endocrinol (Oxf) 53:445–451
29. Taussig LM, Braunstein GD (1973) Effects of vasopressin on sweat rate and composition in patients with diabetes insipidus and normal controls. J Invest Dermatol 60:197–202
30. Shimizu H, Obi T, Miyajima H (1997) Anhidrosis: an unusual presentation of diabetes insipidus. Neurology 49:1708–1710

Chapter 5
Parathyroid Disease

Yann Charli-Joseph and Marcela Saeb-Lima

Key Points

- Cutaneous manifestations in parathyroid-related diseases are rare in sporadic cases but not unusual in familial syndromes.
- Familial isolated hyperparathyroidism is usually not accompanied by diagnostic skin manifestations.
- Diagnostic cutaneous signs are found in MEN type 1 (angiofibromas and collagenomas) and MEN type 2 (cutaneous amyloidosis).
- Metastatic calcification is commonly encountered in patients with hyperparathyroidism secondary to renal failure.
- Most cutaneous manifestations of hypoparathyroidism are nonspecific (xerosis, hair and nail abnormalities) or related to the primary causes of the endocrinopathy.
- Hypoparathyroidism presenting in the context of autoimmune polyglandular syndrome type 1 is characterized by mucocutaneous candidiasis.
- Prognosis and treatment depends upon the clinical setting of the sporadic and familial syndromes.

Keywords Hyperparathyroidism • MEN type 1 • MEN type 2 • Metastatic calcification • Hypoparathyroidism • Autoimmune polyglandular syndrome type 1

5.1 Introduction

Parathyroid hormone (PTH) is secreted by parathyroid glands as a polypeptide, which increases calcium (Ca^{2+}) levels in the blood through parathyroid receptors in bones, kidneys, and intestines, while its counterpart calcitonin (a hormone produced by the parafollicular cells of the thyroid gland) decreases Ca^{2+} concentration. In the bone, PTH enhances the expression of RANKL that can bind osteoclast precursors containing RANK, and it stimulates bone resorption (1). In the kidney, PTH stimulates active reabsorption of calcium and magnesium from distal tubules. PTH also enhances the absorption of calcium in the intestine by increasing the renal production of activated vitamin D. PTH reduces the reabsorption of phosphate from the proximal tubules of the kidney and increases its excretion through the urine. The secretion of PTH is controlled by serum-ionized calcium levels through negative feedback, achieved by activation of calcium-sensing receptors located on the parathyroid cells, by the parafollicular cells of the thyroid glands, the proximal and distal tubular cells of the kidney, epithelial cells of the intestines, osteoblasts, and osteoclasts.

The condition of elevated blood levels of PTH is known as *hyperparathyroidism*. If the cause is the parathyroid gland then it is called *primary hyperparathyroidism*, which may be caused by parathyroid adenomas, parathyroid hyperplasia, and parathyroid cancer. In sporadic, nonfamilial parathyroid adenomas, an acquired somatic chromosomal abnormality that involves mutations and rearrangement of the oncogene cyclinD1/PRAD1 has been demonstrated (2). If the elevated levels of PTH do not involve the gland, it is known as *secondary hyperparathyroidism*. *Tertiary hyperparathyroidism* results from hyperplasia of the parathyroid glands with subsequent lack of response to serum calcium levels. Both secondary and tertiary hyperparathyroidism are most often seen in patients with chronic renal failure.

Hypoparathyroidism is mainly characterized by hypocalcemia due to inadequate parathyroid hormone (PTH) secretion, or less often by unresponsiveness to elevated PTH levels (pseudohypoparathyroidism).

5.2 Clinical and Pathological Aspects of Skin Manifestations

5.2.1 *Hyperparathyroidism*

Hyperparathyroidism is characterized by hypercalcemia and inappropriate suppression of PTH, which may present sporadically, associated with familial syndromes (hereditary hyperparathyroidism), or related to renal failure.

M. Saeb-Lima (✉)
Pathology Department, Instituto Nacional de Ciencias Médicas y Nutrición "Salvador Zubirán", Vasco de Quiroga #15, Colonia Sección XVI, Delegación Tlalpan, CP 14000, México City, México
e-mail: marcela.saeblima@gmail.com

F. Rongioletti and B.R. Smoller (eds.), *Clinical and Pathological Aspects of Skin Diseases in Endocrine, Metabolic, Nutritional and Deposition Disease*, DOI 10.1007/978-1-60761-181-3_5,

5.2.1.1 Familial (Hereditary) Forms of Primary Hyperparathyroidism

Familial (hereditary) forms of primary hyperparathyroidism refer to any association of PTH with other endocrine tumors or familial clustering with variable penetrance (3) and include *the multiple endocrine neoplasia syndromes (type 1 and 2A), familial isolated hyperparathyroidism including the jaw tumor syndrome, familial benign hypercalcemic hypocalciuria, and neonatal severe hypercalcemia*. They represent between 5 and 10% of all cases of hyperparathyroidism.

Multiple endocrine neoplasia type 1 (MEN1), also known as Wermer syndrome (4, 5), is an autosomal dominant entity characterized by the combination of tumors of the anterior pituitary, parathyroid glands, and endocrine pancreas. MEN1 is caused by the loss of function germline mutations in the *MEN1* gene mapped to chromosome 11q13, which encodes a protein named menin that acts as a tumor suppressor gene. The earliest and most common manifestation of MEN1 is hyperthyroidism. Clinical manifestations include bone disease, fractures, nephrolithiasis, gastrointestinal symptoms with recurrent multiple ulcers, and amenorrhea or hypogonadism. Cutaneous neoplasms include *collagenomas, angiofibromas, melanomas, and lipomas*. They appear in the second decade of life. Collagenomas are raised dome-shaped flesh color or slightly hypopigmented papules and nodules of firm skin in the neck and trunk (Fig. 5.1a) and are characterized by markedly thickened dermis due to thickened collagen bundles irregularly arranged (Fig. 5.1b) with diminished elastic tissue (Fig. 5.1c) and sometimes, interstitial mucin deposition (Fig. 5.1d). Angiofibromas are papular lesions that can be flesh colored, slightly telangiectatic, or light brown. They are commonly seen in the mid-face (Fig. 5.2a). Increased numbers of stellate fibroblasts are seen coursing between the fibrotic collagen, and ecstatic vessels are often present (Fig. 5.2b–e). Loss of heterozygosity at the MEN1 locus is seen in some angiofibromas and collagenomas (6). Lipomas may be single or multiple. Other cutaneous findings include café-au-lait and hypopigmented macules.

Multiple endocrine neoplasia type 2A (MEN2A) is an autosomal dominant entity consisting of medullary thyroid cancer, pheochromocytoma, and primary parathyroid hyperplasia (3, 5). The initial neoplastic manifestation is usually medullary thyroid cancer. The aggressiveness of this tumor depends upon the germline mutations of RET proto-oncogene. In 36% of cases, patients develop *macular or lichen amyloidosis*, frequently localized to the interescapular areas as macules or pruritic, scaly lichenoid papules with hyperpigmentation (Fig. 5.3a, b). Macular or lichen amyloidosis has been associated with RET proto-oncogene mutation in codon 634 (7). Macular amyloidosis is characterized by globular eosinophilic deposits of eosinophilic material within the papillary dermis (Fig. 5.3c–e). This material stains with anti-keratin antibodies. In lichen amyloidosis, changes of lichen simplex chronicus (hyperkeratosis, hypergranulosis, and acanthosis) overlie similar papillary dermal deposits. Slight basilar hyperpigmentation is often present (see also Chap. 17).

Familial isolated hyperparathyroidism is an autosomal dominant disorder in which hyperparathyroidism develops without any other tumors or endocrine disorders. It may be caused by incomplete expression of MEN1, HRPT2, and CaSR mutations (8). Cutaneous lesions are uncommon with this condition. *Hyperparathyroidism-jaw tumor syndrome* is characterized by the presence of cystic tumors of the parathyroid glands, ossifying tumors of the mandible and maxilla, endometrial neoplasms, and renal lesions and tumors (3, 5). The genetic features are germ-line inactivating mutations in the HRPT2, located on chromosome 1. Hyperparathyroidism occurs in about 80% of patients, with high risk of developing subsequent parathyroid cancer (15%).

Familial benign hypercalcemic hypocalciuria (FHH) and neonatal severe hypercalcemia (NSH) (9, 10) are inherited as autosomal dominant syndromes characterized by heterozygous (FHH) or homozygous (NSH) inactivating mutations in the calcium-sensing receptor. It is usually asymptomatic and presents with mild four-gland hyperplasia, mild benign hypercalcemia (<3.0 mmol/l), and hypocalciuria.

5.2.1.2 Hyperparathyroidism Related to Renal Failure

These patients usually present with fatigue, decreased bone density, fractures, anemia, and hypogonadism. With end-stage disease, they develop renal disease, intractable pruritus, and metastatic calcifications. Calcifications are commonly widespread and affect predominantly lungs, kidneys, stomach, and blood vessels. Skin (calcinosis cutis, see below) and muscle are also affected. The etiopathogenesis of parathyroid glandular hyperplasia is related to diminished ionized-calcium levels stimulating parathyroid secretion and growth, direct stimulation of the parathyroid cells by hyperphosphatemia, and a decrease in the number of calcium-sensing receptors (5).

5.2.1.3 Other Cutaneous Manifestations

Sporadic hyperparathyroidism does not usually result in cutaneous manifestations except for metastatic calcification, and rarely chronic urticaria.

Calcinosis cutis can be classified as dystrophic, metastatic, or idiopathic (see also Chap. 21). In hyperparathyroidism, metastatic calcification occurs as a result of hypercalcemia or hyperphosphatemia. Calcium deposits can be found in the skin, subcutaneous tissues, muscle, tendon,

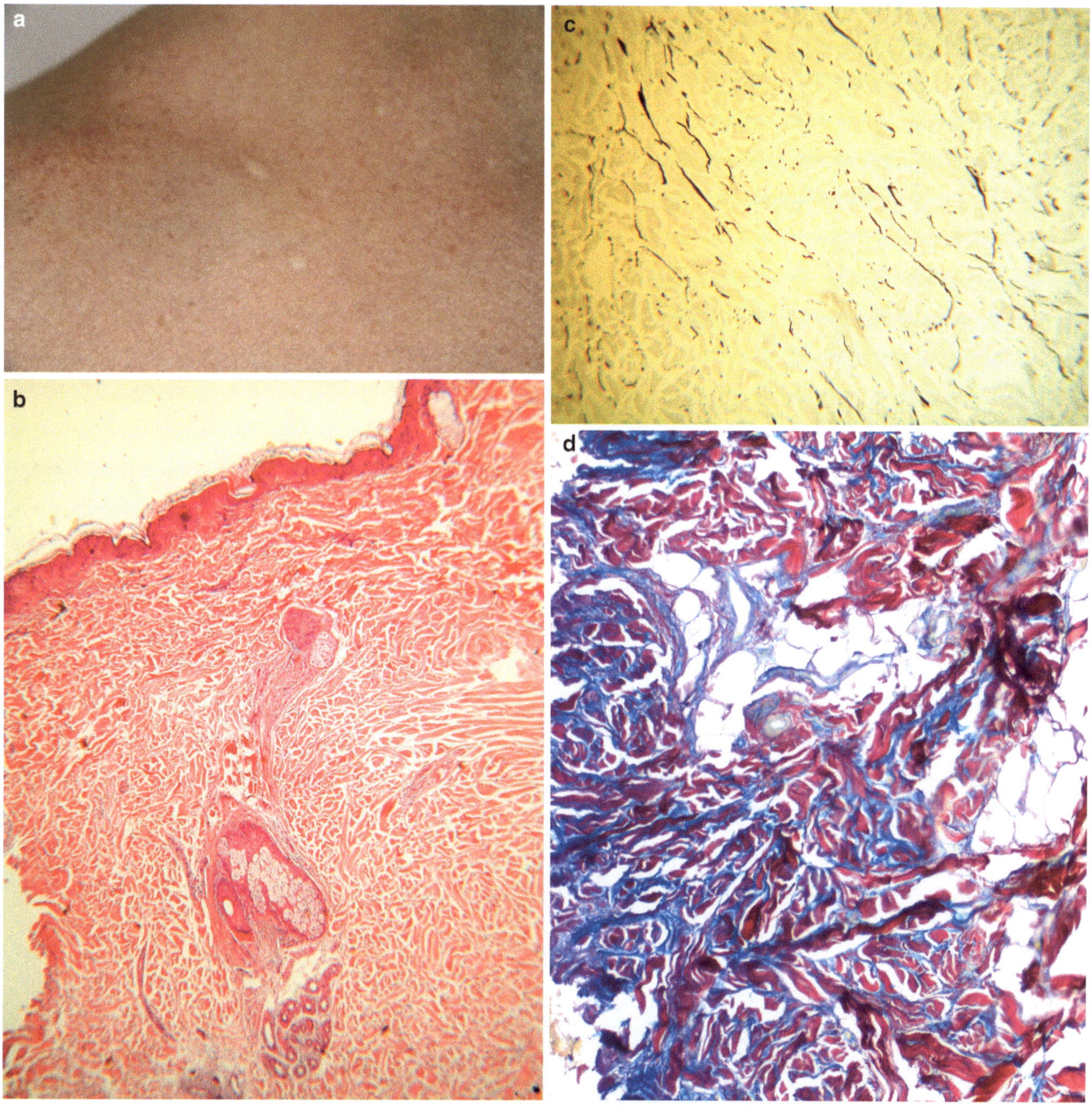

Fig. 5.1 (**a**) Dome-shaped flesh color or slightly hypopigmented papules of multiple collagenomas on the trunk in MEN 1 (courtesy of B. Cribier, Strasbourg, France). (**b**) Histopathology of collagenoma with markedly thickened dermis due to thickened collagen (HE stain) (courtesy of Valentina Caputo, Milan, Italy). (**c**) Decreased elastic tissue in collagenoma (Orcein stain) (courtesy of Valentina Caputo, Milan, Italy). (**d**) Interstitial mucin in collagenoma. Colloidal iron stain (courtesy of P. Romanelli, Miami, USA)

and internal organs. In the skin these are usually seen as hard white papules or subcutaneous nodules or plaques that may ulcerate to liberate a chalky material (Fig. 5.4a–c). Metastatic calcifications are commonly seen over large joints, the iliac crest, or in the flexures. Precipitating factors include skin trauma or injections. Calcium deposits may occasionally resolve spontaneously when calcium and phosphate levels normalize. Metastatic calcification is characterized by the presence of bluish to deep blue deposits seen on routine hematoxylin and eosin stains. These deposits stain black with the Von Kossa stain due to the concomitant presence of phosphate and carbonate. The presence of calcium in the skin elicits a granulomatous foreign body reaction and a chronic inflammatory cell infiltrate (Fig. 5.4d, e). It is not uncommon to find transepidermal elimination of calcified debris.

Vascular calcification with thrombosis can lead to livedo reticularis, ulceration and gangrene, particularly in hands, fingers, toes, lower legs, thighs and abdomen (clinical

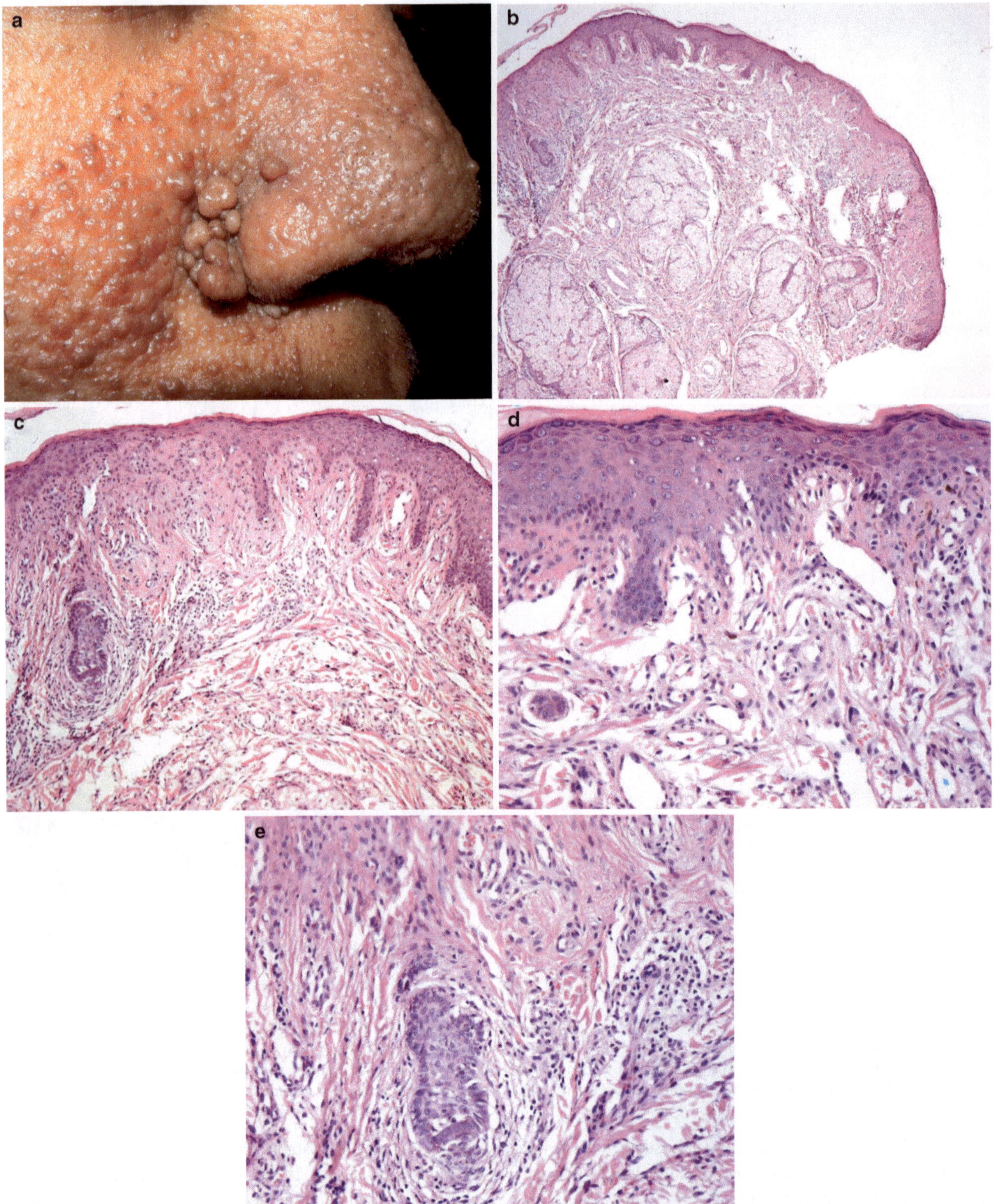

Fig. 5.2 (**a**) Angiofibromas (courtesy of Rocio Orozco Topete, Mexico City). (**b**) Histopathology of angiofibroma with increased cellularity and vascular ectasia (HE stain). (**c**) Angiofibroma with papillary dermal fibrosis, increased stellate cells, and vascular ectasia (HE stain). (**d**) Angiofibroma with prominent dilated vessels and enlarged, stellate cells in a fibrotic background (HE stain). (**e**) Perifollicular fibrosis (HE stain)

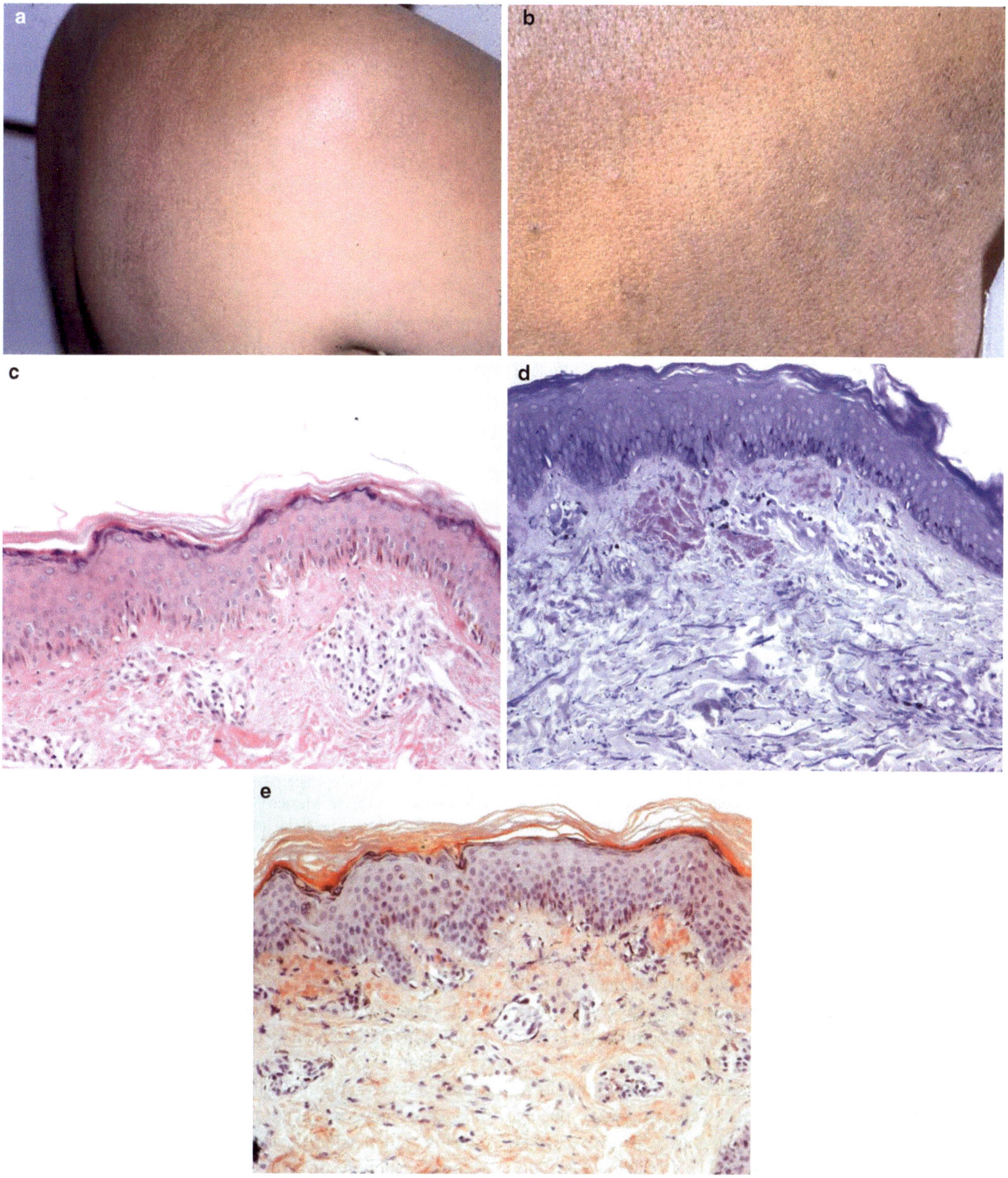

Fig. 5.3 (**a**) Macular amyloidosis seen in prominent bony areas (courtesy of Rocio Orozco Topete, Mexico City). (**b**) Macular amyloidosis (courtesy of Rocio Orozco Topete, Mexico City). (**c**) Histopathology of macular amyloidosis with globular eosinophilic material and a mild lymphohistiocytic infiltrate (HE stain). (**d**) Amyloid in the papillary dermis stained with crystal violet. (**e**) Amyloid in the papillary dermis stained with Congo red

calciphylaxis). *Calciphylaxis* is a syndrome usually fatal due to infectious complications and is seen in the setting of end-stage renal disease in patients on dialysis or post renal transplant. It is usually associated with secondary and tertiary hyperparathyroidism. Its pathogenesis is multifactorial. Local paracrine factors involve bone morphogenetic protein-2, parathyroid hormone-related peptide, osteopontin, osteoprotegerin, Pit-1 (a sodium-dependent phosphate

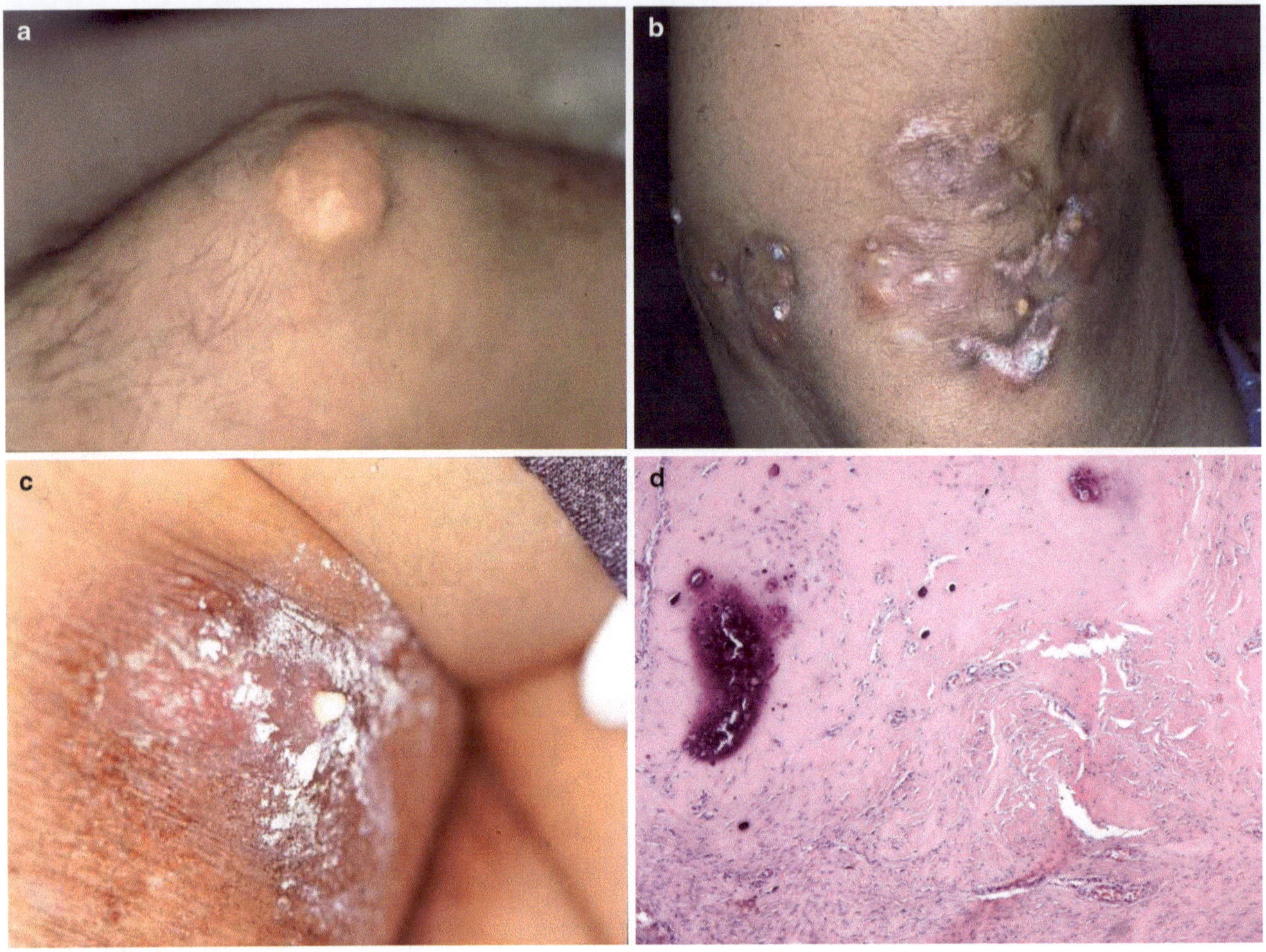

Fig. 5.4 lcinosis cutis. (**a**) Indurated nodule with erythematous yellowish appearance (courtesy of Rocio Orozco Topete, Mexico City). (**b**) Calcinosis cutis associated with scars (courtesy of Rocio Orozco Topete, Mexico City). (**c**) A white chalky material exudes from calcinosis cutis (courtesy of Rocio Orozco Topete, Mexico City). (**d**) Histopathology of calcinosis cutis. An amorphous basophilic material within the dermis

cotransporter), and matrix Gla protein (11). Besides metabolic factors there are also physical factors, which include obesity, reduced cutaneous oxygen tension, and hypercoagulable states. Patients initially develop violaceous, mottled patches and plaques that resemble livedo reticularis on the abdomen, thigh, and hips, which frequently ulcerate (Fig. 5.5a). Occasionally, bullae may be present, ulcerate, and be covered with thick black eschars. Calciphylaxis can also present with acral ischemia of fingers, toes, or penis. Proximal location of the necrosis is associated with a mortality rate of 63%. Besides skin necrosis, skeletal muscle involvement can also occur, resulting in rhabdomyolysis. In calciphylaxis, the essential feature is the calcification of dermal and subcutaneous small blood vessels (venules and arterioles) associated with varying degrees of inflammation and necrosis (Fig. 5.5b, c). Other features include calcification of the subcutaneous adipose tissue accompanied by lipophagic necrosis, an inflammatory infiltrate, and occasional vascular thrombi. The amount of calcium deposition does not correlate with the degree of clinical severity.

5.2.2 Hypoparathyroidism

Hypoparathyroidism is an endocrine disorder characterized mainly by hypocalcemia due to inadequate parathyroid hormone (PTH) secretion, or less often by unresponsiveness to elevated PTH levels (pseudohypoparathyroidism) (12–15). It may be congenital or acquired. Postsurgical hypoparathyroidism is the most frequent acquired form, but other causes include autoimmunity (isolated or as a part of autoimmune polyendocrine syndrome type 1, hemochromatosis, transfusion-dependent thalassemia, Wilson's disease, magnesium depletion or excess, and infiltrative disorders). Genetic diseases include DiGeorge syndrome, autosomal dominant hypocalcemia, familial hypoparathyroidism, the hypoparathyroidism-retardation-dysmorphism syndrome, and mitochondrial gene defects. Signs and symptoms of hypocalcemia are the most prominent features of all forms of hypoparathyroidism; nevertheless, most patients with slowly progressive hypocalcemia remain asymptomatic. Clinical features are primarily neuromuscular (extrapyramidal

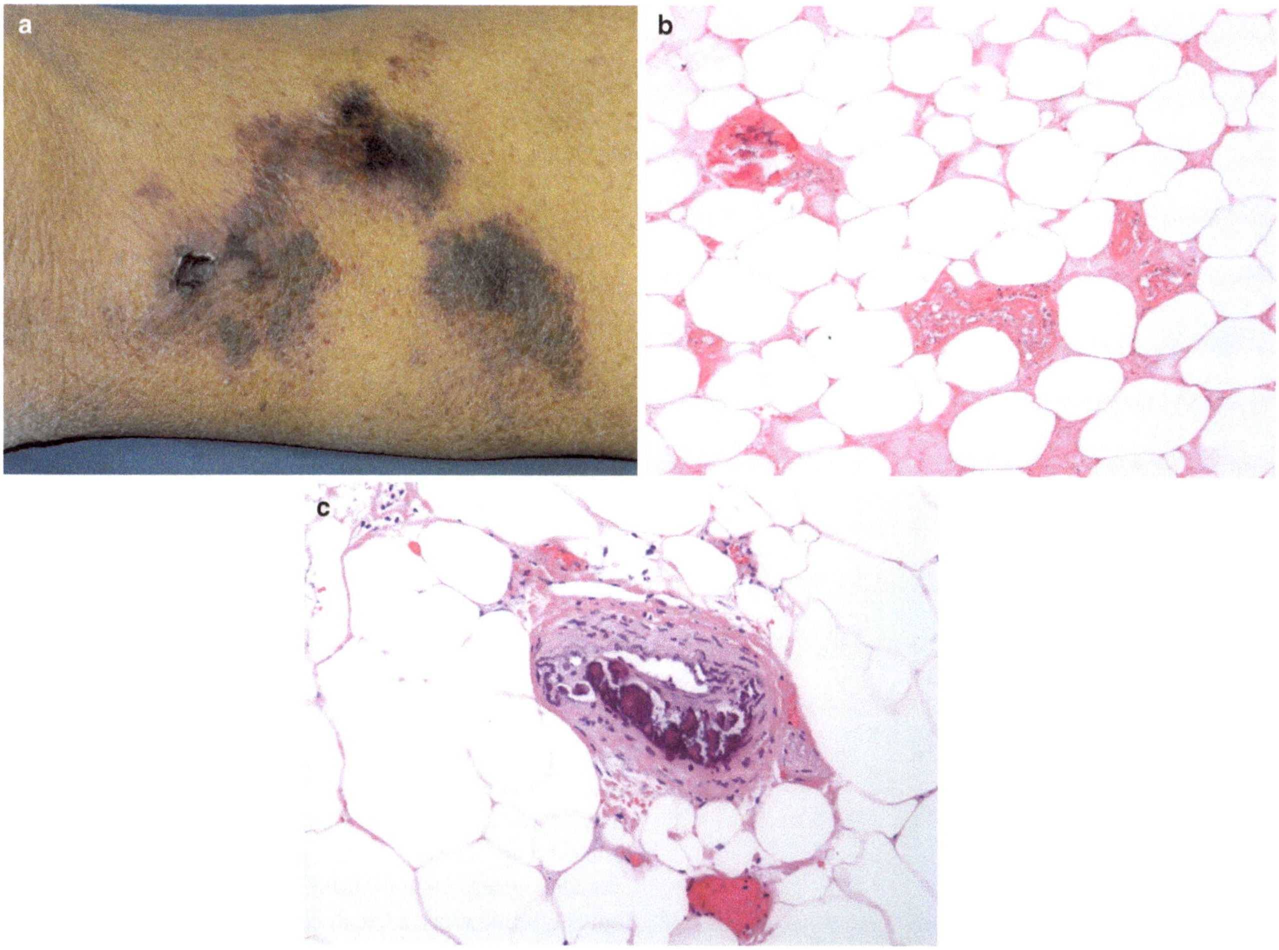

Fig. 5.5 (**a**) Calciphylaxis demonstrates purpura and ulceration in a reticulated pattern (courtesy of Rocio Orozco Topete, Mexico City). (**b**) Calciphylaxis. Calcium deposits within the occluded subcutaneous arterioles demonstrate cracking artifact with little inflammation. (**c**) Calcium deposits delimiting and damaging the vessel wall

signs, paresthesias, cramping, muscular, laryngeal, and bronchial spasm) and cardiovascular (prolonged QT interval, systolic dysfunction). Infrequent manifestations include pseudotumor cerebri, basal ganglia calcifications, abnormal dentition, and premature cataracts. Severe cases may be life threatening, with seizures, altered mental status, tetany, and congestive heart failure.

A detailed medical history with emphasis on family history is paramount for the correct diagnosis and classification of hypoparathyroidism. The diagnosis is based on normal or inappropriately low levels of serum PTH in the context of low ionized calcium levels, elevated phosphate, and no hypomagnesemia, while high PTH levels characterize pseudohypoparathyroidism.

Dermatological findings related to hypoparathyroidism are usually sparse, mild, and nonspecific. These include *xerosis, scaling, edema, rough-fragile hair, alopecia, and mild onychodystrophy* (subtle dyschromia, distal onycholysis, and transverse ridges). Rarely *eczematous dermatitis, hyperkeratotic and maculopapular eruptions* have been described (16, 17). On the other hand, cutaneous signs related to the primary cause of hypoparathyroidism may be quite prominent and diagnostic in a few entities such as hemochromatosis (18), Wilson's disease or hepatolenticular degeneration (19), and autoimmune polyendocrine syndrome type 1 (APS-1).

Hyperpigmentation is the most striking finding in hemochromatosis associated with diabetes and hepatic cirrhosis (see also Chap. 11).

Wilson's disease or hepatolenticular degeneration (toxic accumulation of cooper primarily in the liver and brain) may be suspected in patients with pretibial hyperpigmentation, blue lunulae, and cutaneous signs of cirrhosis (19).

Autoimmune polyendocrine syndrome type 1 (APS-1) has also been described under the names of autoimmune polyendocrinopathy-candidiasis-ectodermal dystrophy (APECED) and Whitaker's syndrome. Its major components are hypoparathyroidism, autoimmune adrenal insufficiency, and *chronic mucocutaneous candidiasis*. Other associated minor diseases of the skin include *vitiligo, alopecia areata and ectodermal* (ungal) *dystrophy. Chronic mucocutaneous*

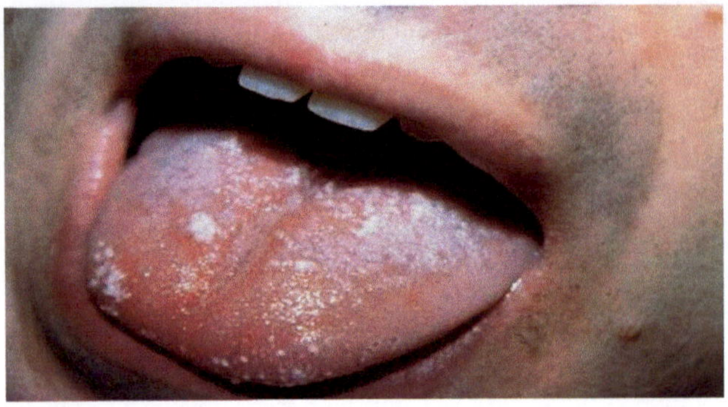

Fig. 5.6 Oral *Candida* infection (thrush) in APECED

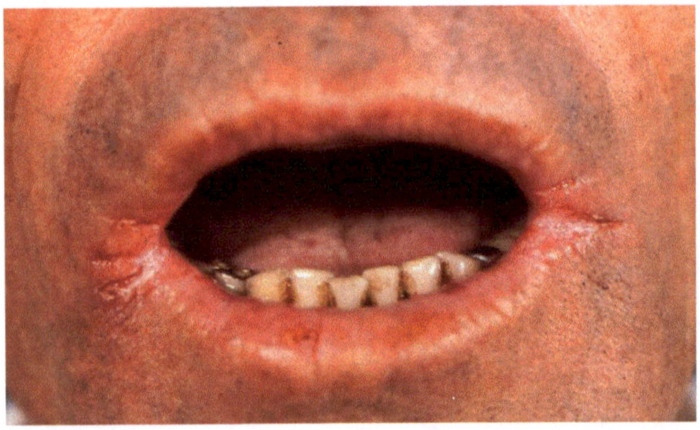

Fig. 5.7 Angular cheilitis

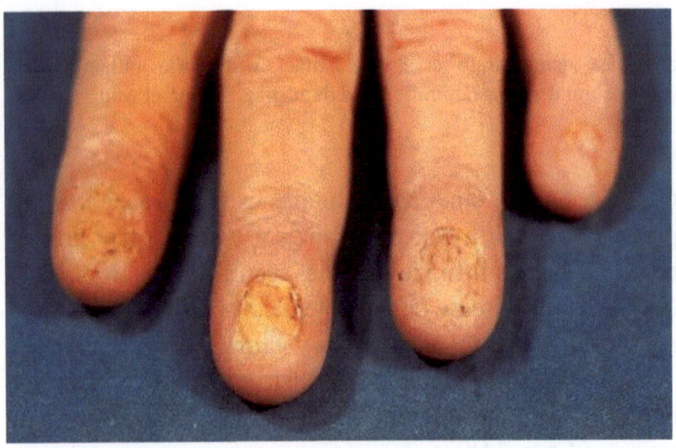

Fig. 5.8 Chronic *Candida* onychomycosis with white-yellow discoloration, marked onychodystrophia, and paronychial swelling

candidiasis is one of the earliest and most frequent disorders of APS-1. It is characterized by progressive and recurrent infections of skin, mucosa, and nails with *Candida albicans,* low propensity for systemic affection, and has a wide spectrum of clinical presentations. Skin lesions are typically erythematous, scaly plaques with serpiginous borders, preferentially intertriginous, periorificial, and on the scalp where there may be scarring alopecia. Infants may present with persistent diaper dermatitis. Mucosal disease may involve genitalia, esophagus, and larynx, but it is more frequently limited to the oral mucous membrane with the pseudomembranous form, or thrush (Fig. 5.6), and angular cheilitis (Fig. 5.7) being the leading presentations. *Candida* onychomycosis is readily diagnosed by marked dystrophy (pachyonychia), white-yellow discoloration, and associated paronychial swelling and erythema (Fig. 5.8) (20).

Albright hereditary osteodystrophy is the leading cause of pseudohypoparathyroidism. It is characterized by myriad, distinctive skeletal and developmental defects consisting of short neck and stature, brachydactyly, round face, and heterotopic calcification that can result in *subcutaneous ossifications* (also reported in congenital hypoparathyroidism), the only distinctive dermatological sign (21, 22).

5.3 Treatment and Prognosis

Parathyroid surgery is the standard treatment for all patients with symptomatic hyperparathyroidism in whom there is a reasonable life expectancy (23). In asymptomatic patients with hyperparathyroidism, surgery is recommended if there is serum calcium of more than 1 mg/dL above the upper limit of normal; marked hypercalciuria; reduced creatinine clearance; reduced bone density ; and age younger than 50 years (24). In sporadic hyperparathyroidism, single gland parathyroidectomy of the identified adenoma is the recommended approach. For patients with familial PHT, there has to be balance between the risk of optimal surgical procedures and the morbidity caused by permanent hypoparathyroidism. In the clinical context of renal failure, parathyroidectomy is recommended for symptomatic patients. Recommendations for the treatment of calciphylaxis include the correction of hypercalcemia and hyperphosphatemia, hyperbaric oxygen, appropriate wound care associated with the adequate use of antibiotics and pain management (5, 12). Benign cutaneous tumors including collagenomas, angiofibromas, and lipomas are excised only for cosmetic purposes. Treatment of hypoparathyroidism focuses on correcting the underlying cause, and pharmacologic treatment depends on the nature and severity of the disease. Severe symptoms require intravenous calcium and additional therapy according to each case (oxygen and diuretics for secondary heart failure, etc.). Oral calcium is appropriate for milder cases along with a low phosphate diet, vitamin D and analogues (13, 16). Correction of the underlying disease and metabolic imbalances may be sufficient therapy for skin manifestations, and dermatological basic interventions may be unnecessary other than routine moisturizing for mild cases of xerosis and pruritus. Therapy of chronic mucocutaneous candidiasis involves long-term systemic antifungals (fluconazole, itraconazole) in view of the inadequate response to standard topical medications (17, 20, 21).

References

1. Poole K, Reeve J (2005) Parathyroid hormone – a bone anabolic and catabolic agent. Curr Opin Pharmacol 5:612–617
2. Arnold A, Shattuck TM, Mallyia SM et al (2002) Molecular pathogenesis of primary hyperparathyroidism. J Bone Miner Res 17(Suppl 2):N30–N36
3. Töke J, Patócs A, Balogh K et al (2009) Parathyroid hormone-dependent hypercalcemia. Wien Klin Wochenschr 121:236–245
4. Brandi ML, Gagel RF, Angeli A et al (2001) Guidelines for diagnosis and therapy of MEN type 1 and type 2. J Clin Endocrinol Metab 86:5658–5671
5. Fuleihan Gel-H, Rubeiz N (2006) Dermatologic manifestations of parathyroid-related disorders. Clin Dermatol 24:281–288
6. Pack S, Turner ML, Shuang A et al (1998) Cutaneous tumors in patients with multiple endocrine neoplasia type 1 show allelic deletion of the MEN1 gene. J Invest Dermatol 11:438–440
7. Ceccherini I, Romei C, Barone V et al (1994) Identification of the Cys634→ Tyr mutation of the RET proto-oncogene in a pedigree with multiple endocrine neoplasia type 2A and localized cutaneous amyloidosis. J Endocrinol Invest 17:201–204
8. Warner J, Epstein M, Sweet A et al (2004) Genetic testing in familial isolated hyperparathyroidism: unexpected results and their implications. J Med Genet 41:155–160
9. Pearce S, Steinmann B (1999) Casting new light on the clinical spectrum of neonatal severe hyperparathyroidism. Clin Endocrinol 50:691–693
10. Toke J, Czirjak G, Patocs A et al (2007) Neonatal severe hyperparathyroidism associated with a novel de novo heterozygous R551K inactivating mutation and heterozygous A986S polymorphism of the calcium-sensing receptor gene. Clin Endocrinol 67:385–392
11. Giachelli CM (2004) Vascular calcification mechanisms. J Am Soc Nephrol 15:2959–2964
12. Marx SJ (2001) Hyperparathyroid and hypoparathyroid disorders. N Engl J Med 344:240, 696
13. Asari R, Passler C, Kaczirek K, Scheuba C, Niederle B (2008) Hypoparathyroidism after total thyroidectomy: a prospective study. Arch Surg 143:132–137
14. Eisenbarth GS, Gottlieb PA (2004) Autoimmune polyendocrine syndromes. N Engl J Med 350:2068–2079
15. Cooper MS, Gottoes NJ (2008) Diagnosis and management of hypocalcemia. BMJ 336:1298–1302
16. Jabbour SA (2003) Cutaneous manifestations of endocrine disorders: a guide for dermatologists. Am J Clin Dermatol 4:315–331
17. Leonhardt JM, Heymann WR et al (2003) Cutaneous manifestations of other endocrine diseases. In: Freedberg IM, Eizen AZ, Wolff K et al (eds) Fitzpatrick's dermatology in general medicine, 6th edn. McGraw-Hill, New York, pp 1662–1670
18. Pietrangelo A (2007) Hemochromatosis: an endocrine liver disease. Hepatology 46(4):1291–1301
19. Schaffer JV, Paller AS (2008) Primary immunodeficiencies. In: Bolognia JL, Jorizzo JL, Rapini RP (eds) Dermatology, 2nd edn. Mosby Elsevier, Philadelphia, pp 801–823
20. Kirkpatrick CH (1994) Chronic mucocutaneous candidiasis. J Am Acad Dermatol 31:s14–s17
21. Aslan Y, Gedik Y, Otken A et al (1999) Congenital primary hypoparathyroidism presented with extensive cutaneous and subcutaneous calcifications. Turk J Pediatr 41:253–257
22. Germain-Lee EL (2006) Short stature, obesity, and growth hormone deficiency in pseudohypoparathyroidism type 1a. Pediatr Endocrinol Rev 3:318–327
23. AACE/AAES Task Force on Primary Hyperparathyroidism (2005) The American Association of Clinical Endocrinologists and the American Association of Endocrine Surgeons position statement on the diagnosis and management of primary hyperparathyroidism. Endocr Pract 11:49–54
24. Bilezikian JP, Potts JT Jr, El-HajjFuleihan G et al (2002) Summary statement from a workshop on asymptomatic primary hyperparathyroidism: a perspective for the 21st century. J Clin Endocrinol Metab 87:5353–5361

Part II
Cutaneous Metabolic Disease

Chapter 6
Dyslipidemia (Hyperlipidemia)

Terrence Katona and Bruce R. Smoller

Key Points

- Skin manifestations can be found in both primary (hereditary) hyperlipidemia and secondary hyperlipidemia (e.g., hyperlipidemia in hypothyroidism or associated with drug intake).
- The major dermatologic manifestations in hyperlipidemia are xanthomas, tumors comprised of lipid-laden histiocytes (foam cells).
- The main types of xanthomas associated with hyperlipidemia disorders are: planar (especially intertriginous and palmar crease xanthomas), eruptive, tuberous, and tendinous.
- Several xanthomatous lesions may be seen in normolipemic patients (e.g., xanthoma disseminatum) or in association with monoclonal gammopathies (normolipemic plane xanthomas).
- Treatment of xanthomas associated with hyperlipidemia requires the identification and therapy of the underlying lipoprotein disorder, as the gravest concern in patients with xanthomatous skin lesions is the risk of long-term cardiovascular consequences from hyperlipidemia.

Keywords Tuberous and tendinous xanthomas • Eruptive xanthomas • Planar xanthomas • Hypercholesterolemia • Hypertriglyceridemia

6.1 Introduction

Skin manifestations can be found in both primary (hereditary) hyperlipidemia and secondary hyperlipidemia (e.g., hyperlipidemia in hypothyroidism or with protease inhibitor administration) [1]. Indeed, many drugs can cause hyperlipidemia, including retinoids such as isotretinoin for acne or bexarotene for mycosis fungoides (and other diseases) [2, 3]. Further, tuberous and tendinous xanthomas have been described in the setting of antiretroviral therapy (ritonavir)-associated hyperlipidemia [4].

The major dermatologic manifestations in hyperlipidemia are xanthomas, tumors comprised, at least in part, of lipid-laden histiocytes. There are multiple histologic and clinical variants of xanthomatous lesions (Table 6.1). The pathogenesis of xanthomatous skin lesions involves excessive levels of plasma lipoproteins that traverse dermal blood vessels and accumulate in dermal macrophages (histiocytes). The macrophages become lipid-rich, taking on a foamy cytoplasm that prompted the appellation "foam cells" [5, 6]. Individuals with paraproteinemia, in particular multiple myeloma, may undergo an interaction of the monoclonal protein with serum lipoproteins that increases the likelihood of xanthoma formation [7]. Several xanthomas are considered pathognomonic for specific hyperlipidemia disorders, e.g., planar xanthomas in an intertriginous distribution, especially finger web spaces, are pathognomonic for homozygous familial hypercholesterolemia (HFH) [1]. Several xanthomatous lesions may also be seen in normolipemic patients. Indeed, some entities such as xanthoma disseminatum and juvenile xanthogranuloma are not associated with an elevation in serum lipids [8]. In the past, xanthomatous lesions, especially tuberous and tendinous xanthomas, were cutaneous clues to an individual with undetected hyperlipidemia. With frequent screening of adults in developed countries, hyperlipidemic conditions may now be detected prior to skin manifestations. Nevertheless, the emergence of a xanthoma should alert the clinician to the possibility of a systemic hyperlipidemia in a patient who has not been previously evaluated.

6.2 Clinical and Pathological Aspects of Skin Manifestations

Cholesterol and triglycerides are the most clinically relevant plasma lipids [1, 5, 6, 9]. Cholesterol is important as a precursor molecule for synthesis of steroid hormones,

T. Katona (✉)
Richfield Laboratory of Dermatopathology, 9844 Redhill Drive, Cincinnati, OH 45242, USA
e-mail: katonter@gmail.com

F. Rongioletti and B.R. Smoller (eds.), *Clinical and Pathological Aspects of Skin Diseases in Endocrine, Metabolic, Nutritional and Deposition Disease*, DOI 10.1007/978-1-60761-181-3_6, © Springer Science+Business Media, LLC 2010

Table 6.1 Xanthomas

Type of xanthoma	Subtype	Lipoprotein in excess	Additional features
Eruptive	n/a	Chylomicrons	Chylomicrons are often secondarily elevated in poorly controlled diabetes mellitus. Ethanol ingestion and exogenous estrogens may also be the etiologies.
Tendinous	n/a	Cholesterol	Although familial dysbetalipoproteinemia, (type III hyperlipoproteinemia) is the most common setting, tendinous xanthomas may present in homozygous or heterozygous familial hypercholesterolemia
Tuberous	n/a	Cholesterol	Most common association is with homozygous familial hypercholesterolemia, for which they are considered a hallmark
Planar	Xanthelasma	Cholesterol or triglyceride	50% Associated with hyperlipidemia
	Xathoma striatum palmare (palmar xanthomata)	Triglyceride (specifically VLDL)	Pathognomonic of familial dysbetalipoproteinemia, type III
	Intertriginous	Cholesterol	Pathognomonic of homozygous familial hypercholesterolemia
Disseminated	n/a	Normolipemic	

vitamin D, and bile acids. Triglycerides are a major source of energy as their primary constituent is free fatty acids. Normal lipid metabolism revolves around transport of lipids in the plasma by several different lipoproteins [9]. The core of a lipoprotein is hydrophobic and can transport triglycerides or cholesterol. The hydrophilic exterior contains phospholipids and apoproteins. The latter have regulatory function including interaction with enzymes or lipoprotein receptors. The exogenous lipid pathway begins as dietary lipids are packaged into chylomicrons as large lipoproteins that enter intestinal lymphatic spaces and ultimately the peripheral blood. Upon arrival in muscle or adipose tissue, the apoC-II lipoprotein on the chylomicron surface interacts with lipoprotein lipase on capillary endothelium. This enzyme splits the chylomicron core of triglyceride into fatty acids and monoglycerides that are then utilized by adipose and muscle tissues, either for storage or for energy. The chylomicron remnants continue in circulation, where they are removed by receptors on hepatocytes. The endogenous pathway operates continuously unlike the exogenous pathway, which is largely a postprandial process. The endogenous pathway is responsible for synthesizing approximately 80% of circulating cholesterol and begins with very low density lipoproteins (VLDL) that are manufactured by the liver and released into the plasma. VLDL, not unlike chylomicrons, reaches adipose and muscles tissue, and its triglycerides are hydrolyzed by lipoprotein lipase. The remnants of VLDL are initially intermediate density lipoproteins (IDLs) that may be taken up by the liver or may transform into low density lipoproteins (LDL), which contain mostly cholesterol and very little triglyceride. The LDL is ultimately removed from circulation by LDL receptors in the liver and other tissues. When any or all of the lipoproteins are in excess, they may be deposited in the tissues [1, 5, 9–11]. If deposited in the corium, subcutis, or tendons, xanthomatous lesions result [1, 5, 6, 12].

Disorders of lipid metabolism, in particular hyperlipidemias, can be organized via two major classification systems. Plasma lipoproteins can be separated by electrophoresis, and therefore, the banding pattern is the basis of one form of lipid abnormality nomenclature. For example, dysbetalipoproteinemia refers to excess of lipids that fall in the beta region of the electrophoretic smear. The resultant phenotypes based upon the electrophoretic pattern of plasma lipids are labeled I–V. The other major classification system focuses on the predominant lipid increased in the plasma, in particular cholesterol and triglycerides (Table 6.2). There is some overlap between the two systems, e.g., familial dysbetalipoproteinemia has increased cholesterol and triglyceride and would be classified as phenotype III based on electrophoresis of plasma lipids. This entity is characterized by an increased beta region of electrophoresis that is very broad ("broad beta") and by increased IDL that contains cholesterol and triglycerides [10, 13].

6.3 Specific Xanthomas

6.3.1 Planar Xanthomas

There are three major subtypes of *planar xanthomas: xanthelasmas, intertriginous xanthomas, and palmar crease xanthomas (xanthoma striatum palmare).* Xanthelasmata are found in the periorbital skin, and 50% of patients have hyperlipidemia, often hypercholesterolemia or type III hyperlipoproteinemia. Intertriginous xanthomas are diagnostic of HFH.

Table 6.2 Classification of lipid disorders [13]

Electrophoretic phenotype	Lipoprotein increased	Region of electrophoretic banding increase	Disorder	Major lipid increased
I	Chylomicrons	Origin	Familial lipoprotein lipase deficiency	Triglyceride
IIa	LDL	Beta	Familial hypercholesterolemia	Cholesterol
IIb	VLDL and LDL	Pre-beta and beta	Apolipoprotein E deficiency	Cholesterol and triglyceride
III	IDL	Beta broadly increased	Familial dysbetalipoproteinemia	Cholesterol and triglyceride
IV	VLDL	Pre-beta	Familial combined hyperlipidemia	Cholesterol and triglyceride
V	VLDL and chylomicrons	Origin and pre-beta	Can be seen in familiar hypertriglyceridemias or Familial apo C-II deficiency	Triglyceride

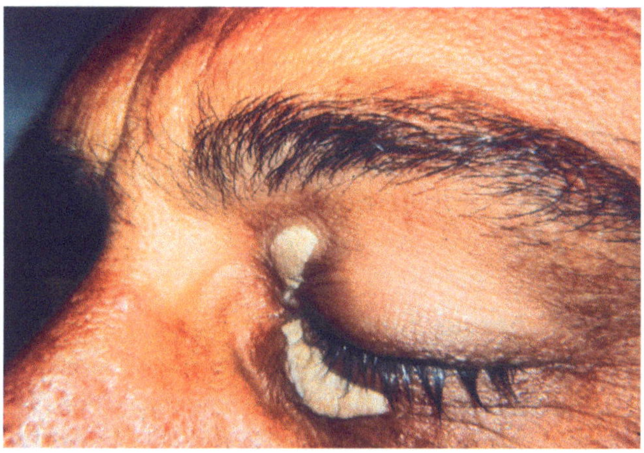

Fig. 6.1 A patient with a large plaque-like xanthelasma near left inner canthus (courtesy of C.M. Davis, Little Rock, AR)

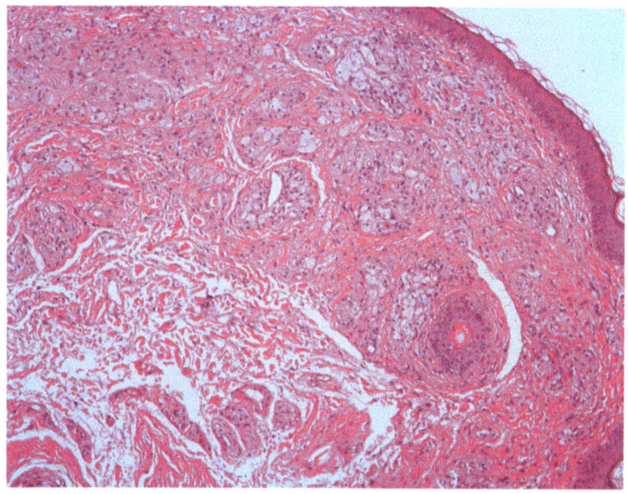

Fig. 6.2 Histopathology of xanthelasma with numerous lipid-laden histiocytes (foam cells) partially filling the dermis

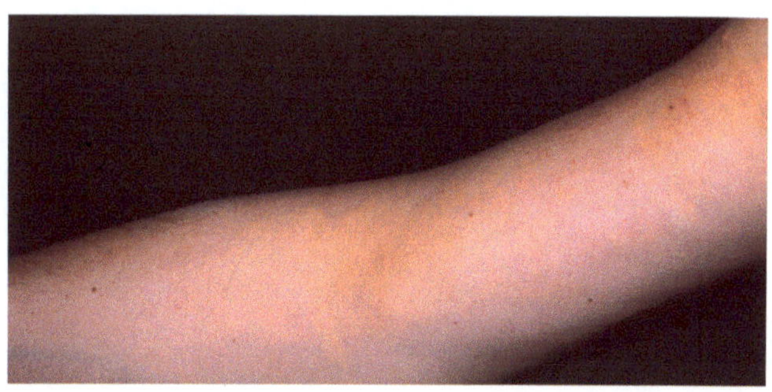

Fig. 6.3 Intertriginous xanthoma of the antecubital fossa

Palmar crease xanthomas are pathognomonic of familial dysbetalipoproteinemia (hyperlipoproteinemia type III, also known as "broad beta disease" due to its pattern on electrophoresis of plasma lipids) [1, 5]. *Xanthelasmas* are soft, yellow plaques situated around the eyes (Fig. 6.1). Often a concurrent arcus senilis is observed on the cornea. One half of the patients have hypercholesterolemia or type III hyperlipoproteinemia. The younger the individual presents with xanthelasmata, the more increased the risk of atherosclerosis, particularly coronary artery disease [5]. Histologically, lipid-laden histiocytes are found within the superficial dermis with mild dermal fibrosis [1] (Fig. 6.2). *Intertriginous xanthomas* are pathognomonic of HFH. They manifest as yellow papules and plaques with a resemblance to cobblestone. The web spaces between fingers are the most frequent site, and less frequently, the axilla, antecubital fossa (Fig. 6.3), and/or popliteal fossa are involved. These lesions are a marker for severe atherosclerosis with early manifestations [1, 5]. Histology is identical to that of xanthelasma. *Palmar crease xanthomas (xanthoma striatum palmare)* are subtle yellow-orange macular lesions of the palmar creases that can be easily overlooked on clinical exam, potentially necessitating optimal lighting for identification. Palmar crease xanthomas are pathognomonic of familial dysbetalipoproteinemia, type III, which is due to aberrant apoprotein ApoE. The abnormality leads to a diminished ability to uptake lipoprotein remnant particles by hepatocytes and macrophages and subsequently hyperlipoproteinemia and atherosclerosis ensue [1, 5, 12].

Of note, some plane xanthomas, particularly diffuse generalized examples, can be associated with monoclonal gammopathies, most frequently multiple myeloma. The monoclonal paraprotein forms complexes with serum lipoproteins, which are typically not elevated, leading to xanthoma formation in a normolipemic setting [7].

6.3.2 Eruptive Xanthomas

Eruptive xanthomas are characteristically associated with secondary hyperlipidemia, particularly elevated chylomicrons (of which triglycerides are the principal element), as may be found in poorly controlled diabetes mellitus. Ethanol ingestion and medications, such as retinoids, glucocorticoids or estrogens, may also be etiologies of eruptive xanthomas [1]. Hyperchylomicronemia can also result from homozygous lipoprotein lipase deficiency, a homozygous condition in which eruptive xanthomas and pancreatitis can be found. Clinically, the lesions are small, yellow papules that may exhibit a red rim or halo. Frequent sites of involvement include the buttocks, shoulder, or extensor surface of the extremities (Fig. 6.4). They may also be located in the axilla, antecubital and popliteal fossae or the lips, eyelids, and ears. The lesions are usually cropped and may vacillate with plasma lipid levels. Classically, they will spontaneously resolve after several weeks. There may be pruritis and at times tenderness. Histologically, the superficial reticular dermis is filled with histiocytes and relatively few foam cells in initial lesions. Lymphocytes and neutrophils may also be found, the latter signifying the acute ("eruptive") nature (Fig. 6.5a, b). More established lesions do contain foamy histiocytes as the dominant cell type. The major intracellular lipid is triglyceride versus most other xanthomas, which are largely comprised of cholesterol. Sometimes, the triglyceride is found outside of the cells; another feature rarely found in other xanthoma variants [1, 5, 14].

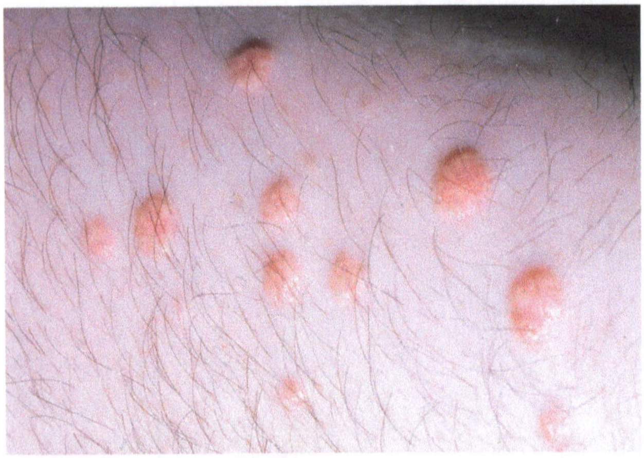

Fig. 6.4 A patient with an eruptive xanthoma manifesting as multiple *yellow-orange* nodules overlying the knee and distal anterior thigh (courtesy of C.M. Davis, Little Rock, AR)

6.3.3 Tuberous Xanthomas

Tuberous xanthomas can vary in size and are felt to form via coalescence of smaller lesions into larger nodular forms. The elbows, knees, and buttocks are most frequent sites, and the lesions often exhibit a yellow hue (Fig. 6.6a, b). Although familial dysbetalipoproteinemia, (type III hyperlipoproteinemia) is the most common setting, tuberous xanthomas may present

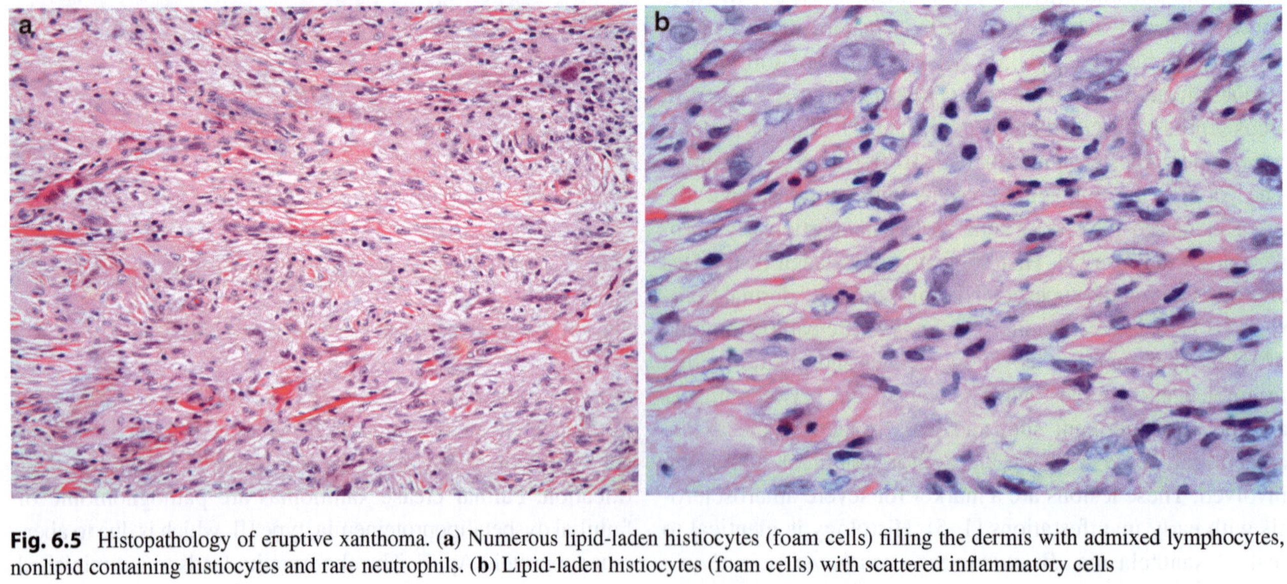

Fig. 6.5 Histopathology of eruptive xanthoma. (**a**) Numerous lipid-laden histiocytes (foam cells) filling the dermis with admixed lymphocytes, nonlipid containing histiocytes and rare neutrophils. (**b**) Lipid-laden histiocytes (foam cells) with scattered inflammatory cells

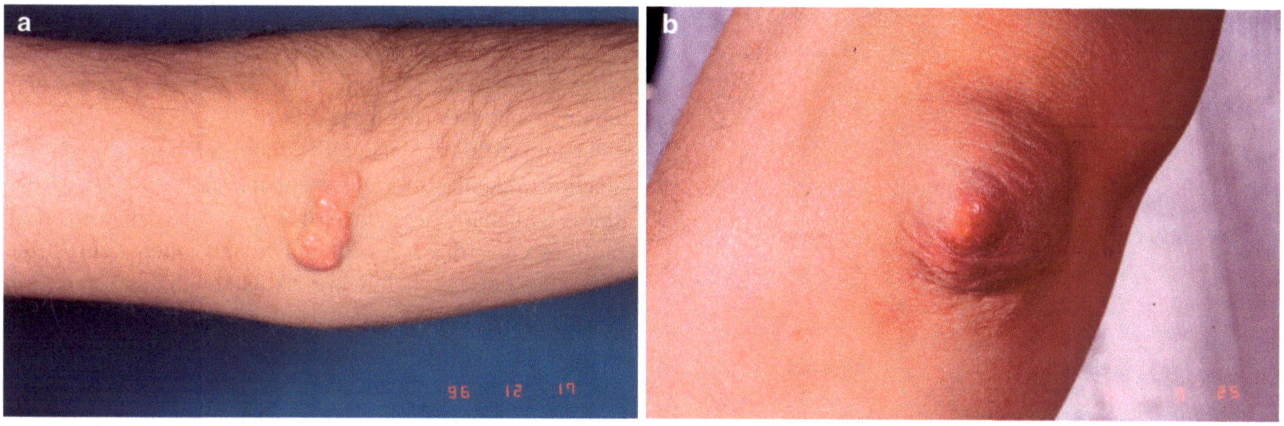

Fig. 6.6 (**a**) Tuberous xanthoma of the elbow. Note the *yellowish* hue. (**b**) Nodular tuberous xanthoma

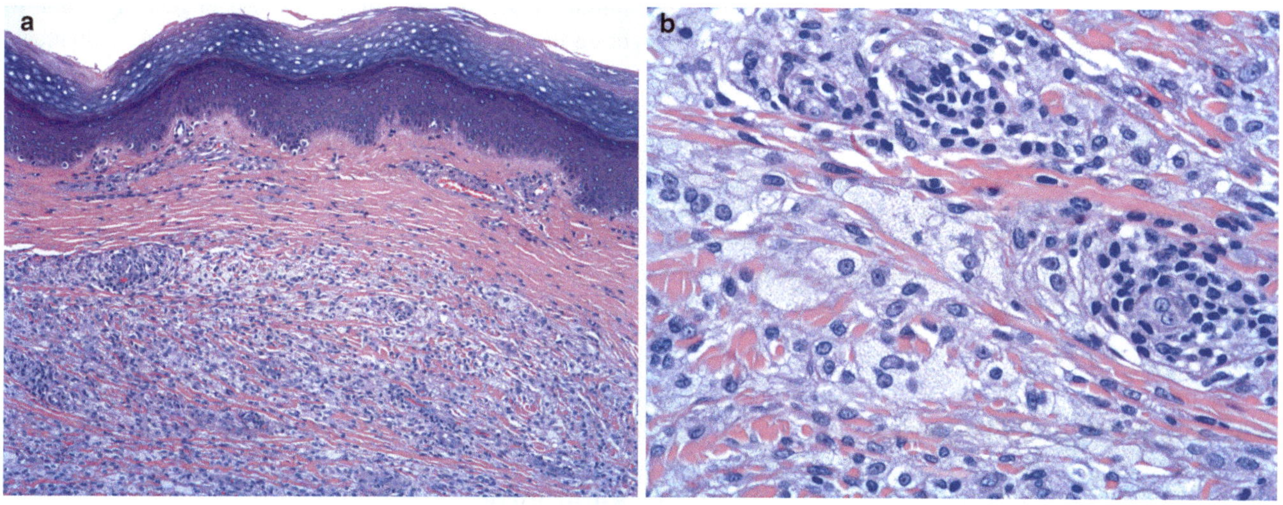

Fig. 6.7 Histopathology of tuberous xanthoma. (**a**) Acral type epidermis with underlying lipid-laden histiocytes (foam cells) filling the reticular dermis. (**b**) Higher magnification displaying frequent lipid-laden histiocytes (foam cells)

in homozygous or heterozygous familial hypercholesterolemia [1]. Although most hyperlipidemic conditions are autosomal dominant, multiple tuberous xanthomas have also been described in the rare autosomal recessive hypercholesterolemia [1, 5, 15]. On histopathology, large collections of foam cells are present within the dermis, while Touton giant cells and other inflammatory cells are typically lacking (Fig. 6.7a, b). As the lesions age, fibroblast numbers increase and collagen is deposited. In the rare specimen obtained fresh or frozen, the lipid within foam cells is oil-red O positive and is doubly refractile on polaroscopic exam [16].

6.3.4 Tendinous Xanthomas

Tendinous xanthomas present as indurated, flesh-colored nodules that arise slowly over years. They involve tendons, ligaments, and fascia, in particular the Achilles' tendon and extensor tendon of the hands and feet. The most common association is with HFH, for which they are considered a hallmark [1]. Presentation in familial dysbetalipoproteinemia (type III) has also been described. The histologic appearance is nearly identical to that of tuberous xanthomas, consisting of sheets of foam cells with minimal contribution from other inflammatory cells (Fig. 6.8) [16].

6.3.5 Cholesterotic Fibrous Histiocytoma

Cholesterotic fibrous histiocytoma is a rare variant of dermatofibroma that contains abundant cholesterol crystals and increased foam cells with otherwise typical features of dermatofibroma, including collagen trapping at the periphery and acanthosis, hyperpigmentation, and/or follicular induction of the overlying epidermis [17]. Only three cases have been described, all in patients with

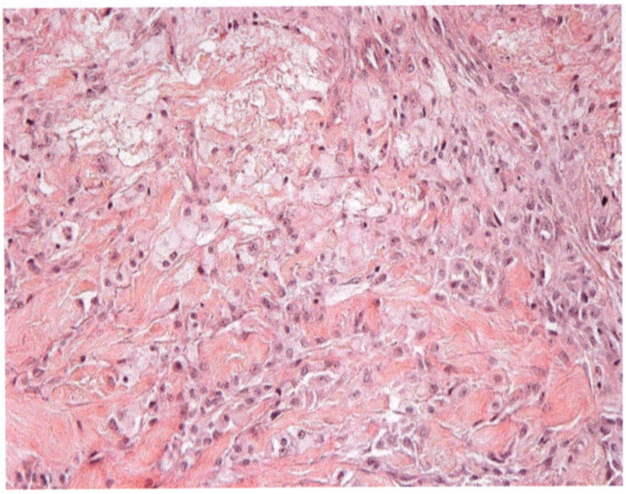

Fig. 6.8 Tendinous xanthomas consisting of sheets of foam cells with minimal contribution from other inflammatory cells

hyperlipidemia [17]. Of note is a case of dermatofibroma with mixed morphology (cholesterotic and sclerotic) that presented in a normolipemic female [18]. Further reports of this rare variant of fibrous histiocytoma/dermatofibroma are needed to clarify its relationship to plasma lipid levels.

6.4 Treatment and Prognosis

Many instances of hereditary hyperlipidemia are associated with severe atherosclerotic cardiovascular disease. Secondary hyperlipidemias often abate with correction of the underlying etiology, e.g., cessation of the offending medication, correction of hypothyroidism, etc. Treatment of xanthomas, in particular xanthelasmata and tendinous or tuberous xanthomas, can be surgical, including laser procedures [19], but additional lesions will likely appear if the underlying hyperlipidemia is not corrected [20].

Nonsurgical treatment of hyperlipidemia involves pharmacologic agents such as HMG-CoA reductase inhibitors (more commonly known as "statins"), fibric acid derivatives, bile acid sequestrates, and nicotinic acid. Statins inhibit the 3-hydroxy-3-methylglutaryl coenzyme A reductase, which is the rate-limiting enzyme for hepatic cholesterol synthesis. This leads to upregulation of LDL receptors and the lowering of plasma LDL cholesterol levels. All statins have this same mechanism of action but vary in their ability to lower LDL [21]. Omega-3 fatty acids are available in a prescription form, which has been approved by the United States Food and Drug Administration for use in patients with very high triglyceride levels (greater than 500 mg/dl). The improvement can be greater than with statin monotherapy [22].

Type III hyperlipoproteinemia (dysbetalipoproteinemia) is typically responsive to pharmacologic therapy, such as fibric acid agents, nicotinic acid, or statins. Therapy may require combination of these drugs [7].

In autosomal dominant HFH, there is marked decrease in function or number of LDL receptors. This results in a severe illness with markedly increased risk for early atherosclerotic cardiovascular disease with individuals often dying from severe heart disease before age 20. Although less severe, 1 in 500 persons is heterozygous for this condition, with cardiovascular disease manifesting in the fourth or fifth decade. Although multiple medications are often used, including high-dose statins, the hypercholesterolemia may persist in homozygous individuals. Other treatments options can include periodic LDL apheresis (apheresis to selectively remove LDL from plasma) or even liver transplantation to bring the hyperlipidemia under control [23]. As individuals with HFH can also develop heart failure from aortic valve stenosis and chronic ischemic heart disease, it has been proposed that liver transplantation is indicated at the point at which heart transplantation has become necessary [24].

It is also important to take note of the genetic counseling ramifications of diagnoses of inherited hyperlipidemia for the individual patient. The potential impact on longevity and family planning can be considerable, and referral to the appropriate genetics specialist, whether a physician geneticist or genetics counselor, should be strongly considered.

References

1. Cruz P, East C, Bergstressor P (1988) Dermal, subcutaneous, and tendon xanthomas: diagnostic markers for specific lipoprotein disorders. J Am Acad Dermatol 19:95–111
2. Abbott R, Whittaker S, Morris S, Russell-Jones R, Hung T, Bashir S, Scarisbrick J (2009) Bexarotene therapy for mycosis fungoides and Sézary syndrome. Br J Dermatol 160:1299–1307
3. Zane L, Leyden W, Marqueling A, Manos M (2006) A population-based analysis of laboratory abnormalities during isotretinoin therapy for acne vulgaris. Arch Dermatol 142:1016–1022
4. Brown C, Lesher JJ, Peterson CM (2005) Tuberous and tendinous xanthomata secondary to ritonavir-associated hyperlipidemia. J Am Acad Dermatol 52:S86–S89
5. Parker F (1985) Xanthomas and hyperlipidemias. J Am Acad Dermatol 13:1–30
6. Parker F (1986) Normocholesterolemic xanthomatosis. Arch Dermatol 122:1253–1257
7. Burnside N, Alberta L, Robinson-Bostom L, Bostom A (2005) Type III hyperlipoproteinemia with xanthomas and multiple myeloma. J Am Acad Dermatol 53:S281–S284
8. Büyükavci M, Selimoglu A, Yildirim U, Ertekin V, Atasoy M (2005) Xanthoma disseminatum with hepatic involvement in a child. Pediatr Dermatol 22:550–553
9. Hegele R (2009) Plasma lipoproteins: genetic influences and clinical implications. Nat Rev Genet 10:109–121
10. Ogedegbe H, Brown D (2001) Lipids, lipoproteins, and apolipoproteins and their disease associations. Lab Med 7:384–388

11. Breslow J (2000) Genetics of lipoprotein abnormalities associated with coronary heart disease susceptibility. Annu Rev Genet 34:233–254
12. Vermeer B, Gevers Leuven J (1991) New aspects of xanthomatosis and hyperlipoproteinemia. Curr Probl Dermatol 20:63–72
13. Mais D (2008) Lipids and carbohydrates. American Society for Clinical Pathology Press, Chicago, IL, pp 56–65
14. Crowe M, Gross D (1992) Eruptive xanthoma. Cutis 50:31–32
15. Siddi G, Pes G, Errigo A, Corraduzza G, Ena P (2006) Multiple tuberous xanthomas as the first manifestation of autosomal recessive hypercholesterolemia. J Eur Acad Dermatol Venereol 20:1376–1378
16. Weedon D (2002) Cutaneous infiltrates – non-lymphoid. Churchill Livingstone, Edinburgh, pp 1075–1078
17. Hunt S, Santa Cruz D, Miller C (1990) Cholesterotic fibrous histiocytoma – its association with hyperlipoproteinemia. Arch Dermatol 126:506–508
18. Zelger BG, Sidoroff A, Zelger B (2000) Combined dermatofibroma: co-existence of two or more variant patterns in a single lesion. Histopathology 36:529–539
19. Katz TM, Goldberg LH, Friedman PM (2009) Fractional photothermolysis: a new therapeutic modalities for xanthelasma. Arch Dermatol 145:1091–1094
20. Ghosh Y, Pradhan E, Ahluwalia H (2009) Excision of xanthelasmata – clamp, shave, and suture. Int J Dermatol 48:181–183
21. Dembowski E, Davidson M (2009) A review of lipid management in primary and secondary prevention. J Cardiopulm Rehabil Prev 29:2–12
22. Mattar M, Obeid O (2009) Fish oil and the management of hypertriglyceridemia. Nutr Health 20:41–49
23. Alkofer B, Chiche L, Khayat A, Deshayes J, Lepage A, Saloux E, Reznik Y (2005) Liver transplant combined with heart transplant in severe heterozygous hypercholesterolemia: report of the first case and review of the literature. Transplant Proc 37:2250–2252
24. Marais A, Firth J, Blom D (2004) Homozygous familial hypercholesterolemia and its management. Semin Vasc Med 4:43–50

Chapter 7
Gout

Uma Sundram

Key Points

- Gout is caused by a deposition of monosodium urate within joints and soft tissues due to supersaturation of body fluids.
- Gout has been increasing in incidence due to increasing risk factors such as obesity, increased alcohol consumption, hypertension, and high purine diet.
- Gout develops in four stages: asymptomatic hyperuricemia, acute gouty arthritis, the intercritical period, and chronic tophaceous gout. The first metatarsophalangeal joint is often affected (podagra).
- Gout is treated in three phases: treatment of the acute attack, prevention of future acute and rebound attacks, and hypouricemic therapy.

Keywords Hyperuricemia • Acute gouty arthritis • Tophaceous gout

7.1 Introduction

Gout has been increasing in incidence over the past 30 years [1]. This may be due to prevalent risk factors in the United States and European population, including obesity [2], increased alcohol intake, and high consumption of purines. Gout is known to be secondary to hyperuricemia, which can be affected by age, sex, body mass index, and renal function. Disease processes can also cause hyperuricemia, including psoriasis and myeloproliferative disorders [3]. Other considerations include lead exposure and exposure to certain drugs such as diuretics. Gout is closely associated with insulin resistance, hypertension, and hypertriglyceridemia [1]. This is often influenced greatly by the addition of a diuretic to the patient's drug regimen. Hemodialysis patients can also be affected due to poor urate clearance [4].

U. Sundram (✉)
Department of Pathology, Dermatopathology & Dermatology, Stanford University School of Medicine, Stanford Hospital and Clinics, 300 Pasteur Drive Room H2110, Stanford, CA 94305, USA
e-mail: sundram@stanford.edu

7.2 Clinical and Pathologic Aspects of Skin Involvement

Gout is a metabolic disorder that occurs when monosodium urate deposits in tissues from supersaturated body fluids. The clinical manifestations include acute gouty arthritis, formation of tophi (accumulation of urate crystals in soft tissues), urate urolithiasis, and rarely gouty nephropathy [3]. Gout develops in four stages: asymptomatic hyperuricemia, acute gouty arthritis (the "gouty attack"), the intercritical period, and chronic tophaceous gout [5]. The typical patient (usually a middle-aged male) presents with a painful swelling of the joint or digit with associated reddening of the overlying skin, prompting considerations of infection or osteomyelitis. Initially, there may be fevers or systemic symptoms. Even if there is no medical intervention, the lesion can resolve on its own within a few weeks. A family history is often present, and it is thought that genetics plays a role in urate renal clearance [6].

Hyperuricemia can be initially asymptomatic. Years of hyperuricemia can precede the first gouty attack, and not everyone with hyperuricemia actually develops gout. The first metatarsophalangeal joint is the first joint affected in approximately half of all patients (podagra). Up to 40% of initial attacks can be polyarticular [7], and common joints of involvement include the knees, ankles, and feet [3]. Both primary and secondary hyperuricemic conditions exist; while secondary hyperuricemia is more common, primary hyperuricemia can be caused by rare genetic disorders that can cause purine overproduction [8]. Other entities within the clinical differential diagnosis include chondrocalcinosis (pseudogout) [9], osteoarthritis, Reiter's syndrome, psoriatic arthritis [10], and rarely multicentric reticulohistiocytosis [11].

F. Rongioletti and B.R. Smoller (eds.), *Clinical and Pathological Aspects of Skin Diseases in Endocrine, Metabolic, Nutritional and Deposition Disease*, DOI 10.1007/978-1-60761-181-3_7, © Springer Science+Business Media, LLC 2010

The intercritical period starts after resolution of the initial gouty attack, during which the joint returns to normal. This period can last from 6 months to 2 years. Gouty attacks tend to become more frequent, involve more joints, and are longer in duration if the condition is left untreated [12].

Chronic tophaceous gout occurs when a significant amount of monosodium urate has deposited around the joint in such a way that resolution between attacks becomes impossible. Its incidence increases with increasing severity of the gout. The dermatologic features of tophi include nodular tophi, draining tophi, chronic ulcers, and panniculitis [13–16]. Tophi are pink and firm upon palpation and are filled with a white pasty substance that consists of compacted monosodium urate crystals. Common sites of involvement include the ears, the olecranon bursae (Fig. 7.1), the knees and digits (Fig. 7.2), and sites of trauma. Tophi can ulcerate, draining a chalky material (Fig. 7.3). Rarely, tophi may be the patient's first manifestation of gout [12, 17]. Bullae are an uncommon manifestation and are thought to occur secondary to trauma and/or underlying tophaceous deposits [18]. Gout can also present as a panniculitis. These are nodular lesions of the anterior or posterior legs that ulcerate and drain opaque fluid. Tophaceous gout can erode into bone cartilage and tendons, and cause significant structural damage [3].

The differential diagnosis for tophaceous gout includes calcinosis cutis, rheumatoid nodules, and xanthoma [3]. Chronic tophaceous gouty arthritis can, on occasion, mimic rheumatoid arthritis or psoriatic arthritis if it is polyarticular [19, 20]. Ultrasound analysis can be useful in distinguishing gout from rheumatoid nodules based on echogenicity, as tophi, unlike rheumatoid nodules, have central echogenic areas [21–23]. In addition, the "double contour sign" produced by the deposition of monosodium urate crystals on the surface of joint synovium and the "snowstorm" appearance of the joint fluid can both be seen on ultrasound and are relatively sensitive for gout [20]. On radiography, gout usually demonstrates an erosive arthropathy with central "punched out" spaces with sclerotic "overhanging" margins [22].

The diagnosis of gout is made upon identification of monosodium urate crystals within synovial fluid or tophi. These are needle-shaped crystals that are negatively birefringent upon polarization. Laboratory studies usually demonstrate hyperuricemia (serum urate level over 7 mg/dL), sometimes accompanied by leukocytosis and an elevated erythrocyte sedimentation rate [3].

Routine biopsies or excisions of gouty tophi do not demonstrate the characteristic brown needle-shaped crystals of monosodium urate, as these crystals are water-soluble. Instead, one sees an area of amorphous fluffy white material within the dermis or subcutaneous tissue with empty needle-shaped fissures inside, surrounded by histiocytes including multinucleated giant cells (Fig. 7.4a–c). These areas represent

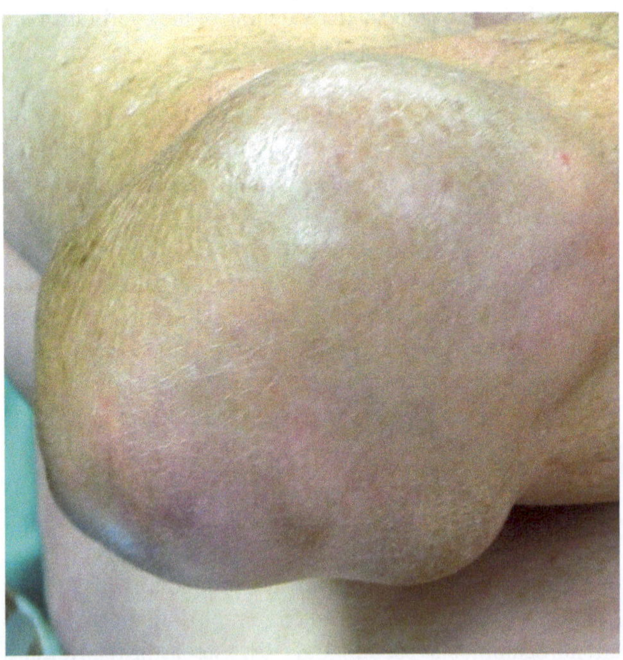

Fig. 7.1 Tophus formation in a common site, the olecranon bursa (courtesy of C. Lee and J. Krygier, Stanford, USA)

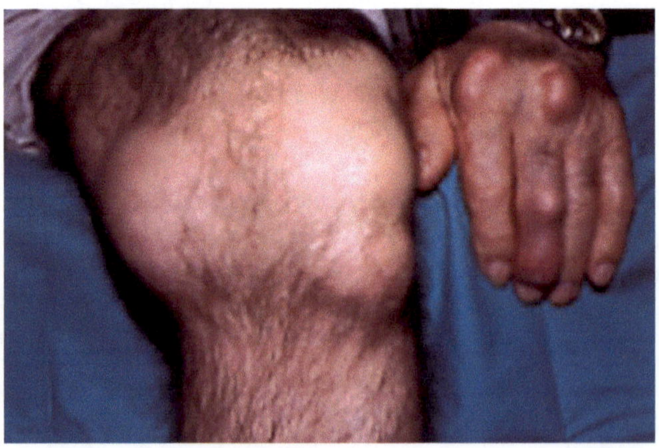

Fig. 7.2 Nodular tophi on knee and hand

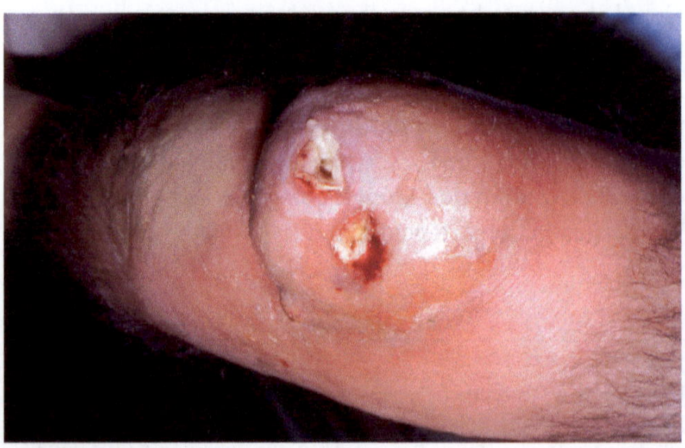

Fig. 7.3 Draining tophus

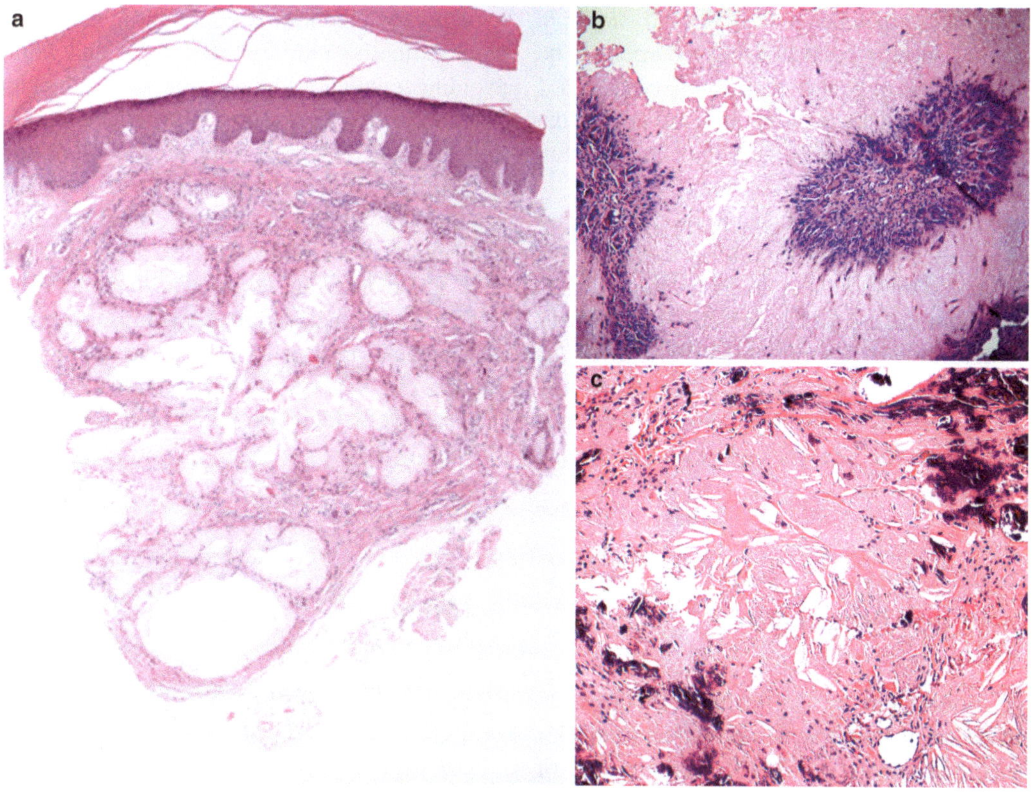

Fig. 7.4 Gouty tophus. (**a**) Typical areas of amorphous fluffy white material within the dermis. (**b**) Deposits of amorphous, hyaline-like, acellular material, surrounded by histiocytes and multinucleated giant cells. (**c**) Needle-like spaces are present within the amorphous deposits (courtesy of P. Romanelli, Miami, USA)

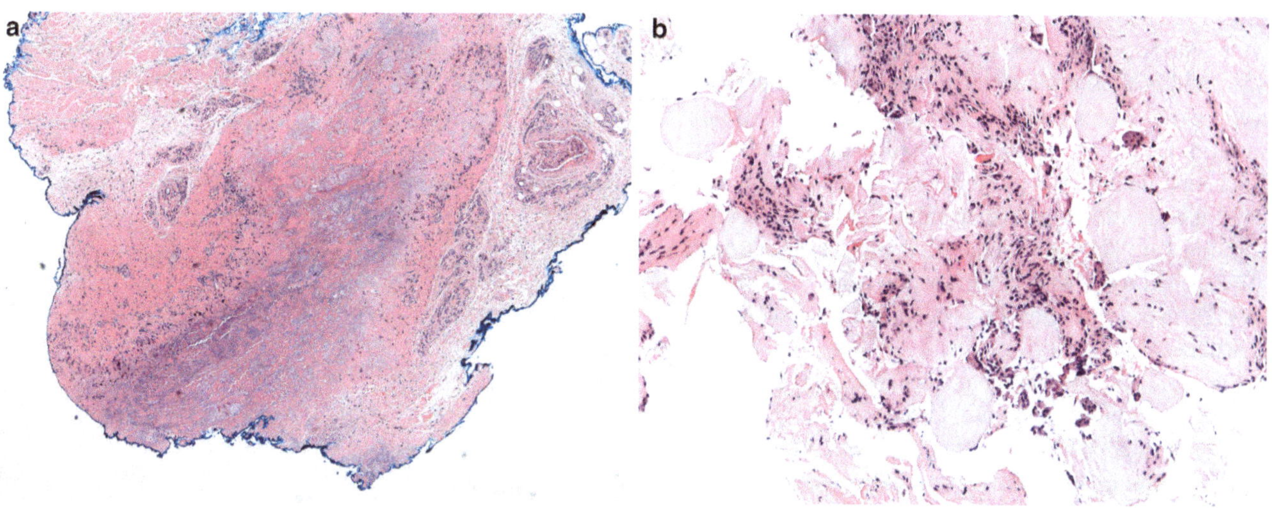

Fig. 7.5 (**a**) Gouty tophus characterized by amorphous basophilic material deposition in the fascia, accompanied by histiocytes and multinucleated giant cells. (**b**) Histiocytes, giant cells, and amorphous material

depositions of urate crystals that have been dissolved by the aqueous formalin solution (Fig. 7.5a, b). If an alcohol fixative is used instead, the brown needles of monosodium urate are seen. These crystals are brightly refractile with polarized light. If a red compensator is added, the crystals turn yellow when they are parallel to the direction of the compensator and blue when they are perpendicular [23]. Recently a simple nonstaining method has been published which purports to be able to detect the crystals of gout in routinely fixed tissues if one cuts and polarizes a thicker section (10 μ rather than the standard 4 μ) [24]. In older lesions, secondary calcification or ossification can occur.

It is thought that the symptoms of gout are precipitated by the deposition of gouty crystals in joint spaces and soft tissues. Crystal deposition stimulates the production of interleukin-2 by tissue macrophages, which then causes inflammation and fever [25]. The presence of IL-2 also activates neutrophils, which then phagocytose the crystals and ultimately cause complement activation. Ingestion of crystals by neutrophils also promotes lysozome rupture and subsequent damage to surrounding tissues.

7.3 Treatment and Prognosis

Gout is treated in three phases: (1) treatment of the acute attack, (2) prevention of future acute and rebound attacks, and (3) hypouricemic therapy [1, 3, 26]. The first line of treatment for the acute attack is usually the use of nonsteroidal anti-inflammatory drugs (NSAIDs), which can be effective if started within 24 h of the attack [26]. NSAIDs can successfully treat the pain and inflammation associated with gouty attacks. Unfortunately, NSAIDs are often contraindicated in a population of elderly patients with cardiovascular disease and poor renal function. Other problems encountered in the elderly population include the development of gastric ulcers and increased platelet dysfunction; the latter is a particular problem for patients who are concomitantly taking warfarin. Colchicine can also be used to treat acute attacks. Colchicine inhibits the phagocytosis of crystals by neutrophils; it also affects leukocyte migration, chemotaxis, and adhesion [3]. Though colchicine is slower in action than NSAIDs and has a narrow therapeutic index, it is safer than NSAIDs in patients with serious comorbidities such as renal insufficiency.

For acute gout, intraarticular corticosteroids can be effective [1], with improvement of affected joints in about 24 h. It is recommended that synovial fluid be sent for culture before administration of steroids, as occasionally septic joints can mimic gout. When polyarticular involvement is present, systemic steroids work well for gouty attacks. Prophylaxis consists of administration of NSAIDs or colchicine during the weeks following the attack. It is necessary to administer these for approximately 2–3 weeks in patients without obvious gouty tophi and possibly longer in those with greater tissue involvement by urate crystals. The third approach, hypouricemic therapy, is important in preventing long-term damage to the joints, soft tissues, and kidneys, and in avoiding continuous gouty attacks. Both allopurinol and probenecid are effective in this regard, but only allopurinol is indicated when the goal is the prevention of nephrolithiasis. Allopurinol reduces serum uric acid levels and increases uric acid excretion in the urine. Tophi usually clear within 6–12 months after the serum levels of uric acid are normalized [27]. These drugs are taken on a lifelong basis. To continue to manage the patients' long-term disease process, medical management approaches should be appropriate, including encouraging patients to manage their weight, increase fluid intake, have a low-purine diet, and desist from excessive alcohol intake [3].

References

1. Falasca GF (2006) Metabolic diseases: gout. Clin Dermatol 24:498–508
2. Yosipovitch G, DeVore A, Dawn A (2007) Obesity and the skin: skin physiology and skin manifestations of obesity. J Am Acad Dermatol 56:1901–1916
3. Touart DM, Sau P (1998) Cutaneous deposition diseases, part II. J Am Acad Dermatol 39:527–544
4. Sarraf P, Kay J, Reginato AM (2008) Non-crystalline and crystalline rheumatic disorders in chronic kidney disease. Curr Rheumatol Rep 10:235–248
5. Lambert WC (1990) Cutaneous deposition disorders. In: Farmer ER, Hood AF (eds) Pathology of the skin. Appleton and Lange, East Norwalk, CT, pp 432–450
6. Wortmann RL, Kelley WN (2005) Chapter 87: gout and hyperuricemia. In: Harris ED Jr (ed) Kelley's textbook of rheumatology, 7th edn. Elsevier, Philadelphia, pp 1402–1429
7. Handleer NM, Franck WA, Bress NM et al (1974) Acute polyarticular gout. Am J Med 56:715–719
8. O'Dufy JD, Hunder GG, Kelley PJ (1975) Decreasing prevalence of tophaceous gout. Mayo Clinic Proc 50:227–228
9. Joseph J, McGrath H (1995) Gout or "pseudogout": how to differentiate crystal-induced arthropathies. Geriatrics 50:33–39
10. Corkill MM (1994) Gout. N Z Med J 107:337–339
11. Santilli D, Lo Monaco A, Cavazzini PL, Trotta F (2002) Multicentric reticulohistiocytosis: a rare cause of erosive arthropathy of the distal interphalangeal finger joints. Ann Rheum Dis 61:485–487
12. Thissen CACB, Frank J, Lucker GPH (2008) Tophi as first clinical sign of gout. Int J Dermatol 47(Suppl 1):49–51
13. Snider AA, Barsky S (2005) Gouty panniculitis: a case report and review of the literature. Cutis 76:54–56
14. Conejo-Mir J, Pulpillo A, Corbi MR et al (1998) Panniculitis and ulcers in a young man. Arch Dermatol 134:501–504
15. Leboit PE, Schneider S (1987) Gout presenting as lobular panniculitis. Am J Dermatopathol 9:334–338
16. Niemi KM (1977) Panniculitis of the legs with urate crystal deposition. Arch Dermatol 113:334–338
17. Wernick R, Winkler C, Campbell S (1992) Tophi as the initial manifestation of gout. Arch Intern Med 152:873–876

18. Khanna D, Shrivastava A (2006) An unusual presentation of polyarticular tophaceous gout. Rheumatology (Oxford) 45:1095
19. Schapira D, Stahl S, Izhak OB, Balbir-Gurman A, Nahir AM (1999) Chronic tophaceous gouty arthritis mimicking rheumatoid arthritis. Semin Arthritis Rheum 29:56–63
20. Le Goff B, Berthelot JM, Andre V, Guillot P, Maugars Y (2008) Ultrasonography for diagnosing atypical gout. Two case reports. Joint Bone Spine 75:610–612
21. Tiliakos N, Morales AR, Wilson CH Jr (1982) Use of ultrasound in identifying tophaceous versus rheumatoid nodules. Arthritis Rheum 25:478–479
22. Nakayama DA, Barthelemy C, Carrera G, Lightfoot RW Jr, Wortmann RL (1984) Tophaceous gout: a clinical and radiographic assessment. Arthritis Rheum 27:468–471
23. DeCastro P, Jorizzo JL, Solomon AR, Lisse JR, Daniels JC (1985) Coexistent systemic lupus erythematosus and tophaceous gout. J Am Acad Dermatol 13:650–654
24. Weaver J, Somani N, Bauer TW, Piliang M (2009) Simple non staining method to demonstrate urate crystals in formalin-fixed, paraffin embedded skin biopsies. J Cutan Pathol 36:560–564
25. Malawista SE, Duff GW, Atkins E, Cheung HS, McCarty DJ (1985) Crystal induced endogenous pyrogen production: a further look at gouty inflammation. Arthritis Rheum 28:1039–1046
26. Schlesinger N (2004) Management of acute and chronic gouty arthritis: present state-of-the-art. Drugs 64:2399–2416
27. Rasaratnam I, Christophitis N (1995) Gout: "a disease of plenty". Austr Fam Phys 24:849–860

Chapter 8
Lipomatosis

Uma Sundram

Key Points

- Lipomas are benign tumors composed of mature lipocytes.
- Lipomatosis is manifested by the deposition of multiple lipomas.
- Lipomatosis can be seen in diffuse lipomatosis, multiple symmetric lipomatosis (Madelung's disease), adiposis dolorosa, and familial multiple lipomatosis.
- Other inheritable disorders associated with lipomatosis include Proteus syndrome and Bannayan–Zonana syndrome.

Keywords Diffuse lipomatosis • Multiple symmetric lipomatosis • Adiposis dolorosa • Familial multiple lipomatosis • Proteus syndrome • Bannayan–Zonana syndrome

8.1 Introduction

While lipomas are benign tumors composed of mature adipocytes and are usually sporadic, in the setting of multiple lesions there can be a hereditary component [1]. Common lipomatoses include diffuse lipomatosis, familial multiple lipomatosis, multiple symmetric lipomatosis (Madelung's disease), and adiposis dolorosa (Dercum's disease).

8.2 Clinical and Pathologic Aspects of Skin Involvement

8.2.1 Diffuse Lipomatosis

This entity is rare and is characterized by nonencapsulated mature fat that involves subcutaneous tissues, muscle, skin, fascia, and bone. It usually presents in childhood, before the age of 2, and can rarely be congenital. It has been seen in association with tuberous sclerosis and poliomyelitis [2–4]. Diffuse lipomatosis usually involves a large portion of the lower extremity or trunk, but the head and neck and upper extremities (Fig. 8.1) can also be involved. The tumor can progressively enlarge and show extension beyond its initial area of presentation. Pelvic involvement may lead to urinary tract, intestinal, and vena cava obstruction [5]. Histologically, the adipocytes of diffuse lipomatosis are those of normal adult-type adipose tissue with no nuclear pleomorphism or other atypia (Fig. 8.2). This infiltration is often in the manner of nevus lipomatosis superficialis, but the clinical presentation is usually useful in excluding this interpretation.

Congenital infiltrating lipomatosis of the face is thought to be a similar entity, namely, diffuse lipomatosis involving only the face [6]. This entity differs from diffuse lipomatosis in its congenital nature and constant association with underlying bone hypertrophy. Congenital infiltrating lipomatosis of the face does not contain lipoblasts, which distinguishes it from both lipoblastomatosis (which can be congenital) and well-differentiated liposarcoma (which largely occurs in adults).

8.2.2 Familial Multiple Lipomatosis

This entity has a variety of other names, including familial multiple lipomas, multiple circumscribed lipomas, hereditary multiple lipomas, and discrete lipomatosis. It is a rare hereditary syndrome of multiple lipomas occurring in a particular distribution [7, 8]. The lesions often present in the third decade of life, with a slight male predominance. The inheritance is thought to be autosomal dominant with incomplete penetrance. The lesions are characterized by tender nodules distributed in the forearms (Fig. 8.3a, b), trunk, and thighs, and spare the scalp, face, neck, and shoulders (in contrast to diffuse lipomatosis and multiple symmetric lipomatosis, respectively). The lesions are discrete, painless, mobile, and have a fibrous capsule.

U. Sundram (✉)
Department of Pathology, Dermatopathology & Dermatology, Stanford University School of Medicine, Stanford Hospital and Clinics, 300 Pasteur Drive Room H2110, Stanford, CA 94305, USA
e-mail: sundram@stanford.edu

F. Rongioletti and B.R. Smoller (eds.), *Clinical and Pathological Aspects of Skin Diseases in Endocrine, Metabolic, Nutritional and Deposition Disease,* DOI 10.1007/978-1-60761-181-3_8, © Springer Science+Business Media, LLC 2010

8.2.3 Multiple Symmetric Lipomatosis

Also known as Madelung's disease, this entity appears to be more common in the regions around the Mediterranean Sea [9]. Familial cases have been reported, but the disease is largely sporadic. It usually begins in adulthood and affects males more commonly than females. It is characterized by symmetric accumulation of fatty tissue in the neck (Madelung's neck), shoulder girdle, and upper arms (Fig. 8.4a, b), and the fat masses tend to be unencapsulated. An association with alcohol has been proposed [10]. The entity has been described in early series by Otto Madelung as well as Pierre Emile Launois and Raoul Bensaude [11]. In a more recent series involving 19 male patients, two different types of multiple symmetric lipomatosis have been described [9]. In MSL type 1, patients are typically underweight and the fatty tumors appear to be circumscribed masses with atrophy of the underlying adipose tissue. In MSL type 2, the patients are overweight and the fatty tumors extensively involve the subcutaneous layer and do not appear outwardly circumscribed. In both the types, the deposits are symmetric, and the distal parts of the forearms and legs are uninvolved. In this study, none of the patients presented with deep visceral involvement, such as involvement of the pelvis or abdomen.

Rarely, mediastinal, tracheal, tongue, and pharyngeal involvement have been reported [11]. Laryngeal involvement is rare but can be striking [12]. Liver function test abnormalities

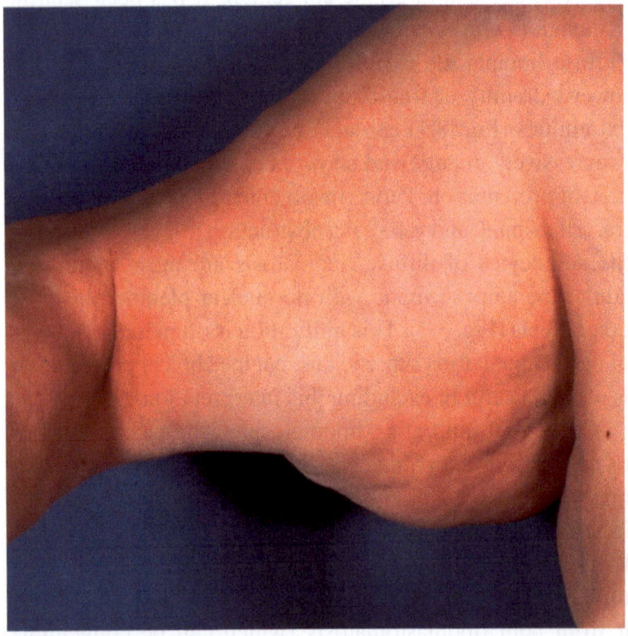

Fig. 8.1 Diffuse lipomatosis

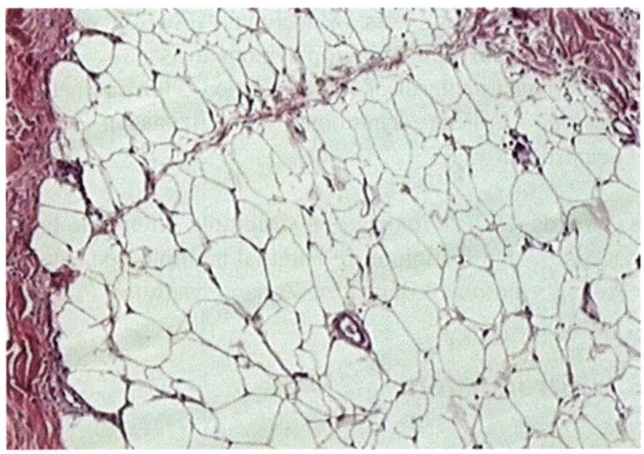

Fig. 8.2 Histopathology of diffuse lipomatosis showing normal adult-type adipose tissue with no atypia

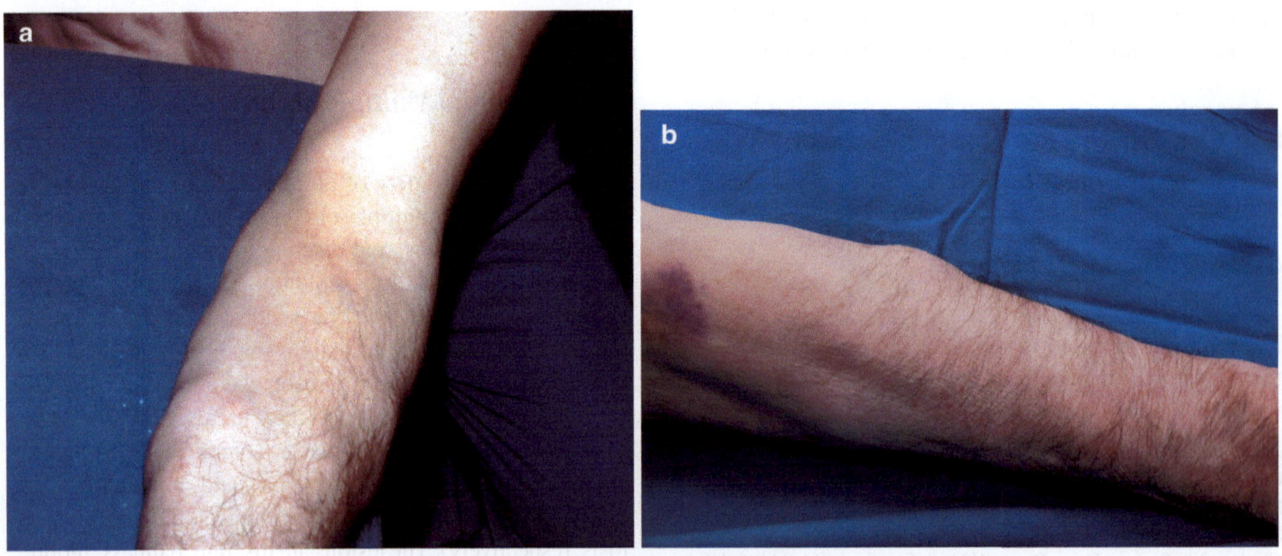

Fig. 8.3 Familial multiple lipomatosis. (**a**) Lipomas on the forearms. (**b**) Counterlateral lipomas in the same patients

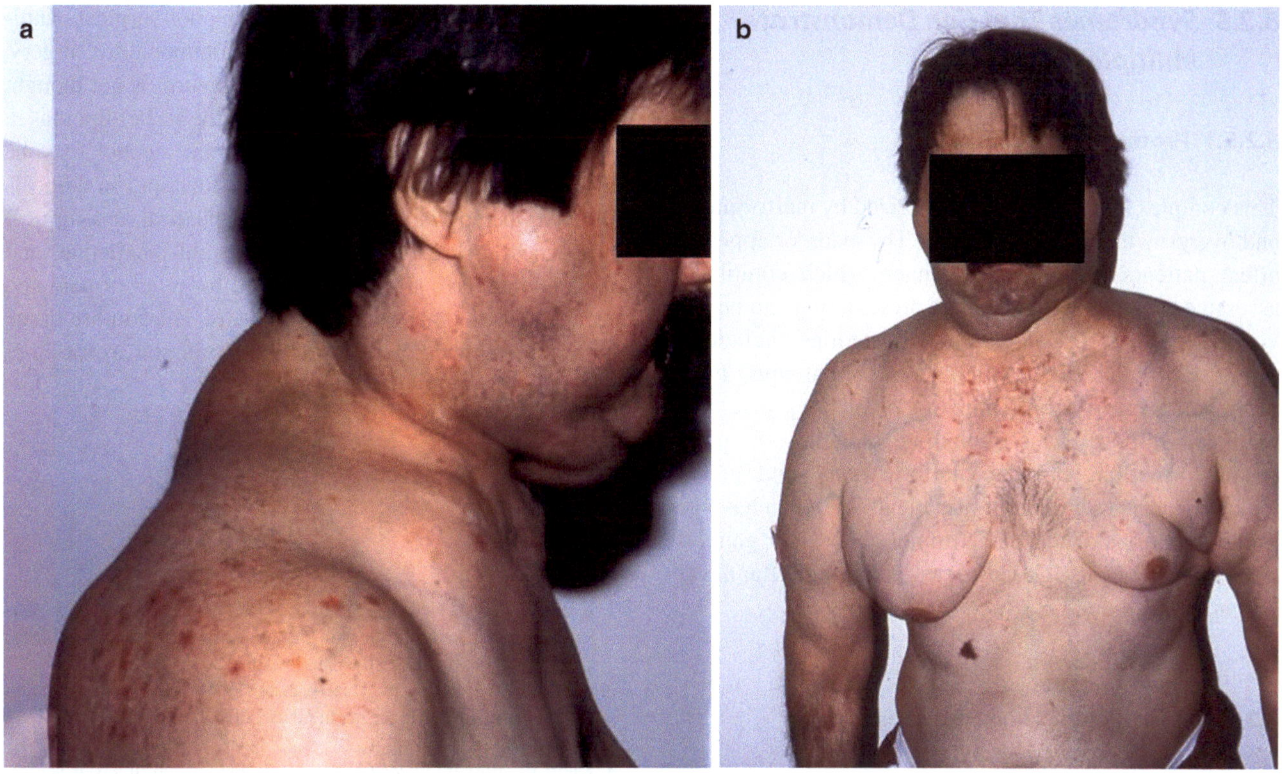

Fig. 8.4 Multiple symmetric lipomatosis in an alcoholic. (**a**) Symmetric accumulation of fatty tissue in the neck, face, and shoulder girdle. (**b**) Pseudoathletic appearance

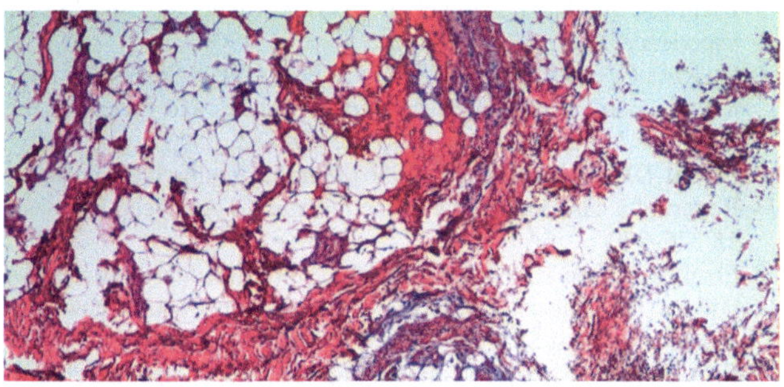

Fig. 8.5 Fat degeneration and fibrosis in adiposis dolorosa

are not uncommon, and polyneuropathies can also be documented. Many recent reports have demonstrated the association of Madelung's disease with metabolic abnormalities such as hyperlipidemia, hyperuricemia, reduced glucose intolerance, and renal tubular acidosis [9]. Disturbingly, it has also been associated with occult upper airway malignant tumors [10]. It is possible that this disease may be related to a primary defect of lipid mobilization in adipose tissue [9] or to excess lipid accumulation in functional defective embryonic brown adipose tissue [11]. Point mutations for mitochondrial DNA (codon 8344), which are important in alcohol metabolism, have been detected in 28% of patients [13].

On histology, the lesional cells look like the adipocytes of classic lipomas but tend to be a little smaller overall [11]. While initially the disorder was thought to be "benign," it is increasingly clearer that the dyspnea, dysphagia, and dysphonia associated with advanced disease, and the risk of neuropathy that all patients have, justify removing the "benign" moniker from this disease.

8.2.4 Adiposis Dolorosa (Dercum's Disease)

Adiposis dolorosa (Dercum's disease) was first described in 1892 and is characterized by progressive, painful, diffuse, and circumscribed fatty tissues, generalized obesity in women of menopausal age, weakness and frequent tendency to fatigue, and mental phenomenon (i.e., emotional instability, depression, epilepsy, and true dementia) [14]. The disorder is thought to be inherited in an autosomal dominant fashion and has been associated with endocrine and lipid metabolism dysfunction. The etiology and pathogenesis of this rare condition is unknown. The lesions often deposit in the pelvic girdle and thighs about the hips and knees. The pain is thought to be due to neuritis obtained from stretching of the peripheral nerves by the expanding lesions. On biopsy, the lesion consists of an increase in adipose tissue associated with increased vascularity, fibroblast proliferation and fat degeneration, and necrosis (Fig. 8.5).

8.2.5 Syndromes That Can Demonstrate Multiple Lipomas

8.2.5.1 Proteus Syndrome

This complex syndrome is characterized by malformations and overgrowth of various tissues. The disorder appears to affect patients in a mosaic manner, which complicates assessment and final diagnosis as presentation can be quite variable [15, 16]. Common manifestations include the presence of connective tissue and epidermal nevi, disproportionate overgrowth of limbs or other body parts, dysregulated adipose tissue (including lipomatosis), specific tumor formation, vascular malformations, and unusual facial phenotypes. A subset of patients seems to have germline mutations of the PTEN tumor suppressor gene, the susceptibility gene for Cowden disease and Bannayan–Zonana syndrome [17].

8.2.5.2 Bannayan–Zonana Syndrome

This rare entity is known by multiple eponyms (i.e., Banayan–Riley–Ruvalcaba syndrome) and belongs to the family of hamartomatous polyposis syndromes, which also includes Peutz–Jeghers syndrome, juvenile polyposis, and Cowden disease. It is characterized by macrocephaly, subcutaneous and visceral lipomas, and hemangiomas [18]. Other related findings include intestinal polyposis and pigmented macules on the penis. Inheritance is by autosomal dominant transmission, and a male predominance is also reported. Individuals frequently present with developmental delay and hypotonia, recognized during the first few years of life. As stated above, Bannayan–Zonana syndrome and Cowden disease both have mutations in the PTEN gene, a tumor suppressor gene located on 10q23. There is clinical overlap between the two syndromes as well, prompting some authors to believe that the two disorders may represent points along the same spectrum of disease [19].

8.3 Treatment and Prognosis

In diffuse lipomatosis, familial multiple lipomatosis, and Madelung's disease, surgical resection and liposuction have been used effectively to reduce the lipomas, but complete removal is not feasible usually due to the extensive nature of the lipomas and (in the case of diffuse lipomatosis and Madelung's disease) their infiltrative propensity [9, 20]. Liposuction is particularly helpful for poor surgical candidates. Unfortunately, recurrences are common after surgery. Drug therapy is not effective. Dietary control is not thought to be particularly helpful in decreasing the size of lipomas in Madelung's disease, but abstinence from alcohol may be helpful in normalizing abnormal liver function. In adiposis dolorosa, therapy is a combination of medical and surgical approaches [14]. Lidocaine, steroids, oral mexiletine, and amitryptyline have all been employed for relief of pain and management of other clinical symptoms. The adipose tissue can also be resected or removed via liposuction, as for other lipomatoses.

References

1. Kohler S (2003) Neoplasms of the skin: muscle, adipose and cartilage neoplasms. In: Bolognia JL, Jorizzo JL, Rapini RP (eds) Dermatology, vol 2. Mosby, London, pp 1888–1890
2. Karademir M, Kocak M, Usal A et al (1990) A case of infiltrating lipomatosis with diffuse, symmetrical distribution. Br J Clin Pract 44:728–730
3. Klein JA, Barr RJ (1986) Diffuse lipomatosis and tuberous sclerosis. Arch Dermatol 122:1298–1302
4. Kindblom LG, Moller-Nielsen J (1975) Diffuse lipomatosis in the leg after poliomyelitis. Acta Pathol Microbiol Scand A 83:339–344
5. Klein FA, Smith MJ, Kasenetz I (1988) Pelvic lipomatosis: 35 year experience. J Urol 139:998–1001
6. De Rosa G, Cozzolino A, Guarino M et al (1987) Congenital infiltrating lipomatosis of the face: report of cases and review of the literature. J Oral Maxillofac Surg 45:879–883
7. Leffell DJ, Braverman IM (1986) Familial multiple lipomatosis. Report of a case and review of the literature. J Am Acad Dermatol 15:275–279
8. Ersek RA, Lele E, Surak GS et al (1989) Hereditary progressive nodular lipomatosis: a report and selective review of a new syndrome. Ann Plast Surg 23:450–455
9. Enzi G (1984) Multiple symmetric lipomatosis: an updated clinical report. Medicine (Baltimore) 63:56–64
10. Ruzicka T, Vieluf D, Landthaler M et al (1987) Benign symmetric lipomatosis Launois-Bensaude. J Am Acad Dermatol 17:663–674
11. Meningaud JP, Pitak-Arnnop P, Bertrand JC (2007) Multiple symmetric lipomatosis: case report and review of the literature. J Oral Maxillofac Surg 65:1365–1369
12. Borges A, Torrinha F, Lufkin RB et al (1997) Laryngeal involvement in multiple symmetric lipomatosis: the role of computed tomography in diagnosis. Am J Otolaryng 18:127–130
13. Murphy MD, Carroll JF, Flemming DJ et al (2004) Benign musculoskeletal lipomatous lesions. Radiographics 24:1433–1466, AFIP Archives
14. Reece PH, Wyatt M, O'Flynn P (1999) Dercum's disease (adiposis dolorosa). J Laryngol Otol 113:174–176
15. Biesecker LG (2001) The multifaceted challenges of Proteus syndrome. J Am Med Assoc 285:2240–2243
16. Biesecker LG, Happle R, Mulliken JB et al (1999) Proteus syndrome: diagnostic criteria, differential diagnosis, and patient evaluation. Am J Med Genet 84:389–395

17. Zhou X, Hampel H, Thiele H et al (2001) Association of germline mutation in the PTEN tumour suppressor gene and Proteus and Proteus-like syndromes. Lancet 358:210–211
18. Gujrati M, Thomas C, Zelby A et al (1998) Bannayan–Zonana syndrome: a rare autosomal dominant syndrome with multiple lipomas and hemangiomas: a case report and review of literature. Surg Neurol 50:164–168
19. Wanner M, Tok Celebi J, Peacocke M, Wanner M, Tok Celebi J, Peacocke M (2001) Identification of a PTEN mutation in a family with Cowden syndrome and Bannayan–Zonana syndrome. J Am Acad Dermatol 44:183–187
20. Boozan JA, Maves MD, Schuller DE (1992) Surgical management of massive benign symmetric lipomatosis. Laryngoscope 102: 94–99

Chapter 9
Obesity

Jessica Linder, Amena Usmani, Maria Miteva, Camillo Ricordi, and Paolo Romanelli

Key Points

- Obesity has a profound impact on the development of skin manifestations.
- Obesity causes abnormalities in skin barrier function, sebaceous glands and sebum production, sweat glands, lymphatics, collagen structure and function, wound healing, microcirculation and macrocirculation, and subcutaneous fat.
- Obesity is implicated in a wide spectrum of dermatologic diseases including acanthosis nigricans, acrochordons, hyperandrogenism, striae distensae, adiposis dolorosa and fat redistribution, lymphedema, plantar hyperkeratosis, bacterial and mycotic infections, hidradenitis suppurativa, and psoriasis.
- Recognizing that obesity can both exacerbate and increase the likelihood of many dermatological conditions will permit earlier diagnosis and treatment of these conditions.

Keywords Obesity • Acanthosis nigricans • Acrochordons • Hyperandrogenism • Plantar hyperkeratosis

9.1 Introduction

Obesity has rapidly become an increasing problem in many countries in which changes in the economy have led to more sedentary lifestyles and consumption of high-calorie diets [1]. Obesity affects all ages, genders, and ethnicities and has many negative health effects. Obesity can be defined as a pathologic state whereby there is too much adipose tissue for the size of the body. The most widely used measurement of obesity is the Body Mass Index (BMI), which is determined by dividing a person's weight by their height squared (kg/m^2). Under current definitions, as adopted by the World Health Organization, men and women are considered of normal weight when they have a BMI less than 25, overweight when they have a BMI between 25 and 29.9, and obese when they have a BMI greater than 30.

Obesity is a risk factor for many diseases, including diabetes mellitus type II, coronary artery disease, hypertension, hypercholesterolemia, osteoarthritis, sleep apnea, and cholelithiasis. Obesity is also associated with higher mortality in many malignancies [2]. In addition to these widely appreciated health consequences, obesity also negatively affects the skin.

The abnormal function of leptin and its receptors in obese individuals may play a role in the increased susceptibility to many skin diseases. Leptin is a hormone secreted by adipocytes and helps to regulate hunger via hypothalamic receptors [3]. The leptin dysfunction seen in obese individual has been implicated in vascular damages [4] and the development of insulin resistance [5].

The proopiomelanocortin (POMC) gene also affects the skin in obesity [6].

Obesity causes imbalances in normal skin physiology, which contributes to the manifestation of disease. Obese individuals have dysregulation of the skin's barrier function characterized by increased transepidermal water loss and erythema [7], and alterations of the skin's surface pH [8]. They have elevated levels of hormones such as androgen, growth hormone, insulin, and insulin-like growth hormone causing dysregulation of sebaceous glands and increase in sebum production [9] and show increase in apocrine and eccrine sweat gland activity due to the large amounts of subcutaneous fat. Obesity alters the normal lymphatic flow, leading to decreased tissue oxygenation and chronic inflammation [10, 11] and also alters the microcirculation of the skin leading to hypoperfusion and poor wound healing. This may be due, in part, to the decreased collagen deposition in the skin of obese individuals. Therefore, in the postoperative period, obese patients are more likely to experience wound dehiscence and infection [12].

P. Romanelli (✉)
Department of Dermatology and Cutaneous Surgery, University of Miami Miller School of Medicine, 1600 NW 10th Avenue, Rosenstiel Building, Miami, FL 33136, USA
e-mail: promanelli@med.miami.edu

F. Rongioletti and B.R. Smoller (eds.), *Clinical and Pathological Aspects of Skin Diseases in Endocrine, Metabolic, Nutritional and Deposition Disease*, DOI 10.1007/978-1-60761-181-3_9, © Springer Science+Business Media, LLC 2010

9.2 Clinical and Pathological Aspects of Skin Manifestations

9.2.1 *Acrochordons*

Acrochordons (fibroepithelial polyps, skin tags) are flesh-colored or brown, soft, pedunculated papules attached to the skin by a thin fibrovascular stalk. They are commonly seen on the neck, axillae, and groin of obese individuals (Fig. 9.1). They are more common in females and are seen in up to 44% of obese patients [13]. The incidence of acrochordons correlates with the severity of obesity. Additionally, these lesions are strongly associated with diabetes and insulin resistance. Occasionally, acrochordons can cause pain due to local irritation or twisting around the stalk, causing ischemia and necrosis. When this occurs, patients may present complaining of a skin tag that has rapidly darkened in color.

Histologically, the epidermis usually lacks rete ridges and has few appendages (Fig. 9.2a). It can be slightly acanthotic and resemble seborrheic keratosis. The dermis contains fine collagen bundles but lacks adnexal structures. Often, there are dilated blood vessels present (Fig. 9.2b). Adipocytes may be present centrally; a subtype known as dermatolipoma (fibroma molle, soft fibroma, lipofibroma) demonstrates abundant adipocytes. An ischemic acrochordon may demonstrate hyperkeratosis, acantholysis, fat necrosis, or macrophage infiltration.

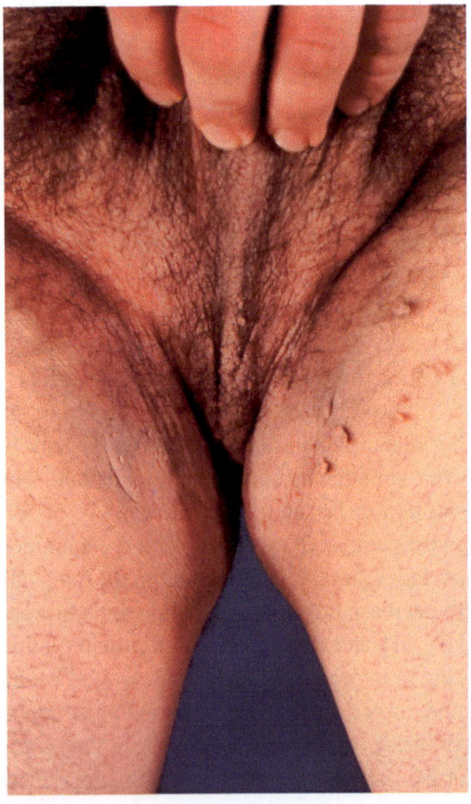

Fig. 9.1 Skin tags with acanthosis nigricans in an obese patient

9.2.2 *Adiposis Dolorosa*

Adiposis dolorosa, or Dercum's disease, is a rare condition that commonly occurs in obese, middle-aged women. It is characterized by multiple, bilateral, painful lipomas that occur more commonly on the trunk and lower extremities, especially around the knees. Other physical exam findings may include hyperalgesia, acral swelling, bruising, and telangiectasias. Patients usually have psychiatric problems (see also Chap. 8). The cause is unknown, and diagnosis can be confirmed by ultrasound (US) and Magnetic Resonance Imaging (MRI) demonstrating diffuse lipomas in the areas causing pain [14].

Histologically, the mature adipocytes of a lipoma are slightly larger than normal adipocytes and vary in size and shape. A sparse collagenous network is present, producing a lobular pattern. Nuclei are uniform but occasional hyperchromatic nuclei may be present. Some cases of adiposis dolorosa have demonstrated lesions similar to angiolipomas which are characterized by a vascular component of greater than 5% and are often painful. Adipocytes stain positive for vimentin and S-100.

9.2.3 *Hidradenitis Suppurativa*

Hidradenitis suppurativa is a painful, chronic disease characterized by folliculitis with abscesses, fistulas, and scarring. It occurs in the apocrine gland-bearing skin of the axillae and groin (Fig. 9.3). Hidradenitis suppurativa affects about 2% of the population [15]. The majority of patients with hidradenitis suppurativa are obese, which likely exacerbates the disease due to high shearing forces and elevated androgens [16]. Hidradenitis suppurativa is associated with nodulocystic acne and dissecting cellulitis of the scalp, and together these three diseases are known as the follicular occlusion triad. Microscopic features of early lesions demonstrate follicular plugging. Later on, folliculitis with extensive infiltration of neutrophils, lymphocytes, and histiocytes is present (Fig. 9.4a). As abscesses extend deeper into the subcutaneous tissue, sinuses lined with squamous epithelium develop and can drain purulent material. This persistent fibroinflammatory state leads to extensive scarring of the dermis and subcutis. A prominent foreign-body granulomatous reaction may develop, with infiltration of lymphoid plasma cells and giant cells surrounding fragments of keratin and hair; granulomas may be seen in up to 25% of cases. Suppurative

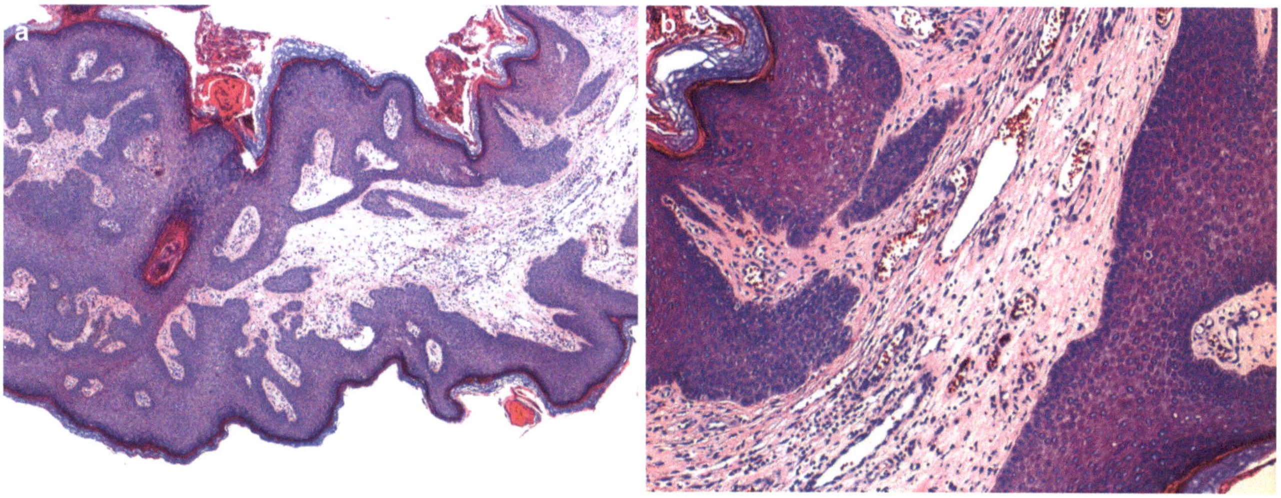

Fig. 9.2 (**a**) Achrocordon. (**b**) Achrochordon with feeding vessels in the stalk

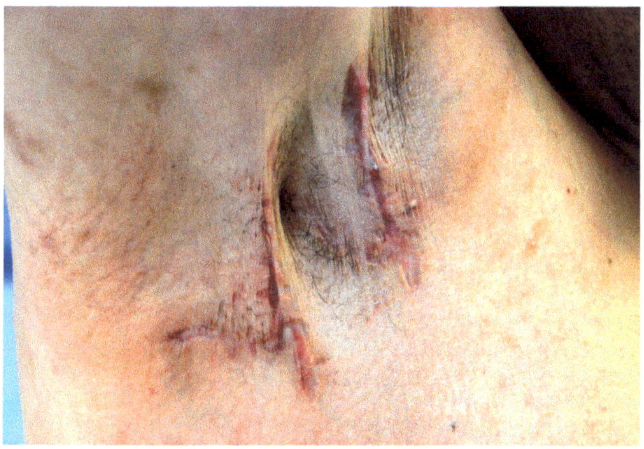

Fig. 9.3 Hidradenitis suppurativa with scar due to surgical treatment

inflammation of the apocrine glands is another pattern present in the minority of cases (Fig. 9.4b).

9.2.4 Lymphedema

Lymphedema is commonly caused by radiation or surgery and is exacerbated by obesity [17]. Lymphedema can also occur secondary to the obesity itself and is seen in the lower extremities (Fig. 9.5a,b) and/or large abdominal pannus of extremely obese individuals. Lymphedema results from impaired lymphatic return. Impaired lymphatic vessels are unable to pump protein-rich lymphatic fluid into the circulation, which leads to decreased blood flow, oxygenation, and wound healing. Lymphedematous tissues are prone to frequent bacterial infections and superimposed cellulitis.

Over time, the skin becomes thickened and fibrotic. In chronic lymphedema, patients may develop hyperkeratosis and papillomatosis of the epidermis, a condition known as elephantiasis nostras verrucosa. A rare but serious complication of chronic lymphedema is development of angiosarcoma, which has been described in the lower extremities and abdominal wall of obese individuals with lymphedema. Massive localized lymphedema is seen in morbidly obese patients and is characterized by a large, ill-defined mass within the skin.

Histologically, adipocytes and connective tissue septa are separated by edema and neovascularization. The dilation of lymphatic spaces can better be appreciated performing immunohistochemical analysis with antibody D2-40 or LYVE-1. The latter is particularly helpful in differentiating lymphedema from lipedema (diffuse, painless, bilateral, and symmetrical swelling of the thighs and lower legs in middle-aged women) in which there is increased interspaces between fat cells without dilation of blood vessels and lymphatics. In elephantiasis nostra verrucosa, a marked irregular epidermal hyperplasia with dermal fibrosis, lymphatic dilation, and inflammatory infiltrate is seen (Fig. 9.6a,b).

9.2.5 Acanthosis Nigricans

Acanthosis nigricans is the most common skin manifestation of obesity [11], and its incidence and severity tends to increase with the degree of obesity. It is often considered a marker for endocrine disease or malignancy. The pathogenesis of acanthosis nigricans is thought to be associated with hyperinsulinemia. This excess insulin is then thought to stimulate insulin-like growth factor (IGF) receptors, which activate keratinocytes and dermal fibroblasts. It is characterized by hyperpigmented, velvety, hyperkeratotic plaques in the axillae, neck, or groin (Fig. 9.1). Other less common

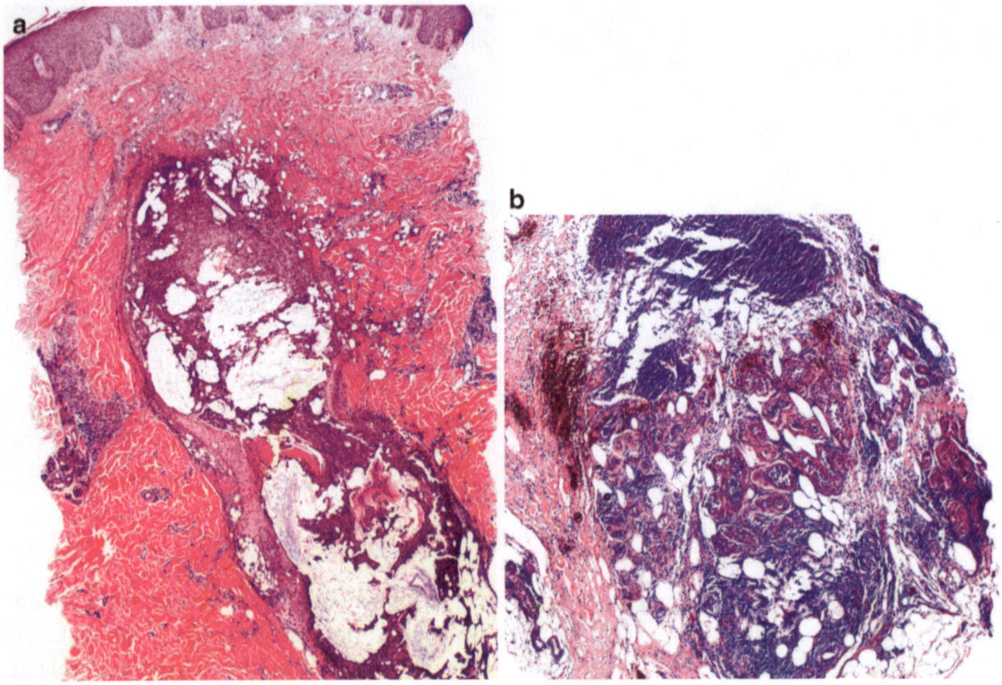

Fig. 9.4 (**a**) Suppurative folliculitis. (**b**) Apocrine gland abscesses in hidradenitis suppurativa

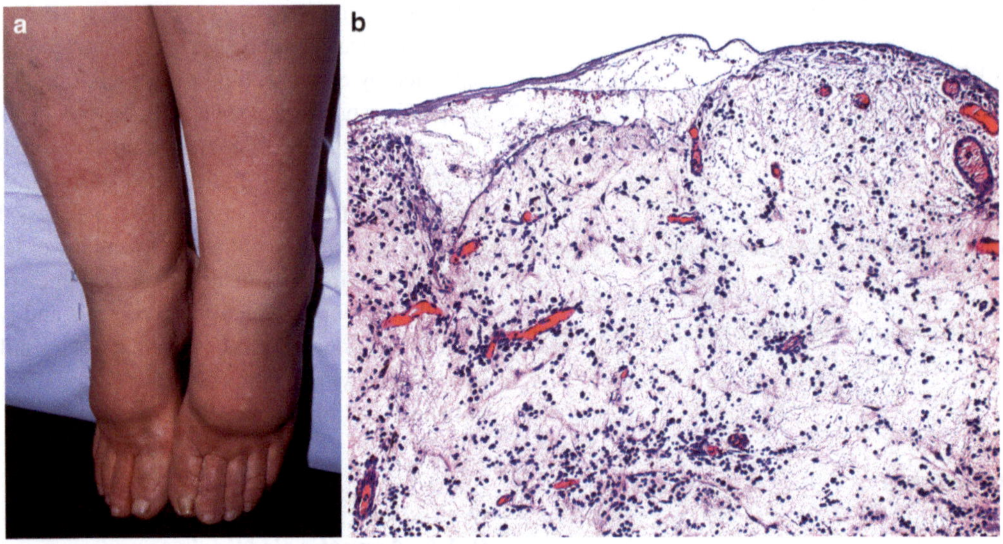

Fig. 9.5 (**a**) Lymphedema in obesity. (**b**) Histopathology of diffuse dermal lymphedema

locations include the elbows, knees, knuckles, scalp, and umbilical areas [18].

Histopathology shows hyperkeratosis and papillomatosis. The hyperkeratosis is responsible for the hyperpigmented appearance of plaques. Between papillae, there are valleys, which show acanthosis and hyperkeratosis. These valleys are often filled with keratotic material. The epidermis is thinned at the tops and sides of the papillae (see also Chap. 2).

9.2.6 Strie Distensae

Striae distensae, often referred to as stretch marks, are most commonly seen on the breasts, buttocks, thighs, and abdomen. Striae are more common in obese individuals, as well as those with Cushing's syndrome and pregnant women (see also Chap. 1) [10]. The pathogenesis of striae distensae is thought to involve an interplay between hormones, mechanical

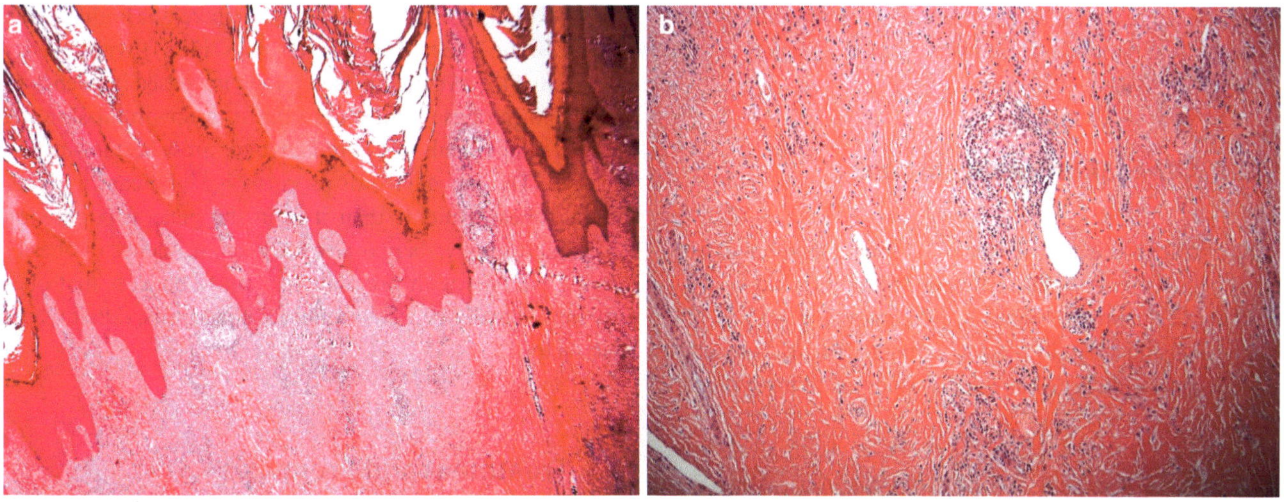

Fig. 9.6 Elephantiasis nostra verrucosa. (a) Marked irregular epidermal hyperplasia with dermal fibrosis. (b) Lymphatic dilation, fibrosis and inflammatory infiltrate

stress, and the physical properties of the skin. Striae may be regarded as a form of dermal scarring. It results from injury to the dermal collagen, leading to synthesis of new collagen in response to local stress [19].

The epidermis appears thin and flattened, with loss of the rete ridge pattern on histopathological grounds. The dermis is thinned, with dermal collagen bundles in a parallel array. In the early phase, fragmented collagen bundles and edema are seen with a mild (predominantly lymphocytic) perivascular infiltrate. In the chronic phase, there is an increase in the number and thickness of elastic fibers highlightened by elastic tissue stains, and elastin and fibrillin in the deep dermis are parallel to the skin surface.

9.2.7 Hyperandrogenism

Adipose tissue is the site of peripheral synthesis of androgen hormones. Thus obese individuals, particularly females, have an increased rate of androgen production. In addition, obese individuals commonly have hyperinsulinemia, which increases the production of ovarian androgens [20]. This excess insulin also acts to decrease the synthesis of sex hormone binding globulins, effectively increasing the level of free circulating testosterone.

Manifestations of cutaneous virilism include hirsutism, acne vulgaris, male-pattern baldness, and hidradenitis suppurativa [11].

9.2.8 Plantar Hyperkeratosis

Plantar hyperkeratosis is a diffuse thickening of the stratum corneum in a horseshoe pattern, affecting the heel (Fig. 9.7),

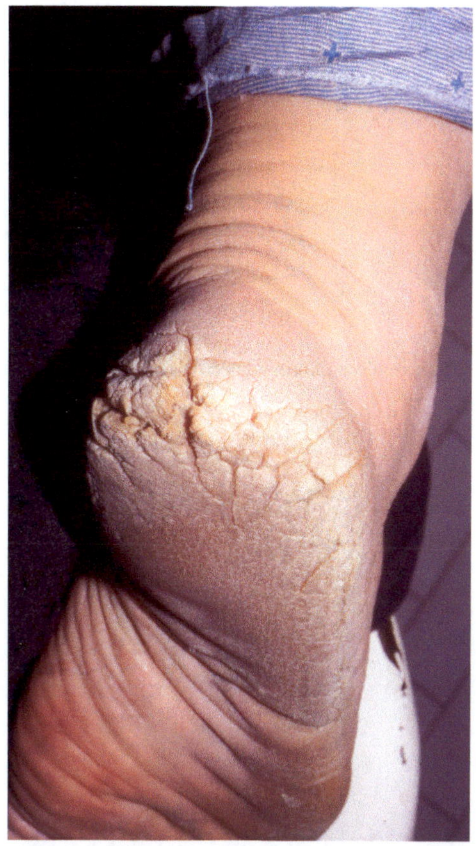

Fig. 9.7 Plantar hyperkeratosis in a horseshoe pattern, affecting the heel of an obese patient

foot arch area, and plantar-medial aspect of the great toe at the level of the interphalangeal join [10]. Plantar hyperkeratosis is the most common skin finding in obese individuals who weighed 176% of ideal body weight or more and is caused by mechanical alterations induced by excess weight in obese individuals [21, 22]. The stratum corneum is thought to thicken in response to this trauma, which presents as thick hyperorthokeratotic layer on histology.

9.2.9 Other Skin Manifestations

Obese patients are at increased risk for development of pressure ulcers (Fig. 9.8) due to higher immobility and poor circulation [23], chronic venous insufficiency (Fig. 9.9a,b) [24], gout, and skin infections such as intertrigo. In fact, obese patients have thicker skin folds and sweat more profusely, due to excess subcutaneous fat, which increases both friction and moisture. The rate of intertrigo rises linearly with severity of obesity [13]. Another reason for the increased incidence of intertrigo in obese patients is related to abnormal skin pH of obese individuals as *Candida* hyphae grow best in an alkaline pH. The prevalence of psoriasis is significantly higher among obese patients than it is in the general population [25]. Interestingly, there is also a higher prevalence of obesity among patients with psoriasis leading to suggest that obesity may actually be a consequence of psoriasis, rather than a risk factor.

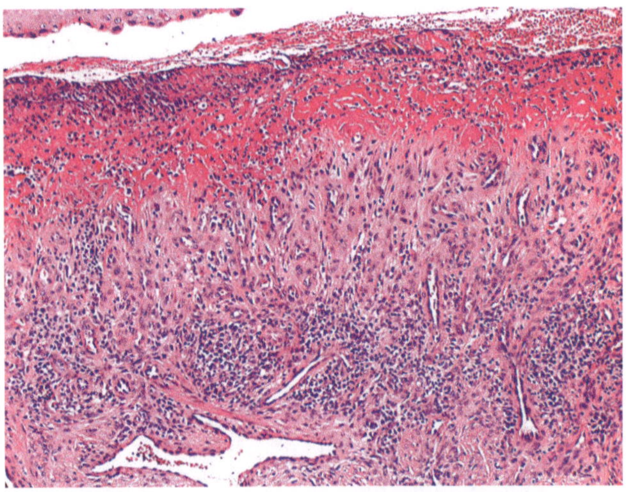

Fig. 9.8 Pressure ulcers, fibrinoid necrosis and dilated vessels

9.3 Treatment and Prognosis

Acrochordons are benign growths and are removed only for cosmetic reasons. Theoretically, a lower rate of recurrence could be seen in patients who achieve a better control of their diabetes and overweight. However, once an achrocordon is present, it does not seem to regress with weight loss [26]. Treatment is by scissor excision, electrodesiccation, or cryotherapy.

Hidradenitis suppurativa is often chronic and relapsing. It has a high degree of morbidity secondary to chronic pain and pustular discharge. Squamous cell carcinoma is a rare consequence in areas of chronic inflammation and scarring. Hidradenitis suppurativa is very difficult to treat. Treatment should include encouraging weight loss. Topical steroids and antibiotics have been tried with minimal success.

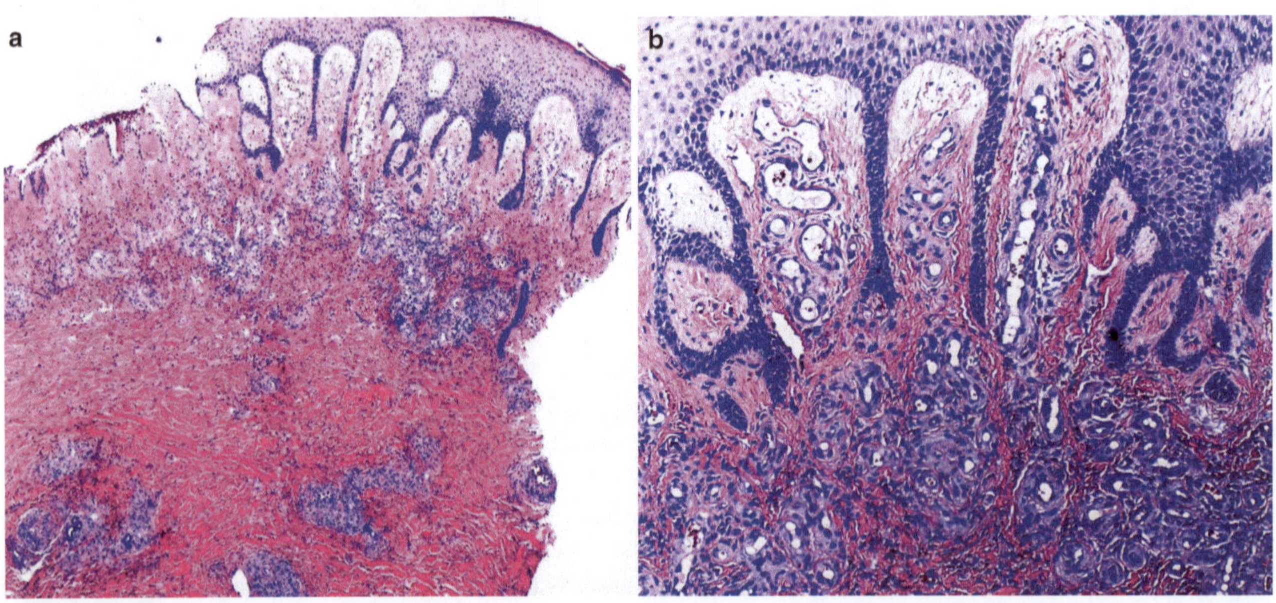

Fig. 9.9 Venous ulcer. (**a**) Clusters of vessels, fibrosis, red blood cell extravasation. (**b**) Angiogenesis and aneurysmatic distortion of the superficial capillary plexus

Retinoids and systemic or intralesional steroids have had variable results. Infliximab has been shown to be effective [27]. However, only surgical excision of all apocrine gland-bearing skin has been shown to effectively treat hidradenitis suppurativa by altering the natural course of the disease [16].

Lymphedema tends to be a chronic and progressive disease and patients usually require lifelong treatment. Treatment consists of elevation, elastic stockings, and applying external compression devices [28]. Weight reduction is extremely important in treatment because excess weight decreases the benefit of therapy and worsens the lymphedema. Infection prevention is also important and is accomplished by daily cleansing with mild soap, followed by a moisturizer.

Treatment of striae distensae includes the application of topical tretinion 0.1% cream early in the course of the disease. Topical tretinoin works by increasing the deposition of collagen and number of fibroblasts. Laser therapy has also shown to be effective in the treatment of striae. Early, erythematous lesions respond best to 585-nm pulsed dye laser, whereas late, hypopigmented scars respond better to the 308-nm excimer laser [29, 30].

Acanthosis nigricans can be managed by controlling hyperinsulinemia. Weight loss and exercise are thus the best treatment options. Metformin has been shown to be effective [31]. Octreotide, which acts by reducing insulin secretion, has also been shown to be effective. Topical antibiotics, retinoids, and keratolytics may also be used for treatment, with variable results.

Treatment of hyperandrogenism focuses mainly on controlling insulin levels. Metformin therapy has been found to lower insulin levels and possibly androgen levels as well. Weight loss, antiandrogenic therapy, and oral contraceptives may also be beneficial in the treatment of hyperandrogenis. Thiazolidinediones may improve insulin resistance and hyperandrogenism in women with polycystic ovarian syndrome [32].

References

1. Kuczmarski RJ, Flegal KM, Campbell SM, Johnson CL (1994) Increasing prevalence of overweight among US adults. The National Health and Nutrition Examination Surveys 1960 to 1991. JAMA 27:205–211
2. Calle EE, Rodriguez C, Walker-Thurmond K, Thun MJ (2003) Overweight, obesity, and mortality from cancer in a prospectively studied cohort of U.S. adults. N Engl J Med 348:1625–1638
3. Friedman JM, Halaas JL (1998) Leptin and the regulation of body weight in mammals. Nature 395:763–770
4. Pardini VC, Victoria IM, Rocha SM et al (1998) Leptin levels, beta-cell function, and insulin sensitivity in families with congenital and acquired generalized lipoatropic diabetes. J Clin Endocrinol Metab 83:503–508
5. Shimomura I, Hammer RE, Ikemoto S, Brown MS, Goldstein JL (1999) Leptin reverses insulin resistance and diabetes mellitus in mice with congenital lipodystrophy. Nature 401:73–76
6. Krude H, Biebermann H, Schnabel D et al (2003) Obesity due to proopiomelanocortin deficiency: three new cases and treatment trials with thyroid hormone and ACTH4-10. J Clin Endocrinol Metab 88:4633–4640
7. Loffler H, Aramaki JU, Effendy I (2002) The influence of body mass index on skin susceptibility to sodium lauryl sulphate. Skin Res Technol 8:19–22
8. Yosipovitch G, Tur E, Cohen O, Rusecki Y (1993) Skin surface pH in intertriginous areas in NIDDM patients. Possible correlation to candidal intertrigo. Diabetes Care 16:560–563
9. Cappel M, Mauger D, Thiboutot D (2005) Correlation between serum levels of insulin-like growth factor 1, dehydroepiandrosterone sulfate, and dihydrotestosterone and acne lesion counts in adult women. Arch Dermatol 141:333–338
10. Garcia Hidalgo L (2002) Dermatological complications of obesity. Am J Clin Dermatol 3:497–506
11. Yosipovitch G, DeVore A, Dawn A, Yosipovitch G, DeVore A, Dawn A (2007) Obesity and the skin: skin physiology and skin manifestations of obesity.[see comment]. J Am Acad Dermatol 56:901–916
12. Derzie AJ, Silvestri F, Liriano E, Benotti P (2000) Wound closure technique and acute wound complications in gastric surgery for morbid obesity: a prospective randomized trial. J Am Coll Surg 191:238–243
13. Garcia-Hidalgo L, Orozco-Topete R, Gonzalez-Barranco J, Villa AR, Dalman JJ, Ortiz-Pedroza G (1999) Dermatoses in 156 obese adults. Obes Res 7:299–302
14. Brodovsky S, Westreich M, Leibowitz A, Schwartz Y (1994) Adiposis dolorosa (Dercum's disease): 10-year follow-up. Ann Plast Surg 33:664–668
15. Jemec GB (2004) Medical treatment of hidradenitis suppurativa. Expert Opin Pharmacother 5:1767–1770
16. Slade DE, Powell BW, Mortimer PS (2003) Hidradenitis suppurativa: pathogenesis and management. Br J Plast Surg 56:451–461
17. Macdonald JM (2001) Wound healing and lymphedema: a new look at an old problem. Ostomy Wound Manage 47:52–57
18. Hahler B (2006) An overview of dermatological conditions commonly associated with the obese patient. Ostomy Wound Manage 52:34–36
19. Guida B, Nino M, Perrino NR, Laccetti R, Trio R, Labella S, Balato N (2010) The impact of obesity on skin disease and epidermal permeability barrier status. J Eur Acad Dermatol Venereol 24: 191–195
20. Wild RA (1995) Obesity, lipids, cardiovascular risk, and androgen excess. Am J Med 98:27S–32S
21. Birtane M, Tuna H, Birtane M, Tuna H (2004) The evaluation of plantar pressure distribution in obese and non-obese adults. Clin Biomech 19:1055–1059
22. Hills AP, Hennig EM, McDonald M, Bar-Or O (2001) Plantar pressure differences between obese and non-obese adults: a biomechanical analysis. Int J Obes Relat Metab Disord 25: 1674–1679
23. Barr J, Cunneen J (2001) Understanding the bariatric client and providing a safe hospital environment. Clin Nurse Spec 15:219–223
24. Beebe-Dimmer JL, Pfeifer JR, Engle JS, Schottenfeld D (2005) The epidemiology of chronic venous insufficiency and varicose veins. Ann Epidemiol 15:175–184
25. Herron MD, Hinckley M, Hoffman MS et al (2005) Impact of obesity and smoking on psoriasis presentation and management.[see comment]. Arch Dermatol 141:1527–1534

26. Mukhtar M (2006) Surgical pearl: tissue forceps as a simple and effective instrument for treating skin tags. Int J Dermatol 45:577–579
27. Adams DR, Gordon KB, Devenyi AG, Ioffreda MD (2003) Severe hidradenitis suppurativa treated with infliximab infusion. Arch Dermatol 139:1540–1542
28. Sieggreen MY, Kline RA (2004) Current concepts in lymphedema management. Adv Skin Wound Care 17:174–178
29. Jimenez GP, Flores F, Berman B et al (2003) Treatment of striae rubra and striae alba with the 585-nm pulsed-dye laser. Dermatol Surg 29:362–365
30. Goldberg DJ, Sarradet D, Hussain M, Goldberg DJ, Sarradet D, Hussain M (2003) 308-nm Excimer laser treatment of mature hypopigmented striae. Dermatol Surg 29:596–598
31. Tankova T, Koev D, Dakovska L, Kirilov G (2002) Therapeutic approach in insulin resistance with acanthosis nigricans. Int J Clin Pract 56:578–581
32. Ortega-Gonzalez C, Luna S, Hernandez L et al (2005) Responses of serum androgen and insulin resistance to metformin and pioglitazone in obese, insulin-resistant women with polycystic ovary syndrome. J Clin Endocrinol Metab 90:1360–1365

Chapter 10
Porphyrias

Jaqueline M. Junkins-Hopkins

Key Points

- Porphyrias are a heterogeneous group of inherited and acquired disorders that result from a deficiency of specific enzymes involved in heme biosynthesis, resulting in accumulation of porphyrins and/or porphyrin precursors.
- Porphyrias may have cutaneous or neurovisceral manifestations, or both and may be further subdivided based on the primary site in which the heme synthesis takes place – erythropoietic and hepatic, or are classified based on the presentation of acute or non-acute (cutaneous) symptoms.
- The erythropoietic porphyrias include congenital erythropoietic porphyria (CEP) and erythropoietic protoporphyria (EPP), while the hepatic porphyrias include acute intermittent porphyria (AIP), δ-aminolevulinic acid dehydratase deficiency (ALA-D) porphyria, variegate porphyria (VP), porphyria cutanea tarda (PCT), hereditary coproporphyria (HCP), and hepatoerythrocytic porphyria (HEP).
- The non-acute (cutaneous) porphyrias include PCT, EPP, CEP, and HEP, and present with a spectrum of cutaneous findings, due to a photosensitivity reaction to porphyrin in the skin. VP and HCP are "mixed" porphyrias, and may have cutaneous and noncutaneous presentations.
- The acute porphyrias (AIP, VP, HCP, ALA-D) present with a wide variety of symptoms that mimic other disorders, often causing a delay in the diagnosis. Cutaneous findings in acute porphyria are only seen in VP and HCP, and are similar to those of PCT.
- Acquired porphyria may be seen in association with lead poisoning, alcoholism, chemicals such as hexachlorobenzene, and hereditary tyrosenemia. Patients with hemochromatosis are susceptible to developing porphyria cutanea tarda, and inheritance of at least one mutation of the HFE gene makes one susceptible to getting PCT.
- Treatment of porphyria includes strict photoprotection and avoidance of triggers. PCT responds to phlebotomy and antimalarials.

Keywords Acute porphyrias • Cutaneous porphyrias • Porphyria cutanea tarda • Erythropoietic protoporphyria

10.1 Introduction

Porphyrias are a heterogenous group of disorders that result from a deficiency of one of eight specific enzymes involved in heme biosynthesis, resulting in accumulation of porphyrins and/or porphyrin precursors [1–4]. Porphyrias may have cutaneous or neurovisceral manifestations, or both. Porphyrias may be further subdivided based on the primary site in which the heme synthesis takes place – erythropoietic and hepatic, or are classified based on the presentation of acute or non-acute cutaneous symptoms [3–5]. There are acquired forms of porphyria, associated with lead poisoning, alcoholism, and hereditary tyrosinemia [4]. In addition, there is a very rare variant that is transient, and occurs in neonates with hemolytic anemia, and is treated with phototherapy.

Porphyrins were named for the Greek root for purple, and the name is credited to a German medical student in 1874. It has been proposed that notable historic people, including King George III of England and Vincent van Gogh suffered from porphyria. The photosensitivity, deforming scars, hyperpigmentation, hypertrichosis, and conspicuous incisors that characterize patients with CEP may have led to the myths about vampires and werewolves [4].

Each subtype of porphyrias has a characteristic biochemical profile, based on the enzymatic deficiency and subsequent porphyrin metabolite accumulation (Fig. 10.1) [1–7].

A diagnosis of porphyria is ultimately made based on documenting abnormally high porphyrin or porphyrin

J.M. Junkins-Hopkins (✉)
Division of Dermatopathology and Oral Pathology, Department of Dermatology, Johns Hopkins Hospital, 600 North Wolfe Street Blalock 907, Baltimore, MD 21287, USA
e-mail: jjunkin1@jhmi.edu

F. Rongioletti and B.R. Smoller (eds.), *Clinical and Pathological Aspects of Skin Diseases in Endocrine, Metabolic, Nutritional and Deposition Disease*, DOI 10.1007/978-1-60761-181-3_10, © Springer Science+Business Media, LLC 2010

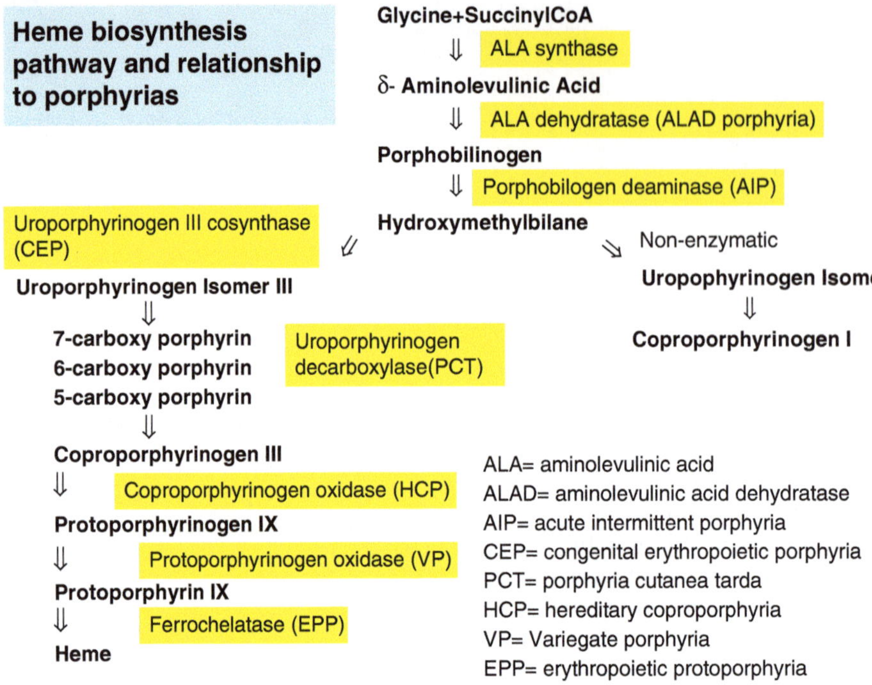

Fig. 10.1 Heme pathway porphyria

precursor levels in the urine, feces, and/or blood. In some instances, overlapping clinical and biochemical features require specialized assays to quantify these enzymatic levels, and genetic analysis may be required to identify the typical mutation (Fig. 10.1).

The acute episodes in porphyrias include abdominal pain, neurological changes, and psychiatric disturbances, and are seen in AIP, VP, HCP, and ALA-D.

Cutaneous manifestations of porphyria may be acute or subacute to chronic. The acute flare pattern presents with rapidly evolving painful and burning lesions with erythema and edema shortly after sun exposure. This typically occurs in EPP, but can occasionally occur in the other porphyrias. The non-acute cutaneous manifestations include skin fragility with the development of tense blisters, erosions, and scars occurring in the sun-exposed skin. This is seen in PCT, HCP, VP, CEP, and HEP. The light sensitivity is attributed to absorption by porphyrins of wavelengths in the Soret band (400–410 nm range), which converts porphyrin from its ground state to a highly reactive excited state, which initiates a cascade of inflammatory events. Only the porphyrins, not the porphyrin precursors are photosensitizing. The more lipophilic porphyrins, such as those in EPP, accumulate in erythrocytes and endothelial lining of vessels, resulting in consequences of vascular damage. The water-soluble uroporphyrins in PCT diffuse to the skin, in the upper dermis, resulting in blistering [8].

10.2 Clinical and Pathological Aspects of Skin Manifestations

The cutaneous porphyrias include: congenital erythropoietic porphyria (CEP) (Günther's disease), porphyria cutanea tarda, erythropoietic protoporphyria, and the so-called pseudoporphyria.

10.2.1 Congenital Erythropoietic Porphyria (CEP)

CEP is a rare autosomal recessive disorder resulting from a deficiency of uroporphyrinogen III synthase (URO–synthase). The URO–synthase gene is located to the chromosomal region 10q. Multiple mutations have been described, including C73R, which is seen in about a third of patients, and associated with a more severe phenotype [6]. It is common in the European patients, and is associated with severe disease. The clinical presentation is variable, and ranges from disfiguring cutaneous manifestations and hemolysis to fetal death. Patients develop photosensitivity-induced chronic recurrent blisters, scarring, skin hyperfragility, sclerodermoid changes, hemolytic anemia with splenomegaly, and massive porphyrinuria. CEP often first presents in infancy as pink or red urine, due to the massive porphyrinuria. Porphyrin deposition in the dentine and enamel results in erythrodontia of the deciduous teeth. Patients usually develop bullae within a day or two of exposure to the sun. Recurrent eruptions can lead to mutilating deformities of the face, especially the nose and mouth, and hands, and sclerodermoid thickening of the affected parts. Other features of this disorder are hypertrichosis, patchy scarring alopecia, nail changes, and ocular scleromalacia. If there is ocular involvement, blindness can occur. Fluorescence with a Woods lamp red reveals the characteristic red color of the teeth, and also accentuates the urine color. The predominant porphyrins found are uroporphyrins I and coproporphyrin I in the urine, stool, plasma, and erythrocytes.

10.2.2 Porphyria Cutanea Tarda

Porphyria cutanea tarda (PCT) is the most common form of porphyria in North America and Europe, with an incidence of approximately 1 in 25,000 in the USA [4]. The disorder results from a reduced activity of the fifth enzyme in heme biosynthesis, uroporphyrinogen decarboxylase (URO–D). There are two main forms of PCT: sporadic or acquired (type I), in which the enzymatic defect is limited to the liver, and familial (type II), where the defect is present in all tissues. In a recently designated type III familial form, the URO-D is deficient only in nonerythroid cells. Thus, patients with type III will have normal blood levels of the enzyme, despite presenting with classic disease and a positive family history.

Type I, the acquired or sporadic form is the most common, with a male predominance, and onset in mid-life. It results from inactivation of URO–D in the liver. More than 70% of cases in the past were associated with alcohol abuse and liver damage. Iron overload, medications, estrogen therapy, oral contraceptive pills, and exposure to polychlorinated aromatic hydrocarbons are triggering factors. Hepatitis C virus, HIV [9], and lupus erythematosus have also been associated with PCT [6].

Type II, the familial form is inherited as an autosomal dominant trait due to mutations in the URO-D gene, which results in decreased URO-D to at least 50–60% of normal in all tissues. The most common exogenous agent associated with PCT is iron [9]. This may be related to the mutations in the hemochromatosis HFE gene, especially C282Y and H63D. Sixty percent of patients with PCT have at least one mutation in the HFE gene. Patients with hemochromatosis are four times more likely to acquire PCT than nonaffected individuals [4, 10]. Other exogenous triggers include excessive alcohol intake, childbirth, hemodialysis for chronic renal failure, and exposure to ultraviolet radiation in tanning parlors. The onset is earlier than the sporadic form.

In all forms of PCT, there is decreased activity of URO-D [9]. The cutaneous changes are associated with photosensitivity; thus are located primarily on the face, arms, and dorsal hands. Blistering and hyperfragility result in erosions, hypo and hyperpigmentation, scarring, and milia. When intact, the blisters range from 0.5 to 3 cm in diameter. Blistering may only be evident as circumscribed crusts or ulcers of unroofed bullae, arising on the background of photo-damaged skin with mottled brown-gray postinflammatory dyspigmentation and milia (Fig. 10.2a,b). Hypertrichosis of the periorbital region and malar cheeks is classic (Fig. 10.3), but not always seen. With chronic disease, sclerodermoid skin alterations occur on the face, neck, thorax, and scalp. The latter may be associated with patchy or diffuse alopecia. Patients with PCT have an increased risk of developing hepatocellular carcinoma [3].

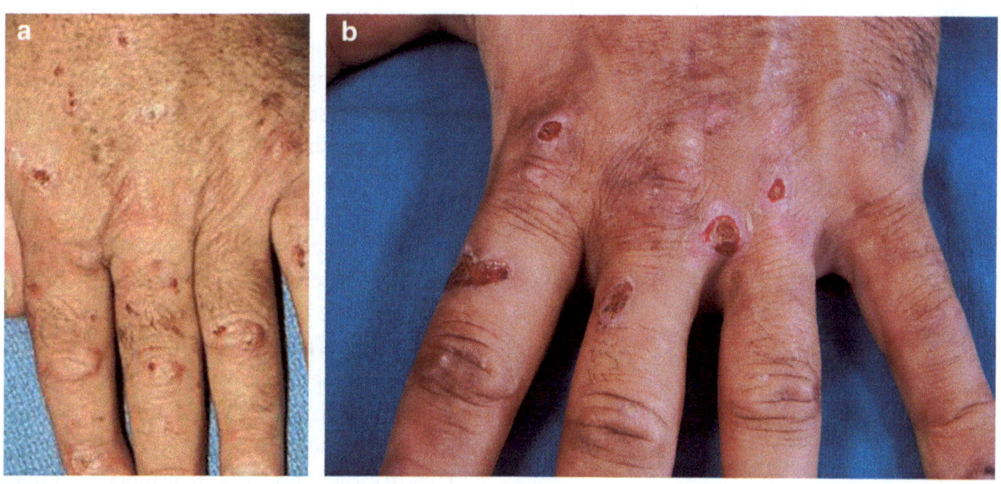

Fig. 10.2 Porphyria cutanea tarda (PCT). (**a**) Typical erosions and crusts on the dorsal hands and fingers, with mottled hyperpigmentation. (**b**) Crusts, ulcers of de-roof bullae and milia

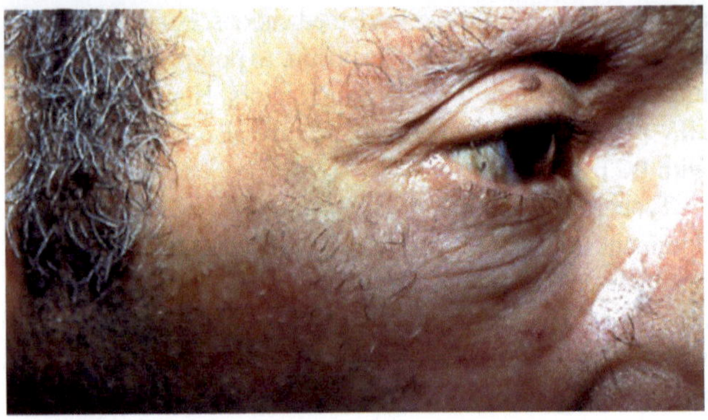

Fig. 10.3 Hyperthicosis of the face in PCT

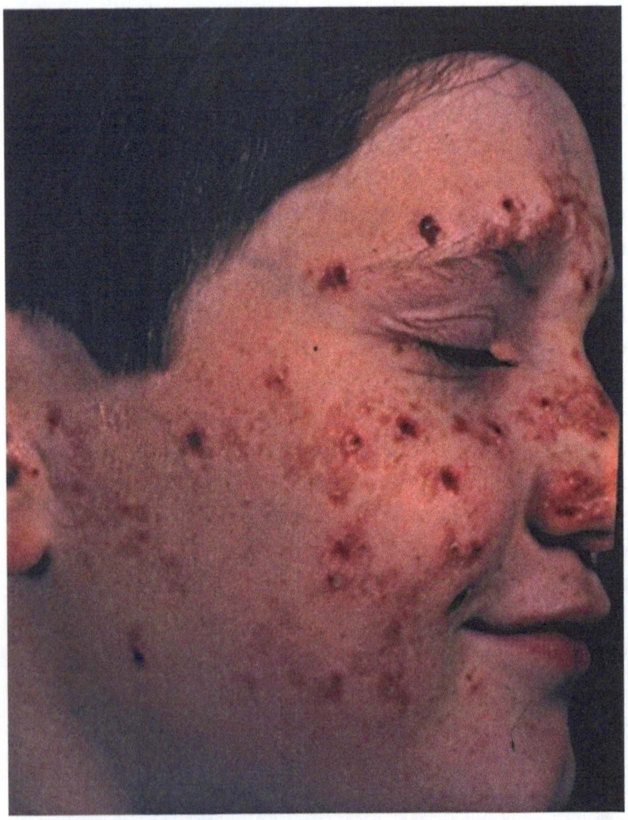

Fig. 10.4 Hemorrhagic crusts on the face in EPP

Laboratory findings in PCT show increased levels of 8-carboxyl porphyrin or uroporphyrin and 7-carboxyl porphyrin in the urine and plasma and increased levels of isocoproporphyrin in the feces.

10.2.3 Erythropoietic Protoporphyria

Erythropoietic protoporphyria (EPP) is the second most common type of cutaneous porphyria, with a prevalence that ranges from 1:75,000 to 1:200,000 [11]. The abnormal porphyrin profile is due to defective ferrochelatase, the eight and last enzyme in the heme biosynthetic pathway. The ferrochetalase gene is on chromosome 18, encoded by the FECH gene. EPP usually manifests in infancy or early childhood, prior to age 5. Within minutes of sun exposure, there is acute stinging, burning, and pruritus, associated with erythema, urticarial plaques, edema, and hemorrhagic crusts on the face (Fig. 10.4) (especially nose and cheeks), dorsal hands, and forearms (Fig. 10.5). Symptoms may persist for hours to several days. With repeated exposure to the sun, characteristic skin alterations ensue, and include yellowish waxy leathery thickening of skin on the face, the knuckles and metacarpophalangeal and interphalangeal joints, varioliform scarring of the nose, perioral furrows and pseudo-rhagades, and pits or scars on the forehead, nose, and cheeks. Blistering is very rare. Nail changes such as photo-onycholysis have been described. EPP may coexist with lupus erythematosus. There are no neurovisceral manifestations in EPP, but a characteristic and rare occurrence is liver disease, cholelithiasis, cirrhosis, and death from accumulation of protoporphyrin in the hepatobiliary system [3].

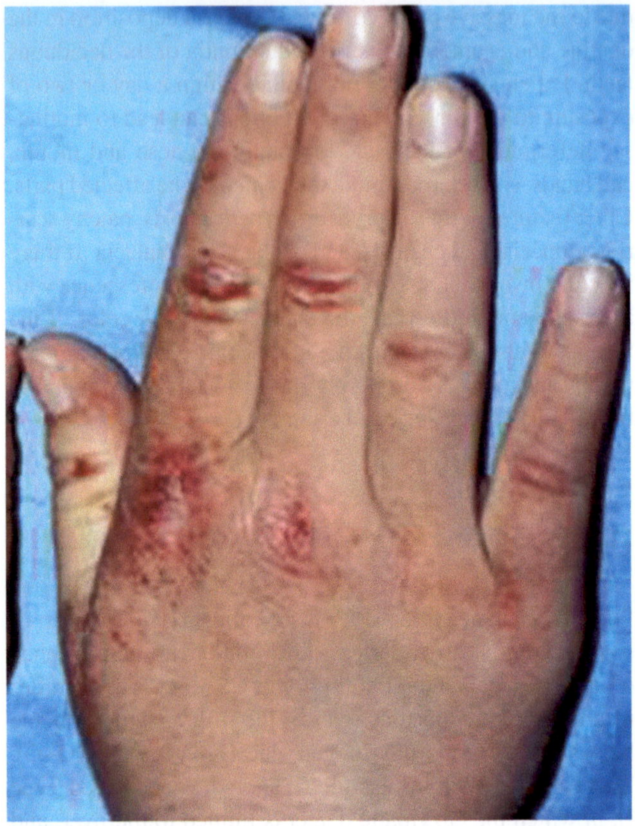

Fig. 10.5 Erythropoietic protoporphyria in a child with erythematous plaques due to repeated sun exposure

This disorder has normal urinary porphyrins. There are elevated levels of protoporphyrin in the feces, bile, erythrocytes, and plasma. The erythrocytes may fluoresce red with Wood's lamp due to the increased protoporphyrin levels. Increased

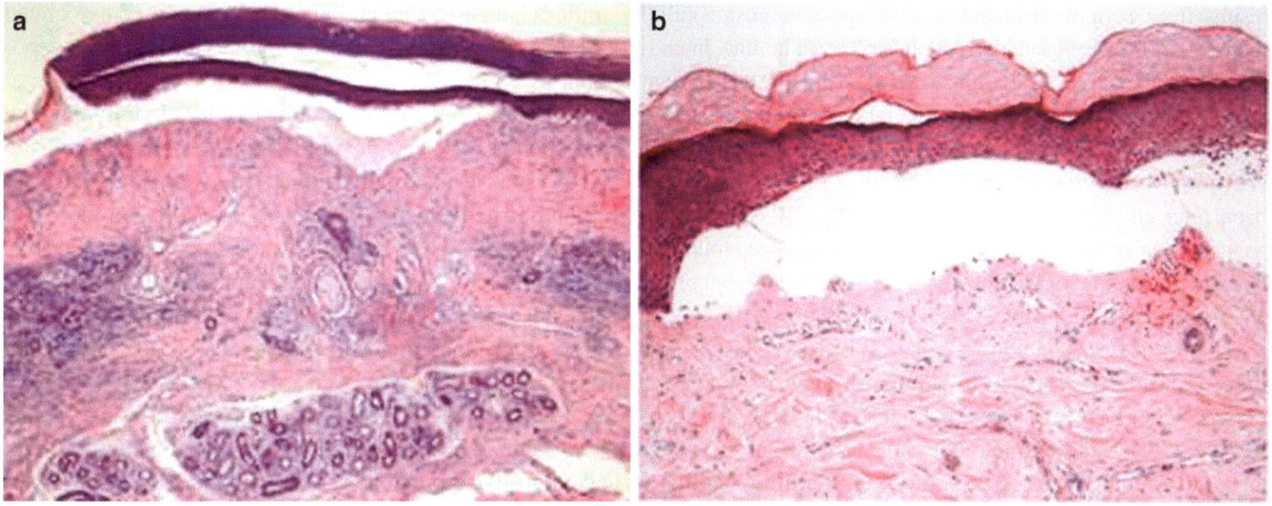

Fig. 10.6 Porphyria cutanea tarda (PCT). (**a**) Acral skin with subepidermal blister. (**b**) Noninflammatory subepidermal blister (H & E stain)

protoporphyrin in the stool also helps secure a diagnosis of EPP.

10.2.4 Hepatoerythropoietic Porphyria

Hepatoerythropoietic porphyria (HEP) is the very rare recessive homozygous variant of PCT, in which there is a profound deficiency (<10% of normal activity) of uroporphyrinogen decarboxylase activity. HEP manifests in early childhood, often as dark urine in the diapers. Severe photosensitivity results in blisters, pruritus, hyperpigmentation, and sclerodermoid scarring. Hypertrichosis,ectropion, erythrodontia, and splenomegaly are also seen. There may be neurovisceral symptoms. Clinically, the patients are similar to CEP, although the enzymatic deficiency of URO-D is similar to PCT, and results in a marked increase of uroporphyrinogen and 7-carboxyporphyrin in the urine and isocoproporphyrin in the feces. In contrast to PCT, zinc protoporphyin may be detected in the erythrocytes [6].

10.2.5 Pseudoporphyria

Pseudoporphyria is usually due to medications. Clinically, it mimics PCT with blisters and hyperfragility of the dorsal hand and neck, but with normal porphyrin and enzyme levels. The lesions may develop from 1 week to several months after commencement of a drug, especially nonsteroidal antiinflammatory agents [12, 13]. Drugs implicated include naproxen, tetracyclines, sulfonamides, furosemide, nalidixic acid, dapsone, pyridoxin, isotretinoin, pravastatin, oxaprozin, mefenamic acid, nabumetone, pyridoxine, chlorthalidone, flutamide, and etretinate. Approximately 4–7% of patients with end-stage renal disease undergoing hemodialysis develop PCT-like cutaneous symptoms, with normal porphyrin levels, and this has been termed pseudoporphyria of end-stage renal disease or bullous dermatosis of hemodialysis. This may be extensive, mimicking toxic epidermal necrolysis [13]. Some cases have been reported after tanning bed exposure.

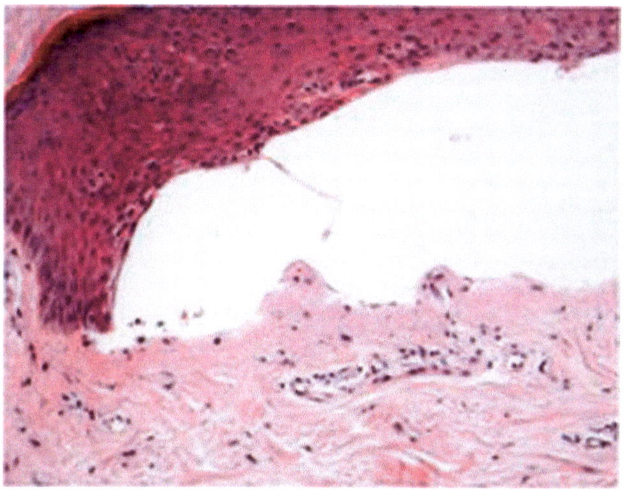

Fig. 10.7 PCT with festooning (H & E stain)

10.2.6 Histologic Features

The porphyrias are similar, but may differ in severity. The acute cutaneous phototoxicity reactions histologically show endothelial cell damage, infiltration of neutrophils, and mast cell degranulation [6]. Blisters of PCT and similar clinical phenotypes present as cell-poor subepidermal bullae (Fig. 10.6a,b) with projection of dermal papillae into the blister cavity, also referred to as "festooning" (Fig. 10.7). These prominent dermal papillae results from periodic acid Schiff (PAS)-positive eosinophilic material, mostly representing reduplicated basal lamina, in and around small vessels in the upper dermis (Fig. 10.8a,b). This vessel wall thickening can be seen in biopsies of non-blistered skin as well (Fig. 10.8c). Elongated and segmented eosinophilic PAS-positive material attached to the roof of the blister has been referred to as "caterpillar bodies." (Fig. 10.9a,b) These are also positive for type IV collagen. These have been found to be a specific feature of PCT, with a specificity of 98%, but present in less than half of cases, with a sensitivity of 43% [14].

The dermis often shows solar elastosis. Classically, there is no or very sparse inflammation, and hemorrhage may be seen. In severe cases of cutaneous porphyrias, such as CEP, the perivascular deposits are extensive in the papillary dermis, and coalesce with those of adjoining capillaries. The deposits form thick cuffs around the vessels, narrowing their lumens. The changes may simulate amyloid, but the deposits are negative for Congo red. Biopsies of EPP show vacuolization of epidermal keratinocytes, and similar changes in the endothelial cells may be associated with lysis of these cells. In EPP, there is also massive deposition of PAS positive homogeneous perivascular material in addition to concentric reduplicated basal lamina, which corresponds on electron microscopy to homogenous and electron dense material, distinct from basal lamina [15]. Immunohistochemistry demonstrates collagen IV and laminin in the basal membrane of the vessels. In EPP, serum amyloid P protein, and kappa and lambda light chains have been demonstrated in the amorphous material. These amorphous deposits help to distinguish EPP from VP and PCT [15].

Direct immunofluorescence (DIF) demonstrates IgG in the thickened vessels. This vascular staining pattern is thick and donut-like around the vessels (Fig. 10.10). Using immunofluorescence mapping, type IV collagen and laminin can be demonstrated at the dermoepidermal junction in the floor of the bulla in PCT. The findings are identical in porphyria and pseudoporphyria.

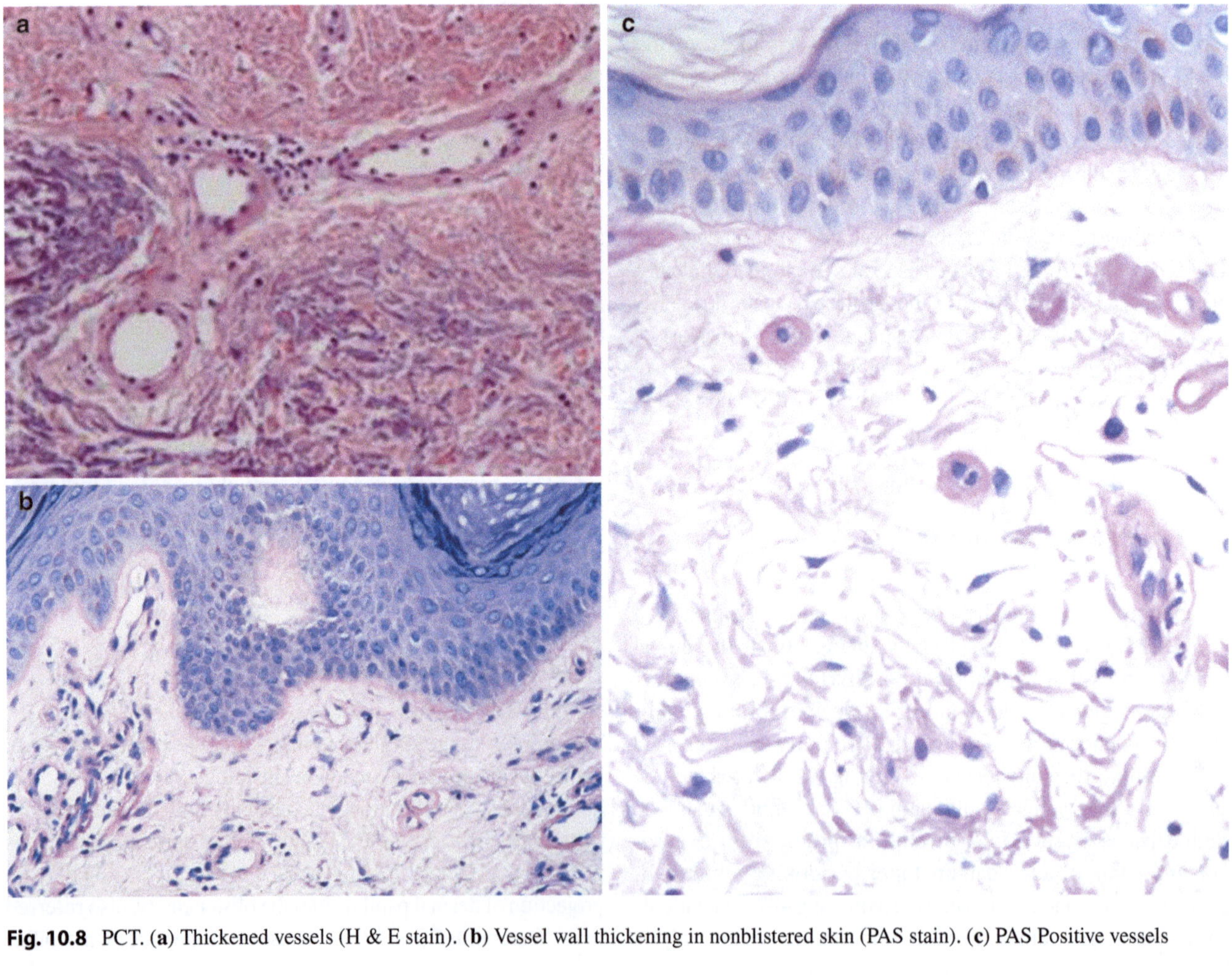

Fig. 10.8 PCT. (**a**) Thickened vessels (H & E stain). (**b**) Vessel wall thickening in nonblistered skin (PAS stain). (**c**) PAS Positive vessels

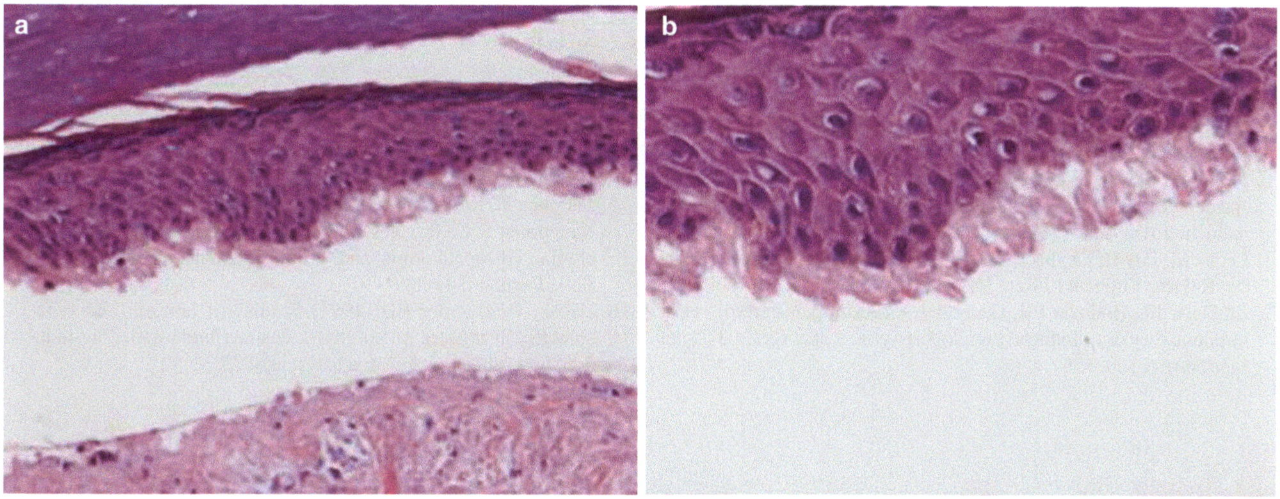

Fig. 10.9 PCT. (a) Caterpillar bodies. (b) Close-up of caterpillar bodies

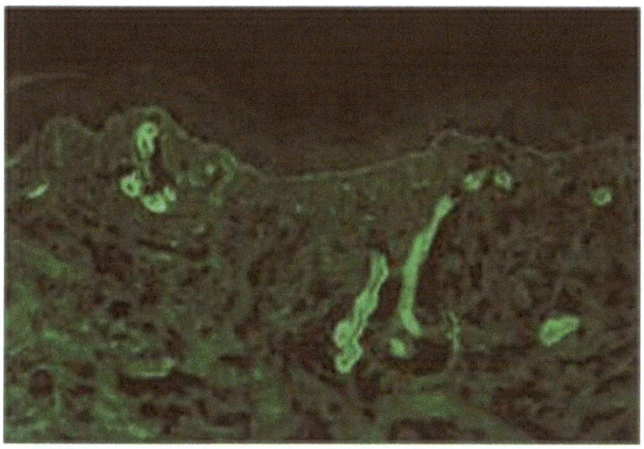

Fig. 10.10 PCT. Direct immunofluorescence showing vascular staining pattern

10.3 Treatment and Prognosis

The prognosis depends on the subtype of porphyria. CEP and EPP have the worst prognoses of the cutaneous porphyrias. CEP has a severe clinical course fraught with mutilating skin and cartilaginous changes and hemolytic anemia. EPP patients are at risk of fatal liver disease and cirrhosis. Patients with PCT and many of the other porphyrias are at risk of developing hepatocellular carcinoma; thus, they should be monitored with liver function tests.

The mainstay in management in all of the porphyrias is strict photoprotection, including protective clothing and use of opaque sunblockers, and avoidance of the triggers such as alcohol ingestion, estrogens, iron overload, polychlorinated hydrocarbons, and various medications, such as sulfonamides, calcium channel blockers, anti seizure medications, diclonfenac, rifampin.

In patients with PCT, phlebotomy and antimalarials are additional common treatment options [3, 6]. These treatments are not helpful in the PCT-like manifestations seen in VP and HCP. In patients with PCT related to hepatitis virus C, treatment of the hepatitis with interferon-α and ribavirin may improve PCT. In patients with PCT and AIDS, improvement of PCT has been reported following treatment with antiretroviral agents.

For patients with EPP, the immediate symptoms may be relieved with cold compresses applied to the affected area. Beta-carotene may be helpful [6].

Patients with drug-induced pseudoporphyria clear within a few weeks of discontinuing the offending medication; however, this response may be delayed for several months in the pediatric population [12].

References

1. Thunell S, Harper P (2000) Porphyrins, porphyrin metabolism and porphyrias. I. Update. Scand J Clin Lab Invest 60:561–580
2. Thunell S, Harper P, Brun A (2000) Porphyrins, porphyrin metabolism and porphyrias. IV. Pathophysiology of erythropoietic protoporphyria – diagnosis, care and monitoring of the patient. Scand J Clin Lab Invest 60:581–604
3. Poblete-Gutiérrez P, Wiederholt T, Merk HF, Frank J (2006) The porphyrias: Clinical presentation, diagnosis and treatment. Eur J Dermatol 16:230–240
4. Foran ST, Ábel G (2003) Guide to porphyrias. A historical and clinical perspective. Am J Clin Pathol 119(Suppl 1):S86–S93
5. Mascaro JM (1995) The porphyrias: A brief overview based on 25 years of experience (1969-1994) by the department of dermatology of the hospital clinic and faculty of medicine of Barcelona, Spain. J Dermatol 22:823–828
6. Lim HW, Cohen JL (1999) The cutaneous porphyrias. Semin Cutan Med Surg 118:285–292
7. Thunell S, Harper P, Brock A, Petersen NE (2000) Porphyrins, porphyrin metabolism and porphyrias. II. Diagnosis and monitoring in the acute porphyrias. Scand J Clin Lab Invest 60:541–560

8. Sarkany RP (2008) Making sense of the porphyrias. Photodermatol Photoimmunol Photomed 24:102–108
9. Thunell S (2000) Porphyrins, porphyrin metabolism and porphyrias. III. Diagnosis, care and monitorying in porphyria cutanea tarda – suggestions for a handling programme. Scand J Clin Lab Invest 60:509–540
10. Mehrany K, Drage LA, Brandhagen DJ, Pittelkow MR (2004) Association of porphyria cutanea tarda with hereditary hemochromatosis. J Am Acad Dermatol 51:205–211
11. Lecha M, Puy H, Deyback J-C (2009) Erythropoietic protoporphyria. Review. Orphanet J Rare Dis 4:19
12. La Duca JR, Bouman PH, Gasperi AA (2002) Nonsteroidal anti-inflammatory drug-induced pseudoporphyria: a case series. J Cutan Med Surg 6:320–326
13. Papadopoulos AJ, Schwartz RA, Fekete Z, Kihiczak G, Samady JA, Atkin SH, Lambert WC (2001) Pseudoporphyria: An atypical variant resembling toxic epidermal necrolysis. J Cutan Med Surg 5:479–485
14. Fung MA, Murphy MJ, Hoss DM, Berke A, Grant-Kels JM (2003) The sensitivity and specificity of "caterpillar bodies" in the differential diagnosis of subepidermal blistering disorders. Am J Dermatopathol 25:287–290
15. Timonen K, Kariniemi A-L, Niemi K-M, Teppo A-M, Tenhunen R, Kauppinen R (2000) Vascular changes in erythropoietic protoporphyria: Histopathologic and Immunohistochemical study. J Am Acad Dermatol 43:489–497
16. Dabski C, Beutner EH (1991) Studies of laminin and type IV collagen in blisters of porphyria cutanea tarda and drug-induced pseudoporphyria. J Am Acad Dermatol 25:28–32

Chapter 11
Hemochromatosis

Aurora Parodi and Franco Rongioletti

Key Points

- Hemochromatosis is an iron-overload syndrome that includes a hereditary and an acquired form
- The main cutaneous manifestations are a brownish bronze to slate gray hyperpigmentation due to hemosiderin deposition, hair loss most commonly involving the pubic region, koilonychias, icthyosiform alterations, and generalized pruritus
- Hyperpigmentation is a very important diagnostic sign, as early treatment with phlebotomy and chelating agents improve the prognosis significantly and even reverses the systemic and skin manifestations

Keywords Hereditary hemochromatosis • Acquired hemochromatosis • Iron-overload syndrome • Skin hyperpigmentation

11.1 Introduction

Iron-overload disorders are characterized by an excessive accumulation of iron in various organs. This condition can develop either from a genetic defect in the regulation of intestinal iron absorption (hereditary hemochromatosis) or from a consequence of transfusional, parenteral, or dietary iron overload (acquired or secondary hemochromatosis) [1, 2].

11.2 Clinical and Pathological Aspects of Skin Manifestations

Hereditary hemochromatosis (HH) is usually inherited in an autosomal recessive manner and is most prevalent in white individuals of European descent. It is characterized by a genetic predisposition to an increased absorption of enteral iron with a consequent increased iron level in the blood [3]. Transferrin saturation and ferritin concentration are raised. Five major categories are considered: HFE-related or type1 hemochromatosis (adult hemochromatosis), which is the most important one, and four rarer diseases which are type 2 (A and B) hemochromatosis (juvenile hemochromatosis), type 3 hemochromatosis (transferrin receptor 2 hemochromatosis), type 4 (A and B) hemochromatosis (ferroportin disease), and a (hypo)ceruloplasminemia. Adult HH type 1 results from a biallele mutation in the gene HFE that encodes an atypical MHC class I protein. The symptoms begin in the fourth or fifth decades of life after sufficient iron storage. The majority of these patients carry a unique missense mutation (C282Y) that alters the protein designated HFE. A liver disease with hyperaminotransferasemia (45–75%) and hepatic iron overload (25–50%), cardiac disease, and endocrine disease with diabetes mellitus (30–65%), loss of libido, amenorrhea, and impotence are typical systemic symptoms. Adult HH is more severe in men since menstruation and pregnancies usually reduce the iron overload in premenopausal women. Hemochromatosis may cause cardiovascular, rheumatological, and psychiatric symptoms including depression, disorientation, or memory problems. Heavy alcohol consumption accentuates the clinical expression of hemochromatosis [4, 5]. Ernest Hemingway, who was known to be a heavy drinker, is reported to have developed hemochromatosis in the years prior to his suicide [6].

The main skin manifestation includes a brownish bronze to slate gray *hyperpigmentation* secondary to hemosiderin deposition, seen in more than 90% of patients. In pigmented skin, the discoloration is brown to black. It is one of the earliest sign of the disease and is more pronounced on sun-exposed skin, particularly on the face (Fig. 11.1) and the hands (Fig. 11.2). External genital pigmentation is seen in one third of patients, while hyperpigmentation of flexural folds, scars, and nipple areolas are present in one fifth of cases. Hyperpigmentation often increases during exacerbations and regresses with therapy [3, 7]. Generalized pruritus is a rare presenting sign [8].

A. Parodi (✉)
Clinica Dermatologica, University of Genova,
Viale Benedetto XV, 7, Genova, Italy
e-mail: aurora.parodi@unige.it

F. Rongioletti and B.R. Smoller (eds.), *Clinical and Pathological Aspects of Skin Diseases in Endocrine, Metabolic, Nutritional and Deposition Disease*, DOI 10.1007/978-1-60761-181-3_11,

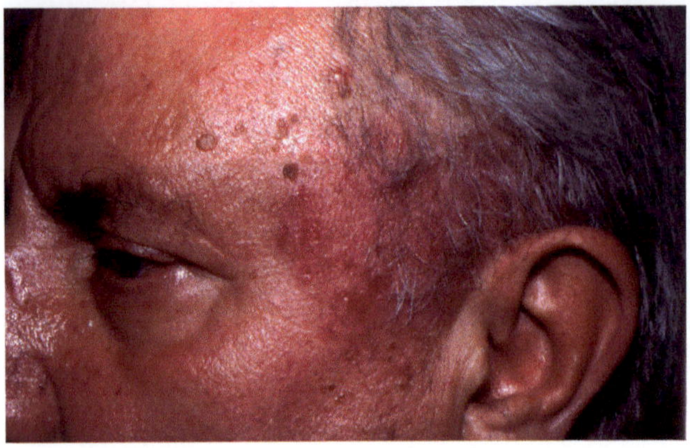

Fig. 11.1 Diffuse skin hyperpigmentation in a patient with hemochromatosis

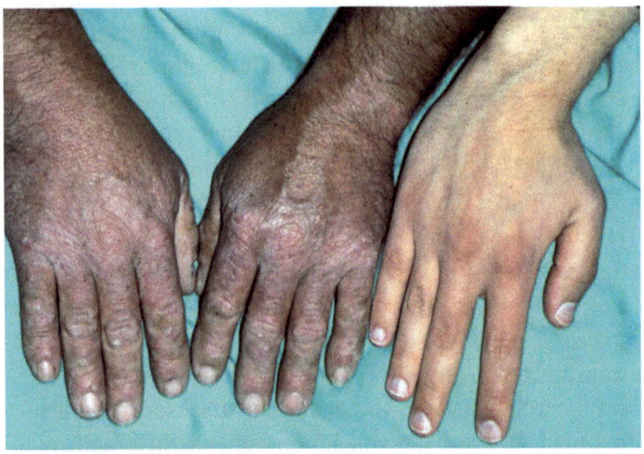

Fig. 11.2 Hyperpigmentation of the hands in hemochromatosis compared with normal hand (courtesy of Kenneth E. Greer, Charlottesville, VA, USA)

Histopathology shows increased melanin within the epidermal basal layers and papillary dermal macrophages containing hemosiderin around the blood vessels (Fig. 11.3) and within the basement membrane zone of sweat glands and the connective tissue cells surrounding them. An iron stain, such as Perl's stain, is used to detect deposits of hemosiderin, which stain as blue-green granules (Fig. 11.4). Siderosis around eccrine glands may be specific for idiopathic hemochromatosis. Skin biopsy should not be performed on the legs because iron deposition in that area may be due to venous stasis.

The cutaneous hyperpigmentation in patients with HH should be differentiated from drug-induced hyperpigmentation (see also Chap. 22), actinic reticuloid, Addison disease (see also Chap. 1), argyria, and postinflammatory hyperpigmentation.

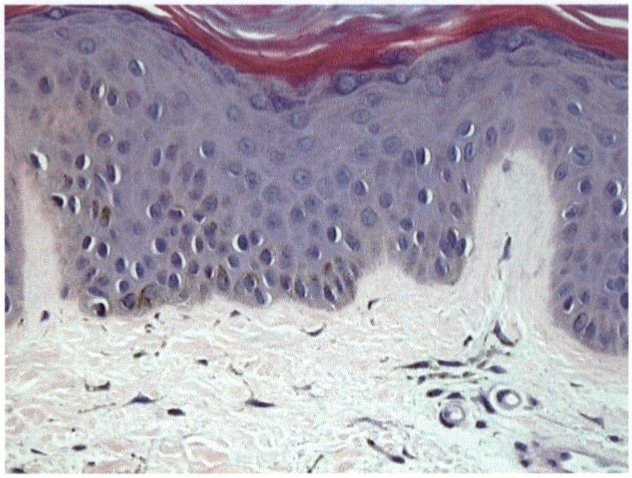

Fig. 11.3 Histopathology of HH shows increased melanin within the epidermal basal layers, and papillary dermal macrophages containing hemosiderin around the blood vessels

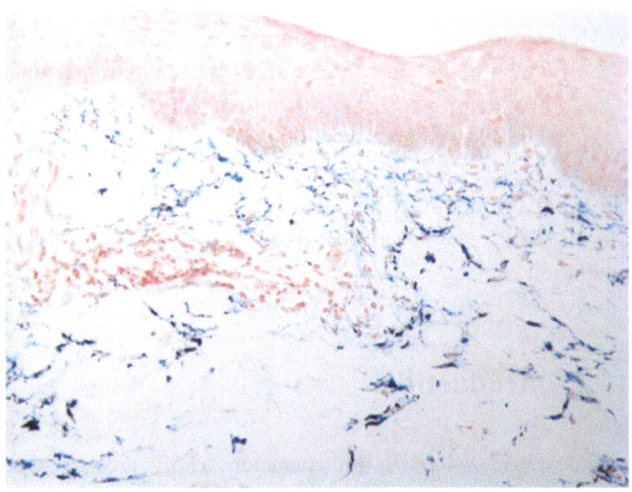

Fig. 11.4 Iron dermal deposition in hemochromatosis (Perl's stain)

Other symptoms of HH are skin atrophy on the anterior surface of the legs (40%), hair loss (62%) most commonly involving the pubic region, koilonychias (50%), icthyosiform alterations (46%), and generalized pruritus resistant to antihistamine treatment. HH can be associated with porphyria cutanea tarda. This may cause fragility and blistering of the skin, especially on the backs of the hands.

Secondary iron-overload syndromes also called *acquired hemochromatosis* occur as a long-term complication of repeated blood transfusions in the context of thalassemia major in children or in myelodysplastic syndromes and leukemias. Hyperpigmentation and pruritus are the most frequent skin symptoms.

11.3 Treatment and Prognosis

When diagnosis is made before organ damage occurs, treatment can prevent manifestations of the disease. Skin pigmentation and some cardiac damage may reverse on depletion of iron stores, but liver and endocrine damage are rarely reversible [9]. Phlebotomy is the treatment of choice for HH and should be started when ferritin levels reach 300 mcg/L in men or 200 in nonpregnant premenopausal woman. It is usually done at weekly intervals until ferritin is reduced below 50 mcg/L. In the maintenance phase, one to six venisections per year are usually needed to maintain adequate iron balance. The frequency is determined by the level of ferritin, which should be lower than 50 mcg/mL [10]. Limiting intake of alcohol, vitamin C (that increases iron absorption in the gut), and red meat is recommended. Increasing intake of substances that inhibit iron absorption such as tea, foods containing oxalic and phytic acids (for example spinach) and calcium are also helpful.

References

1. Andrews NC (1999) Disorders of iron metabolism. N Engl J Med 341:1986–1995
2. Roy CN, Andrews NC (2001) Recent advances in disorders of iron metabolism: mutations, mechanisms and modifiers. Hum Mol Gen 10:2181–2186
3. Alexander J, Kowdley KV (2009) HFE-associated hereditary hemochromatosis. Genet Med 11:307–313
4. Fletcher LM, Powell LW (2003) Hemochromatosis and alcohol liver disease. Alcohol 30:131–136
5. Holder GL (2000) Psychiatric symptoms of hemochromatosis in alcohol dependence. Psychiatr Prax 27:204, Article in German
6. Wagner-Martin L (1998) Ernest Hemingway: seven decades of criticism. Michigan State University Press, East Lansing, MI
7. Chevrant-Breton J, Simon M, Bourel M, Ferrand B (1977) Cutaneous manifestations of idiopathic hemochromatosis. Study of 100 cases. Arch Dermatol 113:161–165
8. Kluger N, Raison-Peyron N, Rigole H, Bessis D, Blanc F, Guillot B (2007) Generalized pruritus revealing hereditary haemochromatosis. Acta Derm Venereol 87:277
9. Angelucci E, Cogoni C, Pettinau M, Pilo F, Targhetta C, Zacchedu F (2008) Organ damage and iron overload. Hematol Meet Rep 2:3–5
10. Brissot P, Troadec MB, Bardou-Jacquet E, Le Lan C, Jouanolle AM, Deugnier Y et al (2008) Current approach to hemochromatosis. Blood Rev 22:195–210

Chapter 12
Metabolic Syndrome in Psoriasis

Paolo Gisondi and Giampiero Girolomoni

Key Points

- Chronic plaque psoriasis is frequently associated with cardio-metabolic disorders including myocardial infarction, stroke, hypertension, diabetes, obesity, dyslipidaemia, metabolic syndrome and non-alcoholic fatty liver disease.
- Common genetic traits, unhealthy lifestyle behaviours as well as common inflammatory mechanisms, such as elevated levels of multifunctional cytokines (i.e. IL-6, TNF-α) may underlie the development of psoriasis and cardio-metabolic comorbidities.
- The metabolic syndrome is a constellation of metabolic changes which collectively confer an inflammatory and pro-thrombotic state and is significantly more common in psoriatic patients than in the general population after the age of 40 years.
- Patients with moderate to severe psoriasis should be treated promptly and effectively and should also be encouraged to drastically correct their modifiable cardio-vascular risk factors, in particular, obesity and smoking habit.

Keywords Chronic plaque psoriasis • Co-morbidities • Psoriatic arthritis

12.1 Introduction

Psoriasis is a chronic inflammatory, immune-mediated skin disease, which affects 2–3% of the general population [1]. Recent evidence indicates that psoriasis and psoriatic arthritis are frequently associated with cardio-metabolic diseases including myocardial infarction, stroke, hypertension, diabetes, obesity, dyslipidaemia, metabolic syndrome, and non-alcoholic fatty liver disease [2–10]. The association between psoriasis and comorbidities is complex as the contributing mechanisms are largely unknown. Some common genetic traits as well as common inflammatory mechanisms, in particular, elevated levels of multifunctional cytokines such as TNF-α and IL-6, may underlie the development of psoriasis and cardiometabolic co-morbidities. In addition, one could speculate that impaired psoriasis-related quality of life may lead to unhealthy lifestyle behaviours such as smoking, alcohol consumption, decreased physical activity, and obesity, which are independent risk factors for cardiovascular diseases [11–13]. The presence of co-morbidities has important implications in the global approach to patients with psoriasis. Traditional systemic anti-psoriatic agents could negatively affect cardiometabolic co-morbidities and may have important interactions with drugs commonly used by psoriasis patients. In contrast, the recent findings that the risk of myocardial infarction is markedly reduced in rheumatoid arthritis patients who respond to anti-TNF-α therapy compared with non-responders support the hypothesis that the anti-inflammatory effect of TNF-α blockers might reduce the cardiovascular risk potentially, also in psoriasis patients [14]. Finally, patients with moderate to severe psoriasis should be treated promptly and effectively and should also be encouraged to drastically correct their modifiable cardio-vascular risk factors, in particular, obesity and smoking habit.

12.2 Clinical and Pathological Aspects of Metabolic Syndrome in Psoriasis

The metabolic syndrome is a constellation of metabolic changes, the most important of which is the insulin resistance, which confers a higher pro-inflammatory and pro-thrombotic risk [15]. The most widely accepted criteria for metabolic syndrome definition are issued by the Adult Treatment Panel III, which defines it as the presence of at least three of the following conditions: abdominal obesity [waist circumference >102 cm (40 in.) men; >88 cm (35 in.) women], elevated serum triglycerides [>150 mg/dl (1.7 mmol/l) or under treatment], low HDL cholesterol [men <40 mg/dl (1 mmol/l); women <50 mg/dl (1.3 mmol/l) or

G. Girolomoni (✉)
Department of Medicine, Section of Dermatology and Venereology, University of Verona, Piazzale Aristide Stefani 1, 37126 Verona, Italy
e-mail: giampiero.girolomoni@univr.it

F. Rongioletti and B.R. Smoller (eds.), *Clinical and Pathological Aspects of Skin Diseases in Endocrine, Metabolic, Nutritional and Deposition Disease*, DOI 10.1007/978-1-60761-181-3_12,

under treatment], elevated blood pressure (>130/85 mmHg or under treatment), and an elevated fasting glucose (>110 mg/dl or under treatment) [16]. Metabolic syndrome is significantly found to be more common in psoriatic patients than in controls (30.1% vs. 20.6%) after the age of 40 years. Psoriatic patients also had a higher prevalence of hypertriglyceridaemia and abdominal obesity, whereas hyperglycaemia, arterial hypertension, and high-density lipoprotein cholesterol plasma levels were similar [17]. Although psoriasis patients were more frequently smokers, the association of psoriasis with metabolic syndrome was independent of smoking.

There was no correlation between severity of psoriasis and prevalence of metabolic syndrome. However, psoriatic patients with metabolic syndrome are usually older and have a longer disease duration compared with psoriatic patients without metabolic syndrome. When looking at individual components of the metabolic syndrome, only hypertriglyceridaemia and abdominal obesity were more significantly prevalent in patients with psoriasis than in controls (Fig. 12.1). In a German study, hospitalised psoriasis patients were found to have increased prevalence of metabolic syndrome compared with hospitalised melanoma patients [18].

Non-alcoholic fatty liver disease (NAFLD) is now regarded as the hepatic manifestation of the metabolic syndrome, as it is largely dependent on the underlying insulin resistance state. NAFLD includes a spectrum of conditions ranging from simple fatty liver, which is relatively benign, to non-alcoholic steato-hepatitis (NASH), which can give rise to cirrhosis. Considering that metabolic syndrome is associated with both psoriasis and NAFLD, it is likely that both entities could coexist in the same patients. Indeed, the frequency of NAFLD in patients with psoriasis is found remarkably greater than that in controls (47% vs. 28%; $p<0.0001$) [19]. Moreover, NAFLD is associated with the severity of psoriasis, independent of potential confounders such as age, gender, BMI, psoriasis duration, and alcohol consumption. NAFLD was unrelated to psoriasis severity, but logistic regression analysis revealed that psoriatic patients with NAFLD are much more likely to have psoriatic arthritis (Fig. 12.2). Interestingly, psoriatic patients with NAFLD also had a significantly higher mean AST/ALT ratio and a higher non-invasive fibrosis scores compared with controls with NAFLD not associated to psoriasis.

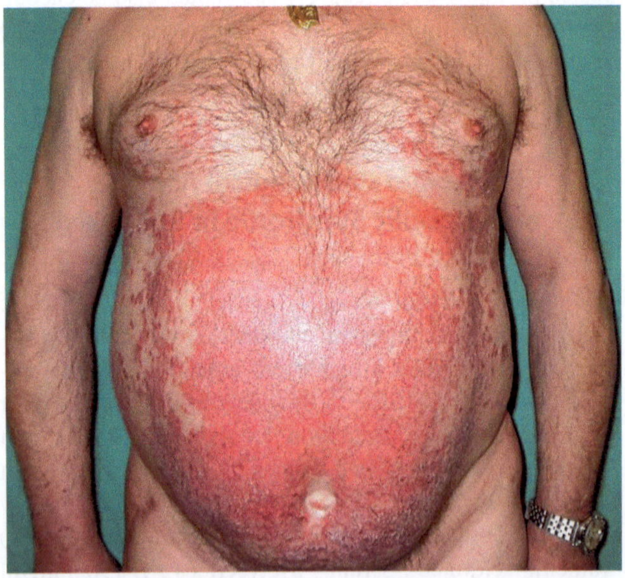

Fig. 12.1 Abdominal obesity in a patient with psoriasis and metabolic syndrome

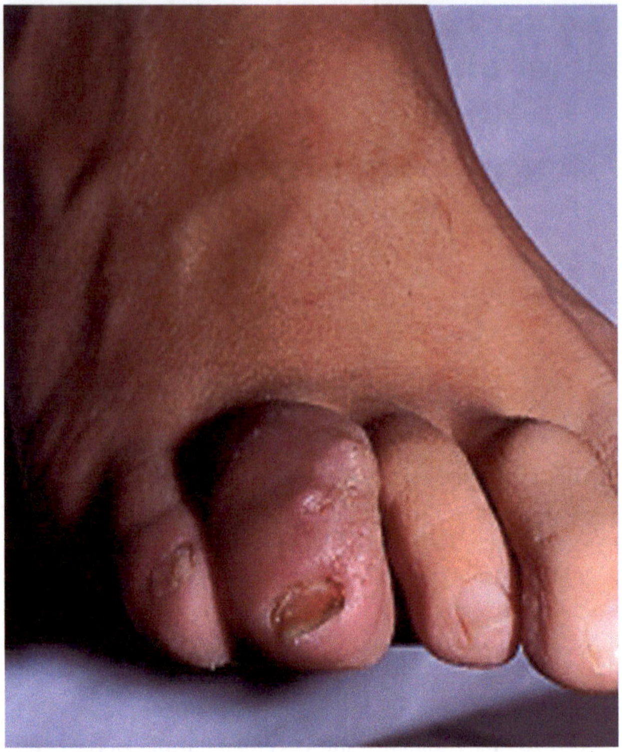

Fig. 12.2 Psoriatic dactylitis in a patient with metabolic syndrome

Histopathologically, there does not seem to be any differences between psoriasis in patients with metabolic syndrome (Fig. 12.3) and psoriasis vulgaris in patients without metabolic syndrome; however, no specific studies have been published on this topic.

12.3 Treatment and Prognosis

Systemic treatments for psoriasis including methotrexate, cyclosporine, retinoids, and biologics may contribute either to reduce or to increase the cardiovascular risk. Indeed, it has been reported that American veterans affected by psoriasis, psoriatic arthritis, and rheumatoid arthritis treated with moderate doses of methotrexate have a reduced risk for major

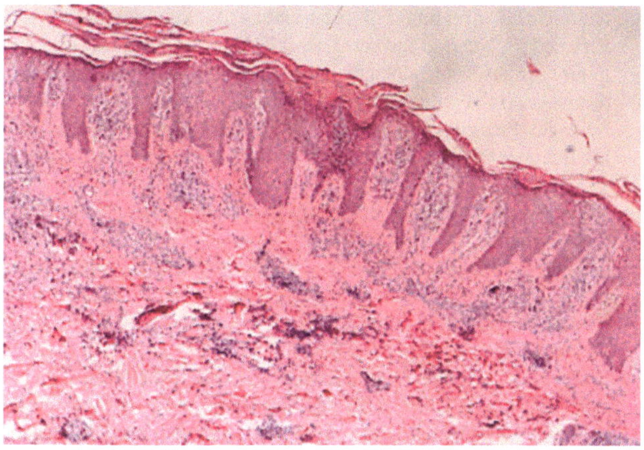

Fig. 12.3 Typical histological features in a psoriatic patient with metabolic syndrome with parakeratosis, reduced granular layer, regular acanthosis, vascular dilatation with superficial perivascular infiltrate

cardiovascular events compared to non-treated patients [20]. This effect is possibly attributable to the anti-inflammatory effects of the drug. On the other hand, methotrexate use can induce hyperhomocysteinaemia, which is an established risk factor for both arterial and venous thrombosis. Moreover, methotrexate should be chosen with caution in cases of overweight patients, high alcohol consumption, diabetes mellitus, or viral hepatitis due to the increased risk of developing liver fibrosis [21]. The presence of fatty liver, which is highly prevalent in patients with psoriasis, should be taken into consideration when choosing therapy, as acitretin and methotrexate are potentially hepato-toxic and consequently could favour the progression from simple steatosis to fibrosis and even cirrhosis. Concerning cyclosporine, the drug can induce or worsen arterial hypertension, alter glucose tolerance, and/or interfere with fatty acid metabolism favouring hyperlipaemia [22]. Pharmacological treatment of dyslipidaemia in psoriasis patients needs attention as statins could favour myolysis when associated with cyclosporine or retinoids. Also, retinoids may increase serum cholesterol and triglycerides [23]. The occurrence of hypertriglyceridaemia and hypercholesterolaemia has been occasionally reported also in patients treated with anti-TNF-α agents, as well as increment of liver transaminases, whereas a true hepatitis has been a more rare but established event [24–26]. In addition, anti-TNF-α agents may increase body weight in patients with psoriasis and Crohn's disease [27–29].

Lifestyle modifications, including a low-calorie diet, may supplement the pharmacological treatment of obese psoriasis patients. Indeed, a moderate weight loss (i.e. 5–10% of body weight) increases the responsiveness of obese patients with moderate to severe chronic plaque psoriasis to low doses cyclosporine [30]. Weight loss through calorie restriction decreases insulin, leptin, C-reactive protein, and MCP-1 levels, and increases adiponectin levels resulting in an anti-inflammatory effect.

Although controversy still exists, the recent findings that the risk of myocardial infarction is markedly reduced at 6 months in rheumatoid arthritis patients who respond to anti-TNF-α therapy compared with non-responders support the hypothesis that anti-inflammatory effect of TNF-α blockers might improve the cardiovascular risk [31]. In particular, anti-TNF-α treatment has been shown to improve endothelial function, as well as reduce C-reactive protein serum levels in patients with rheumatoid arthritis [32]. Whether this effect could be present and relevant in reducing thrombotic events also in psoriasis patients need to be investigated.

References

1. Griffiths CE, Barker JN (2007) Pathogenesis and clinical features of psoriasis. Lancet 370:263–271
2. Gelfand JM, Neimann AL, Shin DB, Wang X, Margolis DJ, Troxel AB (2006) Risk of myocardial infarction in patients with psoriasis. JAMA 296:1735–1741
3. Gelfand JM, Dommasch ED, Shin DB, Azfar RS, Kurd SK, Wang X et al (2009) The risk of stroke in patients with psoriasis. J Invest Dermatol 129(10):2411–2418
4. Ludwig RJ, Herzog C, Rostock A, Ochsendorf FR, Zollner TM, Thaci D et al (2007) Psoriasis: a possible risk factor for development of coronary artery calcification. Br J Dermatol 156:271–276
5. Gisondi P, Fantin F, Del Giglio M, Valbusa F, Marino F, Zamboni M et al (2009) Chronic plaque psoriasis is associated with increased arterial stiffness. Dermatology 218:110–113
6. Ucak S, Ekmekci TR, Basat O, Koslu A, Altuntas Y (2006) Comparison of various insulin sensitivity indices in psoriatic patients and their relationship with type of psoriasis. J Eur Acad Dermatol Venereol 20:517–522
7. Kaye JA, Li L, Jick SS (2008) Incidence of risk factors for myocardial infarction and other vascular diseases in patients with psoriasis. Br J Dermatol 159:895–902
8. Cohen AD, Dreiher J, Shapiro Y, Vidavsky L, Vardy DA, Davidovici B et al (2008) Psoriasis and diabetes: a population-based cross-sectional study. J Eur Acad Dermatol Venereol 22:585–589
9. Wakkee M, Thio HB, Prens EP, Sijbrands EJ, Neumann HA (2007) Unfavorable cardiovascular risk profiles in untreated and treated psoriasis patients. Atherosclerosis 190:1–9
10. Naldi L, Chatenoud L, Linder D (2005) Belloni Fortina A, Peserico A, Virgili AR, et al. Cigarette smoking, body mass index, and stressful life events as risk factors for psoriasis: results from an Italian case-control study. J Invest Dermatol 125:61–67
11. Setty AR, Curhan G, Choi HK (2007) Obesity, waist circumference, weight change, and the risk of psoriasis in women: Nurses' Health Study II. Arch Intern Med 167:1670–1675
12. Després JP, Lemieux I, Bergeron J et al (2008) Abdominal obesity and the metabolic syndrome: contribution to global cardiometabolic risk. Arterioscler Thromb Vasc Biol 28:1039–1049
13. Gisondi P, Girolomoni G (2009) Psoriasis and atherothrombotic diseases: disease-specific and non-disease-specific risk factors. Semin Thromb Hemost 35:313–324
14. Dixon WG, Watson KD, Lunt M, Hyrich KL (2007) Reduction in the incidence of myocardial infarction in patients with rheumatoid arthritis who respond to anti-tumor necrosis factor alpha therapy: results from the British Society for Rheumatology Biologics Register. Arthritis Rheum 56:2905–2912

15. Grundy SM, Brewer HB Jr, Cleeman JI, Smith SC Jr, Lenfant C, American Heart Association; National Heart, Lung, and Blood Institute (2004) Definition of metabolic syndrome: Report of the National Heart, Lung, and Blood Institute/American Heart Association conference on scientific issues related to definition. Circulation 109:433–438
16. National Institute of Health (2001) Third report of the national Cholesterol Education Program Export Panel on detection, evaluation, and treatment of high blood cholesterol in adults (Adult Treatment Panel III). Executive Summary, National Institute of Health, National Hearth, Lung and Blood Institute, Bethesda, MD (NIH publ no 01-3670)
17. Gisondi P, Tessari G, Conti A, Piaserico S, Schianchi S, Peserico A et al (2007) Prevalence of metabolic syndrome in patients with psoriasis: a hospital-based case-control study. Br J Dermatol 157:68–73
18. Sommer DM, Jenisch S, Suchan M, Christophers E, Weichenthal M (2006) Increased prevalence of the metabolic syndrome in patients with moderate to severe psoriasis. Arch Dermatol Res 298:321–328
19. Gisondi P, Targher G, Zoppini G, Girolomoni G (2009) Non-alcoholic fatty liver disease in patients with chronic plaque psoriasis. J Hepatol 51:758–764
20. Prodanovich S, Ma F, Taylor JR, Pezon C, Fasihi T, Kirsner RS (2005) Methotrexate reduces incidence of vascular diseases in veterans with psoriasis or rheumatoid arthritis. J Am Acad Dermatol 52:262–267
21. Rosenberg P, Urwitz H, Johannesson A, Ros AM, Lindholm J, Kinnman N et al (2007) Psoriasis patients with diabetes type 2 are at high risk of developing liver fibrosis during methotrexate treatment. J Hepatol 46:1111–1118
22. Menter A, Korman NJ, Elmets CA, Feldman SR, Gelfand JM, Gordon KB et al (2009) Guidelines of care for the management of psoriasis and psoriatic arthritis: section 4. Guidelines of care for the management and treatment of psoriasis with traditional systemic agents. J Am Acad Dermatol 61:451–485
23. Vahlquist C, Olsson AG, Lindholm A, Vahlquist A (1995) Effects of gemfibrozil (Lopid) on hyperlipidemia in acitretin-treated patients. Results of a double-blind cross-over study. Acta Derm Venereol 75:377–380
24. Antoniou C, Dessinioti C, Katsambas A, Stratigos AJ (2007) Elevated triglyceride and cholesterol levels after intravenous antitumour necrosis factor-alpha therapy in a patient with psoriatic arthritis and psoriasis vulgaris. Br J Dermatol 156:1090–1091
25. Stinco G, Piccirillo F, Patrone P (2007) Hypertriglyceridaemia during treatment with adalimumab in psoriatic arthritis. Br J Dermatol 157:1273–1274
26. Dominique L (2008) Liver toxicity of TNFalpha antagonists. Joint Bone Spine 75:636–638
27. Gisondi P, Cotena C, Tessari G, Girolomoni G (2008) Anti-tumour necrosis factor-alpha therapy increases body weight in patients with chronic plaque psoriasis: a retrospective cohort study. J Eur Acad Dermatol Venereol 22:341–344
28. Saraceno R, Schipani C, Mazzotta A, Esposito M, Di Renzo L, De Lorenzo A et al (2008) Effect of anti-tumor necrosis factor-alpha therapies on body mass index in patients with psoriasis. Pharmacol Res 57:290–295
29. Franchimont D, Roland S, Gustot T, Quertinmont E, Toubouti Y, Gervy MC et al (2005) Impact of infliximab on serum leptin levels in patients with Crohn's disease. J Clin Endocrinol Metab 90:3510–3516
30. Gisondi P, Del Giglio M, Di Francesco V, Zamboni M, Girolomoni G (2008) Weight loss makes obese patients with moderate to severe chronic plaque psoriasis highly responsive to low dose cyclosporine: a randomized, controlled, investigator blinded, clinical trial. Am J Clin Nutr 88:1242–1247
31. Dixon WG, Watson KD, Lunt M, Hyrich KL, Silman AJ, Symmons D, British Society for Rheumatology Biologics Register Control Centre Consortium, British Society for Rheumatology Biologics Register (2007) Reduction in the incidence of myocardial infarction in patients with rheumatoid arthritis who respond to anti-tumor necrosis factor alpha therapy: results from the British Society for Rheumatology Biologics Register. Arthritis Rheum 56: 2905–2912
32. Bosello S, Santoliquido A, Zoli A, Di Campli C, Flore R, Tondi P et al (2008) TNF-alpha blockade induces a reversible but transient effect on endothelial dysfunction in patients with long-standing severe rheumatoid arthritis. Clin Rheumatol 27:833–839

Part III
Cutaneous Nutritional Disease

Chapter 13
Acquired Nutritional Deficiencies

Martina Montinari, Aurora Parodi, and Franco Rongioletti

Key Points

- Alcoholism, several gastrointestinal diseases, intestinal bypass procedures, psychiatric disturbances such as anorexia nervosa, restrictive diets, long-term tube feeding, and perceived or real food allergy may lead to acquired nutritional deficiency in developed nations.
- Cutaneous changes occur in deficiency states of many nutritional elements such as vitamin C, zinc, niacin, iron, retinol, protein-energy, vitamin B12, vitamin K, biotin, riboflavin, pyridoxine, essential fatty acids.
- Skin manifestations are the diagnostic clue in scurvy, acrodermatitis enteropathica, and pellagra.
- Although not strictly specific and pathognomonic, oral mucosal alterations such as glossitis and cheilitis associated with hair and nail changes are extremely common in iron and vitamin deficiencies.
- Nutritional supplementation induces complete regression of systemic and skin symptoms.

Keywords Scurvy • Acquired acrodermatitis enteropathica • Pellagra • Iron deficiency • Skin manifestations • Oral alterations

13.1 Introduction

Nutritional deficiencies are uncommon in developed nations. However, alcoholism, several gastrointestinal diseases (such as Crohn's disease or celiac disease), intestinal bypass procedures, psychiatric disturbances such as anorexia nervosa, restrictive diets, long-term tube feeding, and perceived or real food allergy may lead to lack or malabsorption of various micronutrients, proteins, and vitamins. The skin is commonly affected and may be the presenting sign of nutritional deficiency disorders, especially those caused by deficiency of vitamin C (scurvy), zinc (acrodermatitis enteropathica), and niacin (pellagra).

Iron deficiency is the result of inadequate absorption in conditions of poor availability, excessive antacid therapy, excess dietary bran, tannin, phytates or starch, competition from other metals, bowel resection, celiac disease, chronic inflammatory bowel diseases, intrinsic enterocyte defects, or is due to increased blood loss through the gastrointestinal tract, trauma, or large vascular malformations [1]. Iron deficiency is also present in chronic inflammatory diseases. In chronic diseases, iron is plentiful in bone marrow macrophages, but this iron is not available to erythroid precursors. New evidence suggests that the syndrome is the result of the body's production of hepcidin, a master regulator of human iron metabolism. Hepcidin is produced by the liver in response to inflammatory cytokines, in particular IL-6 [2]. When iron stores are depleted, the iron saturation of transferrin decreases and patients begin to show evidence of iron-deficient erythropoiesis with microcytic anemia.

13.2 Clinical and Pathological Aspects of Skin Manifestations

13.2.1 Scurvy

Scurvy occurs as a consequence of decreased vitamin C consumption or absorption. Though scurvy is a very rare disease, it still occurs in some patients such as elderly people, alcoholics, or those who live on a diet devoid of fresh fruits and vegetables, even in industrialized societies. Similarly, infants or children who are on special or poor diets for any economic or social reasons may be prone to scurvy. Historically, scurvy was the result of long sea voyages, where sailors did not bring along enough foods with vitamin C [3]. Vitamin C or ascorbic acid is a hydrosoluble vitamin derived from glucose metabolism [4]. It acts as a reducing agent required for synthesis of collagen fibers through hydroxyla-

F. Rongioletti (✉)
Department of Endocrinological and Medical Sciences (DISEM)
Section of Dermatology and Department of Pathology
University of Genova, Genova, Italy
e-mail: franco.rongioletti@unige.it

F. Rongioletti and B.R. Smoller (eds.), *Clinical and Pathological Aspects of Skin Diseases in Endocrine, Metabolic, Nutritional and Deposition Disease*, DOI 10.1007/978-1-60761-181-3_13,

tion of proline and lysine. Some tissues such as skin, gums, mucous membranes, and bones contain a greater concentration of collagen and thus are more susceptible to deficiencies. Ascorbic acid also protects the body against damage caused by the free radicals. Humans cannot synthesize ascorbic acid and can obtain daily requirements primarily from natural sources, such as citrus fruits and some vegetables. The current recommendation of daily intake of vitamin C is 90 mg/day for men and 75 mg/day for women. Patients with chronic diseases, such as cancer or diabetes, or those who smoke need higher doses in their usual diet. Clinical manifestations of scurvy can be seen within 8–12 weeks of irregular or inadequate intake.

Presentation varies by individual. Early stages are often characterized by malaise, appetite loss, poor weight gain, and diarrhea. One to 3 months of inadequate intake can lead to anemia with congestive heart failure, myalgias, bone pain with tenderness and discomfort in legs, easy bruising, swelling over long bones, rapid breathing, fever, and mood changes. As the disease progresses, symptoms become more severe and life threatening; common manifestations include generalized edema, severe jaundice, hemolysis, acute spontaneous bleeding, proptosis of the eyeball, costochondral beading, neuropathy, convulsions, and death.

Scurvy causes changes in the skin as a result of faulty collagen synthesis [3]. Classic changes on the legs and buttocks, where hydrostatic pressure is greatest, are *hyperkeratotic papules, corkscrew hairs, and perifollicular hemorrhages* (Fig. 13.1). Petechiae evolving into confluent plaques, into large ecchymoses and even hemorrhagic pseudovasculitis may occur on the lower legs due to blood-vessel fragility. The nails may develop splinter hemorrhages. *Alopecia* may occur as a result of defective disulfide bonding. Because of defective collagen production, wounds heal poorly and even old scars can break down. Sjögren-like symptoms have also been noted. Patients with scurvy also develop *oral complications*. The gums often bleed with minor trauma, becoming red, smooth, swollen, and shiny. Eventually, the gums may retreat or become necrotic. As alveolar bone absorption occurs, tooth loss may occur.

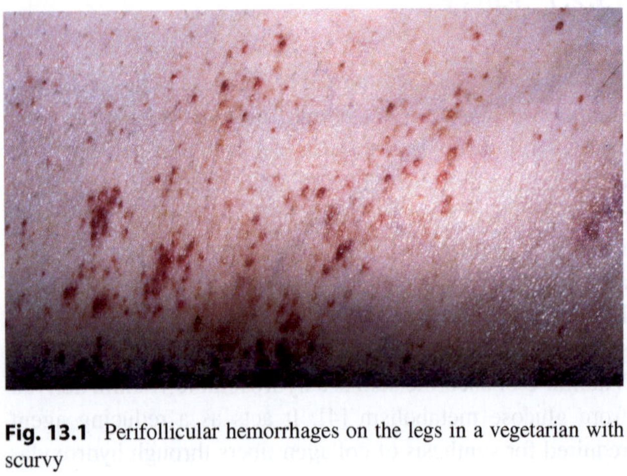

Fig. 13.1 Perifollicular hemorrhages on the legs in a vegetarian with scurvy

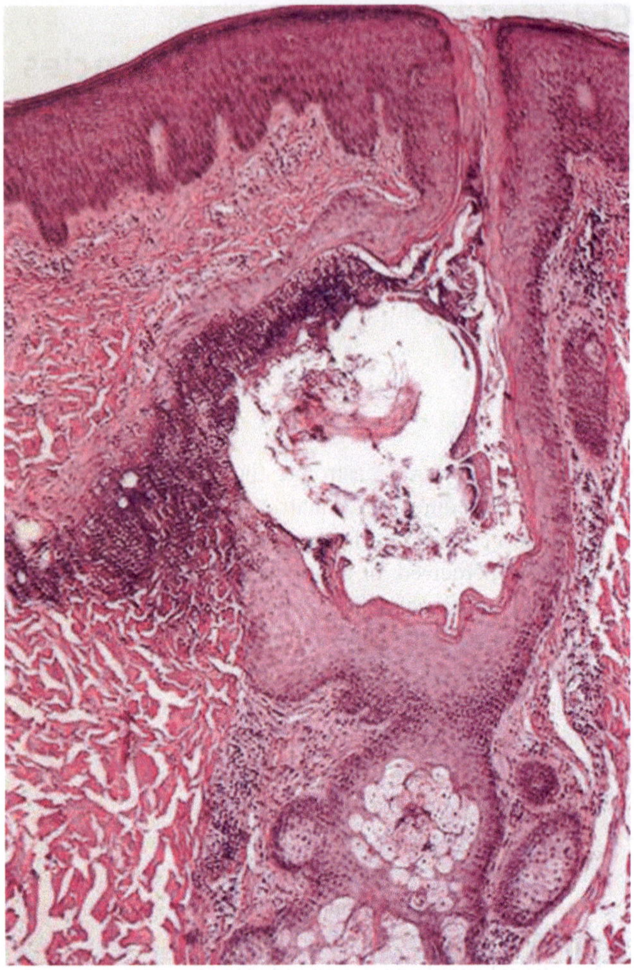

Fig. 13.2 Histopathology of a follicular lesion in scurvy showing dilatation and keratin plugging of the infundibular ostium (HE stain)

Biopsy of a follicular lesion typically shows dilatation and keratin plugging of the infundibular ostium and disruption of the hair follicle (Fig. 13.2). Biopsy of purpuric lesions shows extravasation of red cells in the perifollicular dermis with no vasculitis [5, 6].

13.2.2 Acquired Acrodermatitis Enteropathica (Dermatitis Associated with Zinc Deficiency)

Acrodermatitis enteropathica (AE) is a rare genetic or acquired disorder of hypozincemia caused by impaired intestinal absorption of zinc or by reduced consumption of the mineral [7]. Acquired AE has been reported in numerous conditions like anorexia nervosa, alcoholism, inflammatory bowel disease, total parenteral nutrition, defect of mammary zinc secretion (lactogenic AE), sprue, and other intestinal malabsorption syndromes.

Zinc is one of the most important trace elements vital to humans, playing a key role in the formation and maintenance of all tissues including the skin. It is present in nuts, whole grains, leafy vegetables and shellfish. Zinc deficiency manifests itself with the clinical triad of: (1) skin lesions with localization around the body orifices and on the extremities, (2) alopecia, and (3) diarrhea or other obscure gastrointestinal dysfunctions.

The skin lesions are characterized by *eczematous scaly plaques* (Figs. 13.3 and 13.4) which can develop into *vesicular, bullous* (Fig. 13.5), or *pustular lesions*. The lesions involve the extremities and periorificial areas, including the anogenital region (Fig. 13.6a, b). Secondary infection with bacteria and *Candida albicans* occurs. *Angular cheilitis* is a common early manifestation (Fig. 13.7) followed closely by *paronychia*. In the absence of treatment, skin lesions slowly evolve into erosions and patients develop generalized *alopecia* and diarrhea. Hair shafts have been reported to display alternating dark and bright bands on polarized light microscopy [8]. Patients with advanced disease also exhibit poor wound healing, anemia, photophobia, hypogeusia, anorexia, and hypogonadism [9].

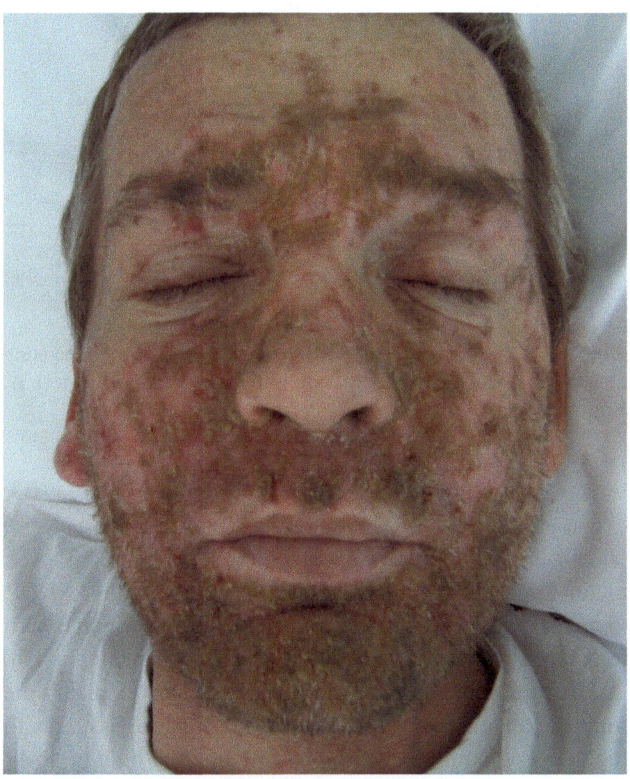

Fig. 13.3 Eczematous scaly plaques on the face in acrodermatitis enteropathica due to alcoholism

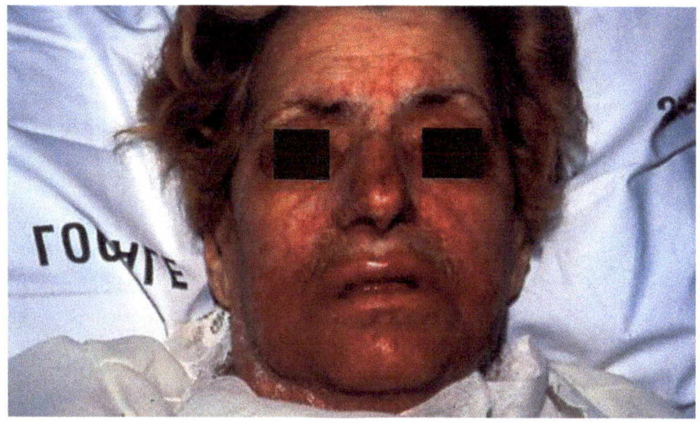

Fig. 13.4 Acrodermatitis enteropathica of the face due to severe long-standing inflammatory bowel disease. Note perioral involvement

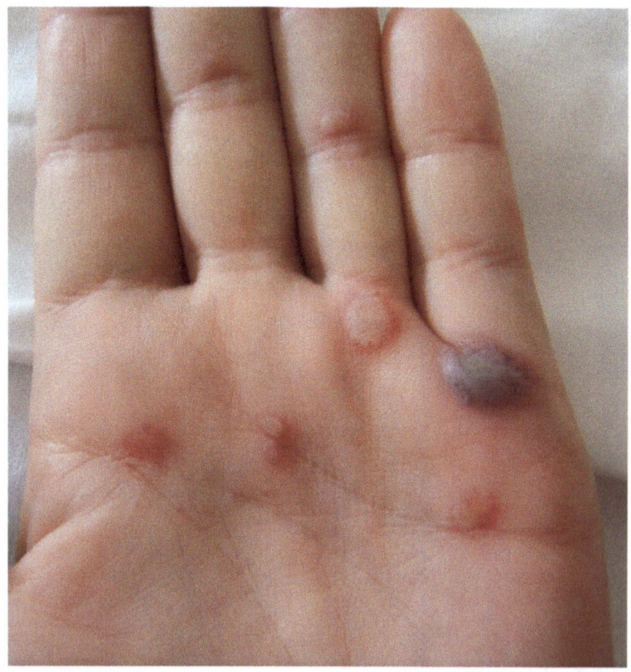

Fig. 13.5 Vesicular and bullous lesions in acrodermatitis enteropathica due to alcoholism

Chronic lesions of AE display a *psoriasiform* pattern with accompanying *nail dystrophy*, and the differential diagnosis with psoriasis is difficult.

The histopathologic features of AE, pellagra, and necrolytic migratory erythema are generally regarded as indistinguishable from one another [9]. The most relevant microscopic clue is the presence of "necrolysis," a term describing cytoplasmic pallor, vacuolization, ballooning degeneration (Fig. 13.8), and subsequent confluent necrosis of keratinocytes in the upper part of the epidermis [9]. The affected keratinocytes often have pyknotic nuclei. Parakeratosis is present in the early reddish patches and is typically confluent rather than focal, usually associated with loss of the granular layer

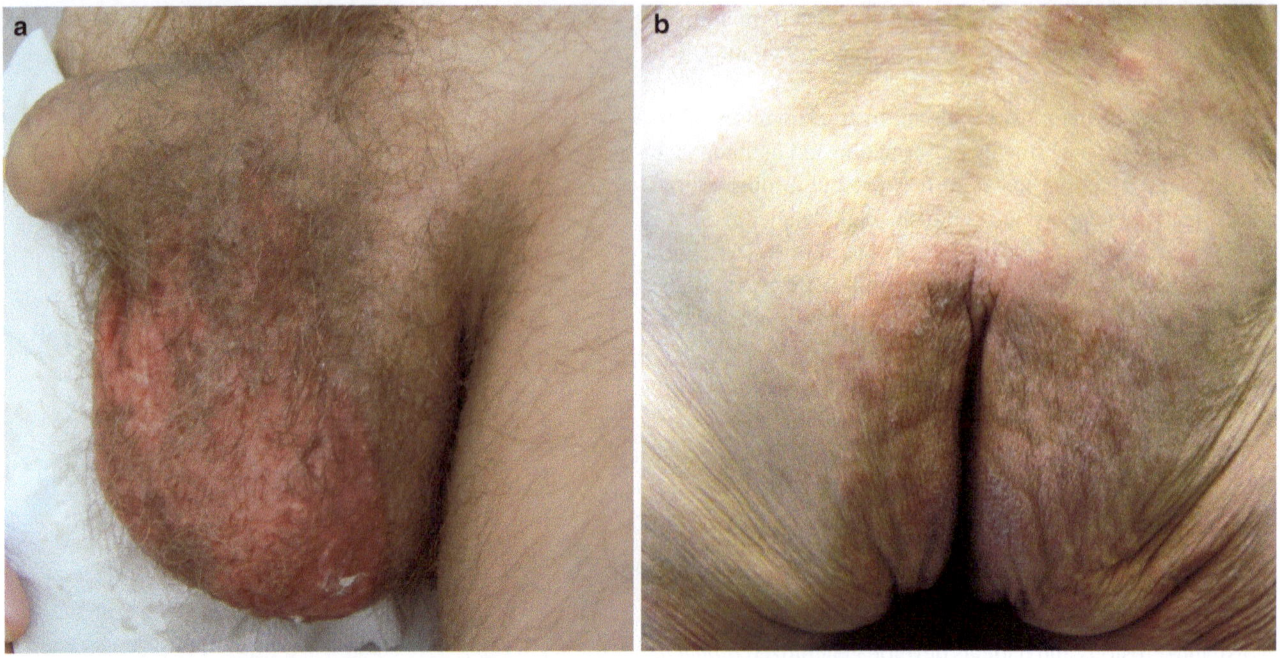

Fig. 13.6 Acrodermatitis enteropathica. (**a**) Eczematous scaly plaques on the genital area. (**b**) Eczematous scaly plaques on the perianal area

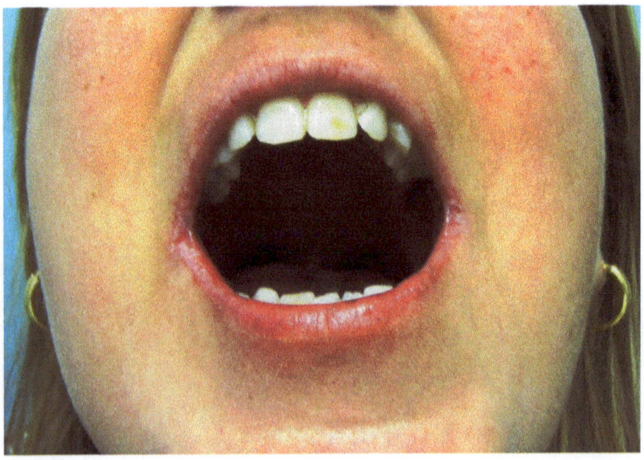

Fig. 13.7 Angular cheilitis

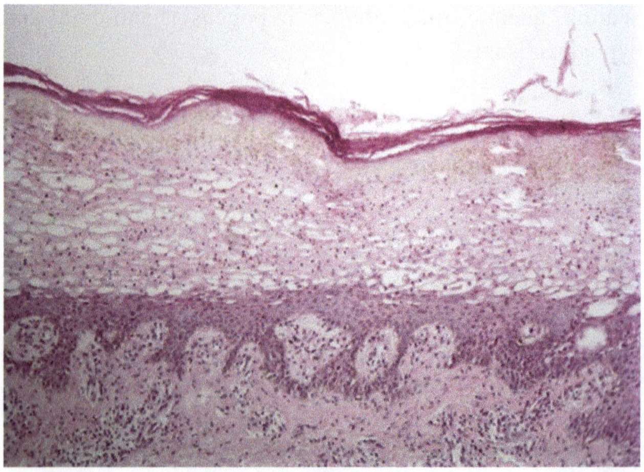

Fig. 13.8 Cytoplasmic pallor, vacuolization, ballooning degeneration in acrodermatitis enteropathica (HE stain) (courtesy of Jameel A. Brown, Little Rock, AR, USA)

and dermal edema. Subcorneal vesicle formation in the pale areas, and rarely, acantholysis may be observed. Associated neutrophilic crust is a variable finding. Scattered dyskeratotic keratinocytes are often present within all levels of the epidermis. Late or chronic AE lesions mimic psoriasis, showing confluent parakeratosis and psoriasiform hyperplasia, while necrolysis and pallor of keratinocytes are minimal or absent.

13.2.3 Pellagra

Pellagra is a systemic disease resulting from a marked cellular deficiency of niacin or its precursor tryptophan. Niacin is a water-soluble vitamin, also known as vitamin B3. Tryptophan, an essential amino acid, is converted into niacin. Niacin is an important constituent of coenzyme 1 (NAD, nicotinamide adenine dinucleotide) and coenzyme 2 (NADP, nicotinamide adenine dinucleotide phosphate), which in turn intervenes in essential oxidation–reduction reactions [10]. The ubiquitous presence of these coenzymes explains the multi-organ afflictions associated with pellagra. Tissues with high energy requirements such as the brain or high turnover rates such as gut or skin are primarily affected [11, 12]. High niacin contents are found in meat, poultry, fish, dry beans, mushrooms, nuts, dairy products, and eggs.

Pellagra is rare in developed nations. It is caused not only by a poor diet but also can be secondary to conditions that interfere with niacin intake, absorption, or processing, such as inflammatory bowel disease, prolonged diarrhea, gastrectomy, hepatic cirrhosis, chronic alcoholism, malabsorption, or anorexia nervosa. Metabolic imbalances, such as carcinoid syndrome, may also lead to pellagra which diverts tryptophan to serotonin synthesis causing niacin deficiency. Pellagra has been increasingly reported in HIV patients. Drugs such as isoniazid and anticonvulsants have also been implicated, interfering with niacin or tryptophan metabolism [13].

The classical triad of pellagra is *dermatitis*, diarrhea, and dementia. The symptoms do not appear necessarily in this order. Although the skin is inevitably the key to the diagnosis of pellagra, usually the first symptoms are gastrointestinal, with loss of appetite, abdominal pain, vomiting, and later watery diarrhea, accompanied by fatigue and irritability. Few patients display the full triad; indeed, 33% of patients have dermatitis alone. The skin eruption is characteristically a rash related to sunlight, heat, friction, or pressure, affecting the dorsal surfaces of the hands, face, neck, arms, and feet. In the acute phase, it resembles sunburn with erythema and bullae (wet pellagra) progressing to a chronic, symmetric, scaly rash that exacerbates following reexposure to sunlight (Fig. 13.9). The typical locations are the front of neck (Casal's necklace) and hands and forearms (pellagra gauntlet). On the face, a "butterfly" rash similar in appearance to that of lupus erythematosus may be seen. On the forehead, there may be a narrow border of normal skin between the erythema and the anterior hairline.

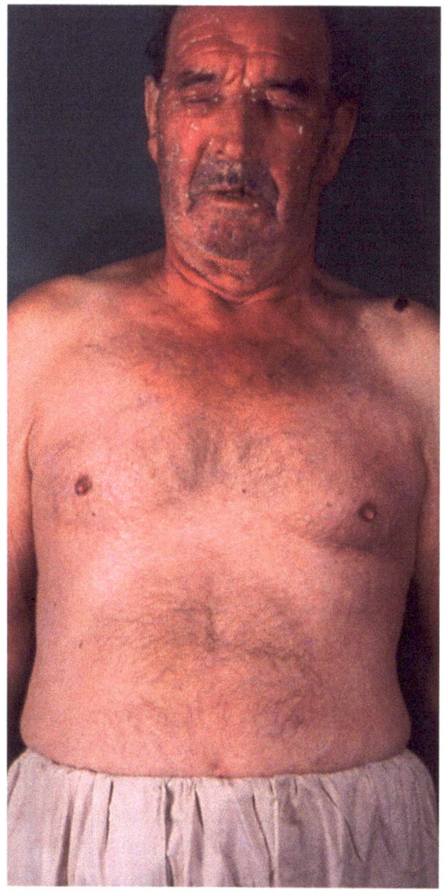

Fig. 13.9 Pellagra. Chronic, symmetric, scaly rash that exacerbates following reexposure to sunlight

One-third of patients have *oral findings*. The tongue and oral cavity may be painful and erythematous as a result of mucous membrane inflammation (Fig. 13.10); the tongue is hypertrophic with pseudo-membranous furrows, erosions, or ulcers, and later becomes atrophic with diminution of its papillae. Cheilitis, angular stomatitis, and glossitis are characteristic features. Severe glossitis causes dysphagia. As the disease advances, neuropsychiatric symptoms develop and include photophobia, asthenia, depression, disorientation, and memory loss that can evolve into frank psychosis and even death if the disease is not identified and treated. Atypical pellagra may be oligosymptomatic or monosymptomatic. Abortive forms are known as erythema pellagroides [14].

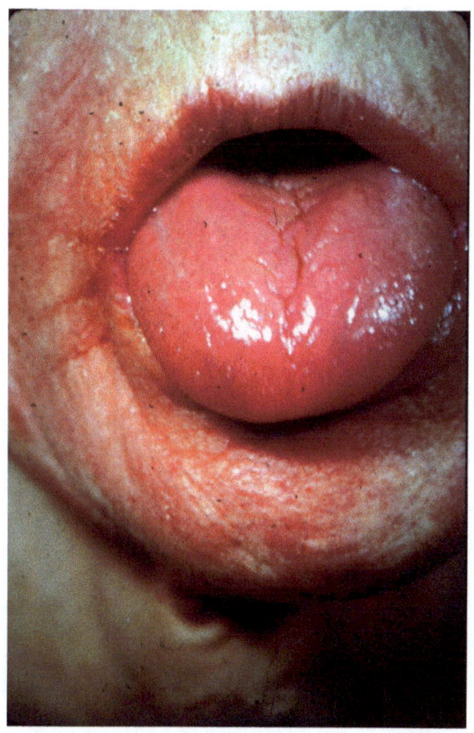

Fig. 13.10 Red beefy hypertrophic tongue with cheilitis in pellagra

The diagnosis of pellagra is based on the characteristic clinical presentation and rapid response to oral niacin supplementation. Biopsy findings can support the diagnosis but are relatively nonspecific due to the resemblances to AE and necrolytic migratory erythema. Histologically, the acute stage may show a variety of changes including exocytosis of neutrophils and intracellular edema. Vesicles, if present, arise subepidermally as a result of vacuolar degeneration of the basal layer, or intraepidermally as a result of intense spongiosis. There is also perivascular lymphocytic infiltrate of the superficial vascular plexus. Older lesions may present with hyperkeratosis, parakeratosis, and variable acanthosis, with increased basal layer melanin. In the chronic phase, epidermal atrophy overlying dermal fibrosis, sebaceous gland atrophy, and a chronic lymphohistiocytic perivascular infiltrate are observed [14].

13.2.4 Iron Deficiency

Women are at higher risk than men particularly in middle age. Skin manifestations [15–17] of iron deficiency include *pallor* and *koilonychias* (Fig. 13.11). This aspect is usually associated with a severe and long-standing iron deficiency. Plummer–Vinson syndrome, also called Paterson–Brown–Kelly syndrome or sideropenic dysphagia presents as a triad of dysphagia, glossitis and iron deficiency anemia. This condition is now very rare in clinical practice. Patients with this syndrome complain of *glossitis* with a burning sensation of the tongue and oral mucosa and atrophy of lingual papillae, which produces a beefy red tongue associated with *cheilitis and angular stomatitis* (Fig. 13.12). This condition is also one of the risk factors for developing squamous cell carcinoma of the oral cavity. Iron deficiency has been associated with generalized *pruritus* including documentation of improvement with replacement of iron [18] and with noncicatricial *hair loss* with or without alterations of the shaft [19].

13.2.5 Other Nutritional Deficiencies

A few other vitamin deficiencies may result in cutaneous lesions. Vitamin B12 plays a significant role in DNA synthesis. The common cause of vitamin B12 deficiency is malabsorption.

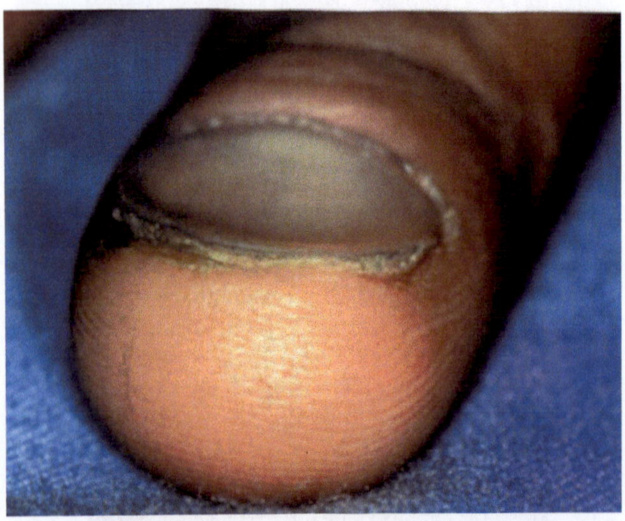

Fig. 13.11 Koilonychia (courtesy of G.E. Cannata, Imperia, Italy)

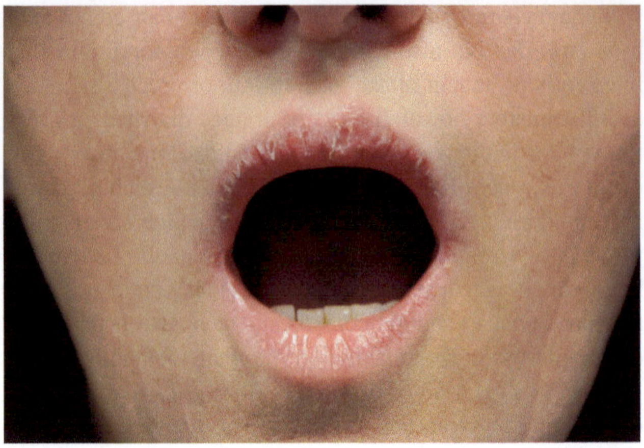

Fig. 13.12 Cheilitis with cracked and fissured lips in an anorexic patient with severe iron and multivitamin deficiency

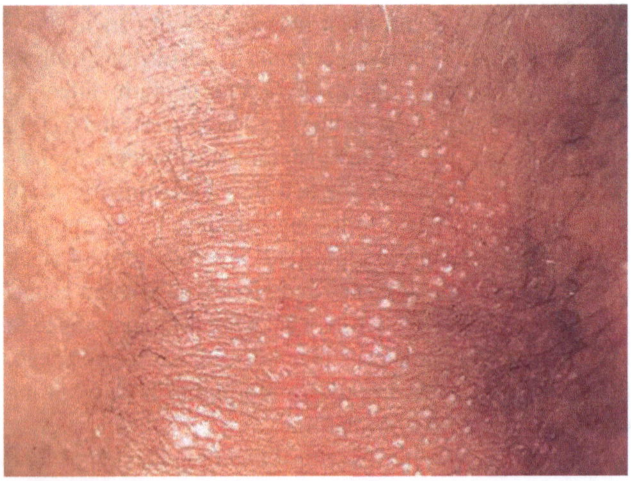

Fig. 13.13 Phrynoderma

Megaloblastic anemia and pancytopenia are characteristic manifestations of vitamin B12 deficiency. Neurological symptoms include peripheral neuropathy, subacute combined degeneration of the spinal cord, ataxia, optic atrophy, psychosis, depression, and dementia [20].The mucocutaneous manifestations of vitamin B12 deficiency are less frequent and include *skin hyperpigmentation, vitiligo, recurrent angular stomatitis, glossitis with linear and band-like lesions, and hair changes.* Hyperpigmentation of the extremities, especially over the dorsum of the hands and feet, with accentuation over the interphalangeal joints and terminal phalanges, associated with pigmentation of oral mucosa is characteristic of vitamin B12 deficiency [21, 22].

Phrynoderma is a rare form of follicular hyperkeratosis associated with vitamin A or essential fatty acids deficiency (Fig. 13.13) [23]. In addition to follicular hyperkeratosis, vitamin A deficiency causes xerosis, generalised hyperpigmentation, and sparse and fragile hair [24]. Ocular involvement is common, frequently causing night blindness.

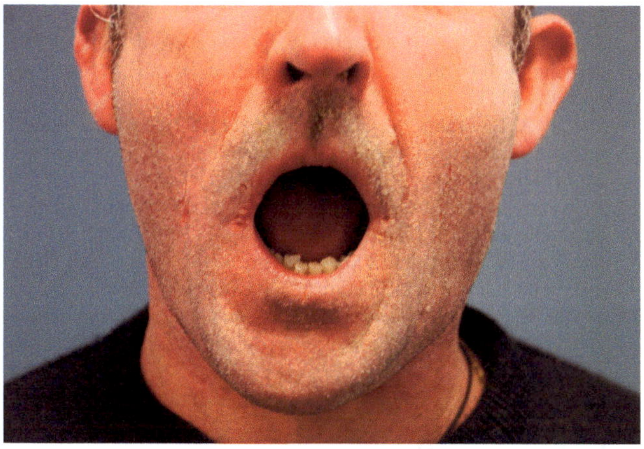

Fig. 13.14 Seborrheic dermatitis-like eruption and angular cheilitis due to nutritional deficiency in an alcoholic cirrhotic patient

Vitamin K deficiency is associated with disorders of the coagulation cascade and may manifest as increased tendency of bleeding.

The skin is very rich in biotin (vitamin H) and its deficiency leads to mucous membrane alterations with dryness and redness. The lips are cracked and fissured. In children, two clinical forms are described. In the early infantile form, skin lesions resemble ichthyosis or diffuse seborrheic dermatitis. This form is usually lethal. The later infantile form resembles acrodermatitis enteropathica. One of the most important causes of biotin deficiency is total parenteral nutrition. However, deficiencies can be caused by consuming raw egg whites for months to years, as egg whites contain high levels of avidin, a protein that binds biotin strongly. When cooked, avidin is denatured.

The skin manifestations due to Vitamin B1 deficiency include an orogenital dermatitis; however, the most important alterations are those of the heart and nervous system. Today the main cause of Vitamins B1 deficiency is alcoholism.

A deficit in vitamin B2 (riboflavin) is responsible for mucosal manifestations such as dry red and fissured lips, angular cheilitis and red, atrophic tongue and conjunctivitis. Cutaneous alterations are less specific and resemble seborrheic dermatitis (Fig. 13.14). Hyperpigmentation of the scrotum or vulva can also occur. Vitamin B2 deficiency usually occurs in cases of relative protein deficiency in the diet. Chronic alcoholism and cirrhosis of the liver are important causes.

Experimental deficiency of B6 (pyridoxine) produces a perioral dermatitis similar to that found in zinc deficiency. A low level of pyridoxine often produces nicotinic acid deficiency and pellagra-like cutaneous, gastrointestinal, and polyneuritic manifestations.

Skin manifestations due to folic acid deficiency are similar to the manifestations of vitamin B12 deficiency. Pigmentation is found on the tongue or genital area. Mucous manifestations are glossitis and angular cheilitis. Nutritional deficiency of folic acid is not frequent and is due to ingestion of foods boiled for a long time, alteration of digestive absorption, or an increased need in pregnancy. It occurs also in infants who are fed solely with goat's milk. The use of drugs such as methotrexate and anticonvulsants that inhibit folate metabolism requires folic acid supplementation.

Kwashiorkor is one of the severe forms of protein malnutrition caused by the inadequate intake of protein with reasonable caloric (energy) intake. The other form of protein-energy malnutrition is the condition known as *marasmus*, which is characterized by inadequate intake of both protein and calories. It is associated with extreme poverty in developing countries and with chronic malabsorptive conditions such as cystic fibrosis or nutritional ignorance and perceived food intolerance in developed countries. Characteristic skin and hair changes occur in kwashiorkor and develop over a few days. *Edema* is universally present, and the skin changes range from erythematous and hyperpigmented scaly plaques involving the flexures and the diaper areas to the classic *flaky paint dermatitis*. Hairs are sparse, dry, and brittle and may turn reddish yellow to white in color [25].

13.3 Treatment and Prognosis

The treatment of scurvy relies on vitamin C supplementation. One to two grams of vitamin C administered daily for the first 2–3 days followed by 500 mg/day for the next week is adequate to replenish the total body pool. Afterward, a daily intake of 100 mg of vitamin C should be given for 1–3 months. Symptoms of fatigue, lethargy, pain, anorexia, and confusion improve within 24 h of supplementation. Bruising, perifollicular hemorrhages, and gingival bleeding usually improve within 1–2 weeks. Corkscrew hairs return to their normal appearance by 4 weeks. Complete improvement should be expected after approximately 3 months of regular vitamin C supplementation [5].

Therapy of acrodermatitis enteropathica requires supplementation with oral zinc. Skin lesions respond within 2–7 days of administration and resolve within 2–4 weeks [26].

The treatment of pellagra includes oral nicotinamide supplementation 100–300 mg daily in three to four separate doses until major acute symptoms resolve, followed by the oral administration of 50 mg every 8–12 h until all skin lesions heal. Usually neuropsychiatric symptoms subside first, after a few days. Resolution of dermatitis occurs in 3–4 weeks [12].

Oral iron therapy (ferrous sulfate) is given for iron deficiency. Common recommendations are to treat with 150–200 mg elemental iron daily. The cause of the iron deficiency must be found, especially in older patients who face the greatest risk for gastrointestinal cancers.

The treatment of vitamin B12 deficiency is 1,000 μg of vitamin B12 by intramuscular injection every day or every other day for 1–2 weeks, followed by monthly injections for 3 months, and thereafter every 3 months for life. The skin manifestations respond rapidly to vitamin B12 therapy [21].

The treatment of vitamin A deficiency consists of high-dose vitamin A replacement therapy. Visual disturbances resolve within days, although corneal scarring is permanent. The skin lesions usually take 1–4 months to heal [24].

References

1. Andrews NC (1999) Disorders of iron metabolism. N Engl J Med 341:1986–1995
2. Roy CN, Andrews NC (2001) Recent advances in disorders of iron metabolism: mutations, mechanisms and modifiers. Hum Mol Gen 10:2181–2186
3. Olmedo JM, Yiannias JA, Windgassen EB et al (2006) Scurvy: a disease almost forgotten. Int J Dermatol 45:909–913
4. Valdés F (2006) Vitamina C. Actas Dermosifiliogr 97:557–568
5. Nguyen TD, Cowley DM, Muir JB (2003) Scurvy: a cutaneous clinical diagnosis. Australas J Dermatol 44:48–51
6. Léger D (2008) Scurvy: reemergence of nutritional deficiencies. Can Fam Physician 54:1403–1406
7. Sanchez JE, Barham KL, Sangueza OP (2007) Acquired acrodermatitis enteropathica: case report of an atypical presentation. J Cutan Pathol 34:490–493
8. Traupe H, Haple R, Grobe H et al (1986) Polarization microscopy of hair in acrodermatitis enteropathica. Pediatr Dermatol 3: 300–303
9. Maverakis E, Fung MA, Lynch PJ et al (2007) Acrodermatitis enteropathica and an overview of zinc metabolism. J Am Acad Dermatol 56:116–124
10. MacDonald A, Forsyth A (2005) Nutritional deficiencies and the skin. Clin Exp Dermatol 30:388–390
11. Karthikeyan K, Thappa DM (2002) Pellagra and skin. Int J Dermatol 41:476–481
12. Jen M, Shah KN, Yan AC (2008) Cutaneous changes in nutritional disease. In: Wolff K, Goldsmith LA, Katz SI et al (eds) Fitzpatrick's dermatology in general medicine, 7th edn. McGraw Hill, New York, pp 1209–1211
13. Darvay A, Basarab T, McGregor JM et al (1999) Isoniazid induced pellagra despite pyridoxine supplementation. Clin Exp Dermatol 24:167–169
14. Hegyi J, Schwartz RA, Hegyi V (2004) Pellagra: dermatitis, dementia and diarrhea. Int J Dermatol 43:1–5
15. Pitambe HV, Schulz EJ (2005) Life-threatening dermatoses due to metabolic and endocrine disorders. Clin Dermatol 23:258–266
16. Kostler E, Porst H, Wollina U (2005) Cutaneous manifestations of metabolic diseases: uncommon presentations. Clin Dermatol 23:457–464
17. Nairz M, Weiss G (2006) Molecular and clinical aspects of iron homeostasis: from anemia to hemochromatosis. Wien Klin Wochenschr 118:442–462
18. Polat M, Oztas P, Ilhan MN, Yalçin B, Alli N (2008) Generalized pruritus: a prospective study concerning etiology. Am J Clin Dermatol 9:39–44
19. Trost B, Bergfeld WF, Calogeras E (2006) The diagnosis and treatment of iron deficiency and its potential relationship to hair loss. J Am Acad Dermatol 54:824–844
20. Oh R, Brown DL (2003) Vitamin B12 deficiency. Am Fam Physician 67:979–986
21. Graells J, Ojeda RM, Muniesa C, Gonzalez J, Saavedra J (2009) Glossitis with linear lesions: an early sign of vitamin B12 deficiency. J Am Acad Dermatol 60:498–500
22. Kannan R (2008) Cutaneous lesions and vitamin B12 deficiency-An often-forgotten link. Can Fam Physician 54:529–532
23. Girard C, Dereure O, Blatière V et al (2006) Vitamin A deficiency phrynoderma associated with chronic giardiasis. Pediatr Dermatol 23:346–349
24. Chia MW, Tay YK, Liu TT (2008) Phrynoderma: a forgotten entity in a developed country. Singapore Med J 49:160–162
25. Liu T, Howard MR, Mancini AJ et al (2001) Kwashiorkor in the United States: fad diets, perceived and true milk allergy, and nutritional ignorance. Arch Dermatol 137:630–636
26. Jensen SL, McCuaig C, Zembowicz A et al (2008) Bullous lesions in acrodermatitis enteropathica delaying diagnosis of zinc deficiency: a report of two cases and review of the literature. J Cutan Pathol 35:1–13

Chapter 14
Anorexia Nervosa

Jameel Ahmad Brown and Bruce R. Smoller

Key Points

- Anorexia nervosa is primarily a psychosocial disorder with secondary dermatologic manifestations.
- Cutaneous sequelae of anorexia nervosa are the result of malnutrition, self-induced vomiting, drug ingestion, and/or concomitant psychiatric disorder.
- Russell's sign, i.e., the development of calluses over the dorsum of the dominant hand as a result of repeated friction against the front teeth during self-induced emesis, is the most pathognomonic skin sign in anorexia nervosa.
- A number of other dermatological conditions such as xerosis, alopecia due to telogen effluvium, development of lanugo hairs, carotenoderma, pruritus, cheilitis, acne, and nail lesions may be associated with anorexia nervosa, although none are specific for it.
- Most cutaneous sequelae of anorexia nervosa abate upon reestablishing normal body weight and nutritional status, but the prognosis is guarded and patients should be encouraged to consult a psychiatrist or psychotherapist.

Keywords Anorexia nervosa • Anorectic hand • Xerosis • Effluvium • Nail lesions • Cheilitis

14.1 Introduction

Famed vocalist, the late Karen Carpenter, has served as the "poster child" for eating disorder awareness since her premature death in 1983 at the age of 32 years. Her tragic death evoked a rebirth of the discussion regarding eating disorders, namely, anorexia nervosa (AN), bulimia nervosa (AN), and eating disorder not otherwise specified (EDNOS). There exists a significant degree of behavioral, diagnostic, and clinical overlap among these subtypes; hence, this chapter will be limited to the well-defined restrictive and binge-purge forms and the cutaneous manifestations thereof.

Anorexia nervosa is characterized by a refusal to maintain body weight ≥85% of expected body weight for an age- and height-matched peer. The parameter most often measured to evaluate ideal body weight is the body mass index (BMI) [1]. These patients have a deeply seated fear of weight gain and becoming obese despite the fact that they are significantly underweight. Self-perception plays a role in the diagnosis of AN in that patients with AN perceive their weight, size, and shape in a distorted fashion. In female patients, amenorrhea is a component of the diagnostic criteria as well [2].

The lifetime prevalence of anorexia nervosa in American women and men is 0.9 and 0.5% respectively [3]. These statistics suggest that AN is an important medical entity and justify its inclusion in medical literature and texts. Anorexia nervosa carries with it significant morbidity and mortality. The secondary complications associated with this primary psychological disorder have multisystem effects, in particular cutaneous manifestations, which are often the heralding sign of disordered eating behavior. A classification scheme has been proposed which stratifies the cutaneous signs of eating disorders into four categories. These categories are etiologically derived: those due to caloric restriction/malnutrition, those caused by automatous emesis, those caused by the ingestion of drugs, and those caused by superimposed psychiatric illnesses [4, 5].

14.2 Clinical and Pathological Aspects of Skin Manifestations

14.2.1 *Xerosis*

Xerosis is one of, if not the most common, cutaneous signs of anorexia nervosa with a prevalence in this specific population of 97% [5]. The trunk and extremities are most frequently affected, and the severity of the condition spans the gamut from minimally xerotic and pruritic to severely

J.A. Brown (✉)
Faculty at the University of Arkansas for Medical Sciences in the Department of Pathology and the Division of Dermatopathology, 4301 West Markham, Slot 517, Little Rock, AR 72205, USA
e-mail: JABrown@uams.edu

F. Rongioletti and B.R. Smoller (eds.), *Clinical and Pathological Aspects of Skin Diseases in Endocrine, Metabolic, Nutritional and Deposition Disease*, DOI 10.1007/978-1-60761-181-3_14, © Springer Science+Business Media, LLC 2010

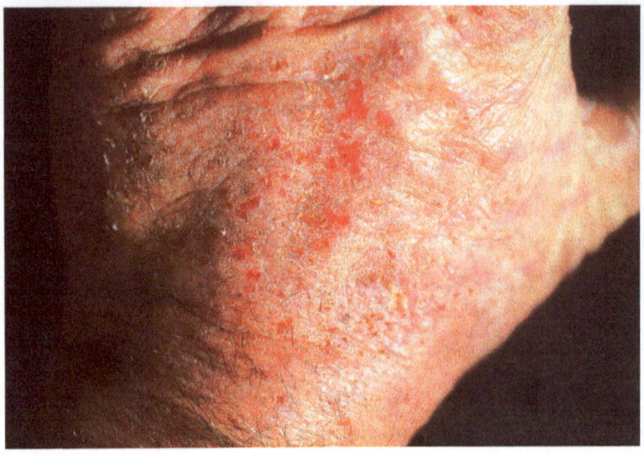

Fig. 14.1 Xerosis of the hand

irritating and visually reminiscent of fish scale (Fig. 14.1). It is hypothesized that xerosis is a secondary phenomenon due to inadequate consumption and uptake of vitamins and trace elements [6]. A metabolically driven hypothyroid state has also been postulated as a contributor to the xerotic state observed in almost all patients with anorexia nervosa. The mechanism by which this is postulated to occur involves a hypothalamic dysfunctional state as manifested by two separate pathways: (1) delayed thyrotropin response to protirelin and (2) defective peripheral conversion of thyroxine to triiodothyroxine with increased conversion of its inactive isomer. When xerosis combined with concomitant obsessive compulsive disorder/disease and excessive washing is present, the condition worsens. There are no xerosis-specific histopathologic changes.

14.2.2 Lanugo-Like Body Hairs

The hypocaloric state of anorexia nervosa specifically induces the new growth of fine, downy, and pale hair called lanugo. It has a predilection for the trunk and distal upper extremities. A distinction should be made between the aberrant hair growth seen in hyperandrogenic states, a sign of virilization, and the pale downy growth observed in AN [1]. In fact, low serum testosterone and gonadotropin levels are frequently noted in male patients suffering from anorexia nervosa. The low androgenic state induced by AN has a behavioral corollary in that these male patients experience a decreased libido and lower potency [7]. Interestingly, lanugo does not occur in other settings of starvation – for example, malabsorption. There is a linear relationship between its arrival during starvation and its subsequent disappearance when normal total body fat has been restored [6].

14.2.3 Alopecia

Hair loss, or alopecia, is among the commonest cutaneous signs observed in the setting of anorexia nervosa. It is most easily recognized and causes greater morbidity in girls and women, as traditionally longer hairstyles are worn which accentuate the paucity of hair growth or excessive hair loss. The principal pattern of alopecia seen in patients with AN is diffuse scalp involvement; however, a frontal predominance has been observed [5].

Telogen effluvium, as a specific mechanism of alopecia, occurs often in patients with anorexia nervosa. It reveals itself by way of global shedding of normal telogen hairs, disrupting the typical ratio of anagen-to-telogen (9:1) hairs in the well-nourished individual. The number of hairs in the anagen or growth phase is decreased, while the number of hairs in the telogen or rest phase is increased. A greater proportion of hairs are pushed into telogen phase in AN, resulting in an overall loss of hair, as fewer hairs are in the growth phase. The scalp exhibits a decrease in hair density; hair thinning at the temples can often be observed (Fig. 14.2a) without evidence of scarring and/or inflammation [6]. A hair-pull test is often positive, and patients report a

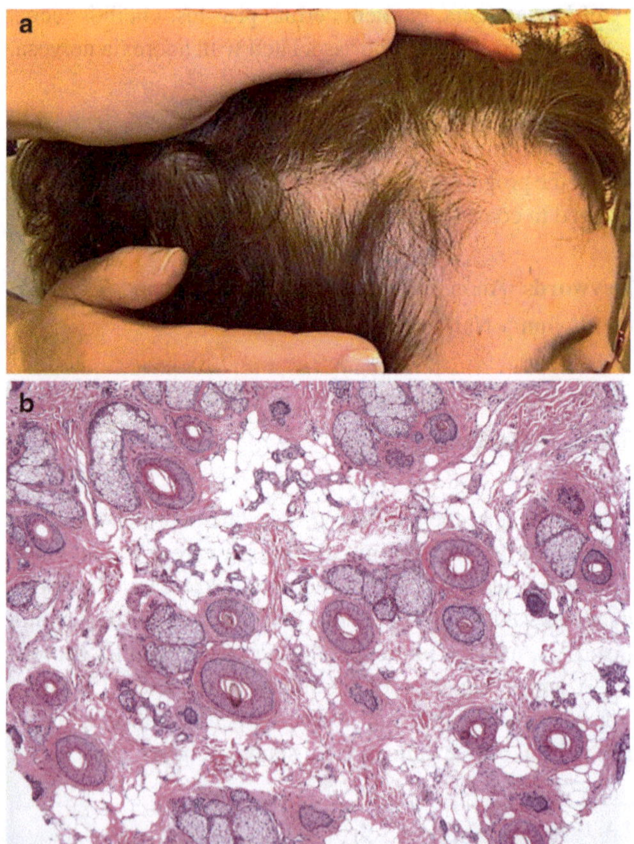

Fig. 14.2 (**a**) Telogen effluvium. (**b**) Histopathology of telogen effluvium (horizontal section)

history that is concordant with clinical examination [1]. The shed hairs appear club-shaped, depigmented, and lack a sheath. Histopathology demonstrates a noninflammatory, nonscarring, alopecia with the presence of a disproportionate number of telogen hair follicles (Fig. 14.2b). Alopecia totalis is highly unusual.

14.2.4 Hypercarotenemia/Carotenoderma

Anorexia nervosa incites a decrease in basal metabolic rate (BMR). Generally, all organ systems are affected by the slowed BMR; the liver is impacted greatly. This is evidenced by increased levels of carotene, a fat-soluble provitamin, found in the serum of patients with AN as a result of an inability of the liver to break down the compound rapidly. These patients tend to consume high quantities of low-calorie foods containing carotene in an effort to curtail weight gain, thus exacerbating the condition [6]. Carotene-rich foods include pumpkin, squash, carrots, and spinach; this list is not exhaustive.

Carotenoderma is the clinical cutaneous manifestation of the laboratory finding of hypercarotenemia. It is the yellow appearance of the skin due to deposition of carotene within the tissue [1]. Tyler et al. reported a palmar–plantar accentuation in the absence of scleral changes [6]. These findings highlight the prudent distinction that must be made between the innocuous yellow pigmentation observed in carotenoderma and the potentially harmful pigment alteration in jaundice due to hyperbilirubinemia. Bilirubin has a high affinity for components of the scleral tissue and localizes there, unlike carotene. Hypercarotenemia also occurs in other states of compromised hepatic metabolism of carotene such as hypothyroidism but is not observed in states of malabsorption [6]. Histopathology is nonspecific.

14.2.5 Acne

The prevalence of acne in patients with anorexia nervosa has been reported to be between 41 and 60% in several studies [5, 8]. An etiological or causative relationship between acne and anorexia nervosa is difficult to establish, as the observation of acne in this context is confounded by many factors. An inherent bias may exist in the interpretation of acne in patients with eating disorders. Glorio et al. found that in an evaluation of 200 patients with eating disorders, approximately 73% of them were less than 20 years of age [5], a population with a physiologic predisposition for acne. This suggests that acne may not be a comorbid finding in patients with anorexia nervosa despite its high prevalence in patients with the disease.

Furthermore, it is conceivable that acne may serve as a risk factor for anorexia nervosa and actually precedes disordered eating. A subset of patients report having made dietary modifications with the intent to clear their acne and inadvertently developed anorexia nervosa by way of excessive restriction. Lee and colleagues describe a series of presumed acne-evoked restriction in girls in which acne is suggested as a valid risk factor [9]. In contrast, other authors observed an acne eruption following recovery from anorexia nervosa in a subset of patients [10]. Anorexia nervosa-associated acne is usually found distributed about the face and back with signs of secondary excoriation, and patients typically have mild-to-moderate disease (Fig. 14.3a) [11]

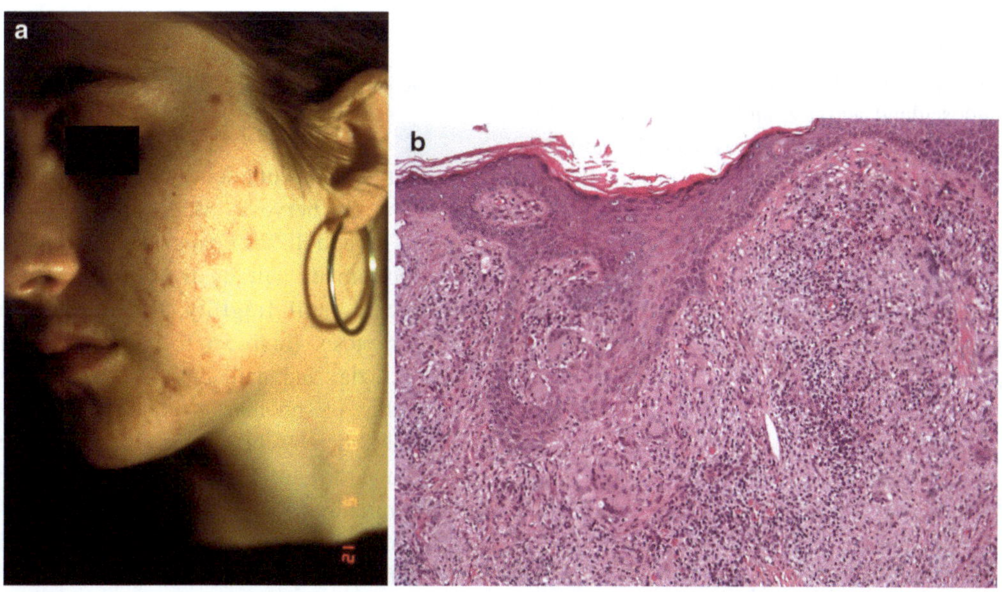

Fig. 14.3 (**a**) Acne in a suffering anorexic patient. (**b**) Histopathology of inflammatory acne

Histopathology reveals the presence of impacted horny cells in the ductules of sebaceous follicles, a variable and mixed inflammatory infiltrate, multinucleated giant cells, pustule formation, trapped and ruptured hair follicles with associated bacteria, and scar formation (Fig. 14.3b).

14.2.6 Acrocyanosis

Acrocyanosis is the blue-to-violaceous hue of the skin acquired under conditions of arterial vasoconstriction and venular vasodilation [6]. The condition frequently involves cold hands and feet by definition, and a concomitant facial and truncal pallor is often observed. The true etiology of acrocyanosis is unknown, but it has been postulated that it may represent a concerted effort by the thermoregulatory system to conserve heat, as many patients with anorexia nervosa battle cold intolerance and poor thermal homeostasis [1]. Schulze observed acrocyanosis in 40% of patients with AN [11], providing additional credence to its high prevalence in the disease process. No disease-specific histopathologic findings are observed, significantly reducing the utility of biopsy.

14.2.7 Pruritus

Itchiness, or pruritus, can be localized or generalized in patients with anorexia nervosa. It is a fairly common symptom, reported to occur in up to 58% of patients [12]. The clinical sign corresponding to the perception of pruritus are lichenification and excoriation in affected areas. The etiologic culprit of pruritus in AN is not well defined; however, it is decidedly multifactorial. Reduction in skin surveillance by the immune system due to starvation, primary xerosis or that induced by excessive hand washing, and elevated concentrations of opioids may all play a role [13]. The presence of eczema, reduced sebaceous gland activity, and regional blood flow variations have also been proposed as causal factors in anorexia nervosa-associated pruritus. The histopathologic correlate to pruritus in this setting has not been explored. Antihistamines have been anecdotally reported as useful [6], suggesting the presence of increased cutaneous mast cell concentration. Morgan and colleagues detected a statistically significant relationship between increased severity of itching and lower BMI. [12]

14.2.8 Purpura

Severe cases of the restricting subtype of anorexia nervosa predispose one to starvation-associated bone marrow suppression and an ensuing thrombocytopenia. In this setting, purpura is the cutaneous sign of a low platelet count and appears as violaceous macules and patches which are nonblanching. One study described diffuse purpura of the trunk and distal upper extremities in patients with severe anorexia [14]. Systemic evidence of poor coagulation has been reported and manifested as purpura, gingival, nasal, and gastrointestinal bleeding [15]. In the purging subtype of AN, purpura can be the result of sudden and repeated increases in pressure induced by retching. Purpura secondary to this mechanism are commonly found in periocular and subconjunctival distributions. Histopathology shows epidermal, dermal, and subcutaneous tissues with extravasated red blood cells, hemosiderin deposition if chronic, and a mild mixed inflammatory infiltrate (Fig. 14.4).

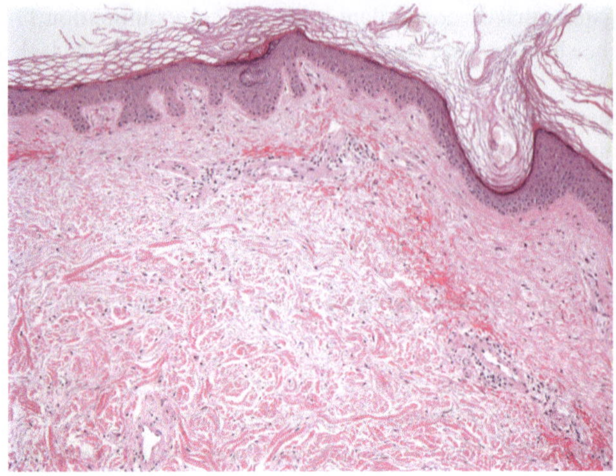

Fig. 14.4 Noninflammatory purpura

14.2.9 Nail Changes

Nail changes are common cutaneous findings in patients with anorexia nervosa. Studies have quoted incidences between 29 and 48% in patients with the disease [14, 16]. The spectrum of nail dystrophy is broad and includes koilonychia, nail fragility, longitudinal ungual striae, onychocryptosis (ingrown toenail), periungual erythema, onychoschizia, and nail alterations due to onychophagia. Koilonychia, or spooning nails, is a morphologic alteration in the nail whereby the nail acquires central concavity and lateral upward reflection. It is one of the many sequelae of iron deficiency [6]. Onychoschizia presents as splitting of the distal nail plate. Asymmetric nail dystrophy occurs frequently and can share clinical features with onychomycosis.

14.2.10 Angular Cheilitis

Angular cheilitis (perleche) is seen in up to 76% of patients with anorexia nervosa and is considered to be a consequence of several vitamin deficiencies. Interestingly, it has been associated most commonly with a dearth of riboflavin [1, 6].

14.2.11 Russell's Sign

In 2005, Strumia developed the concept of the "anorectic's hand" [1]. The idea was based upon the observation that many of the cutaneous manifestations of anorexia nervosa were limited to the hands. Embedded in this concept is the only true pathognomonic sign for AN, Russell's sign (RS). RS is the development of calluses over the dorsum of the dominant hand as a result of repeated friction against the front teeth during self-induced emesis (Fig. 14.5) [17]. Russell's sign is

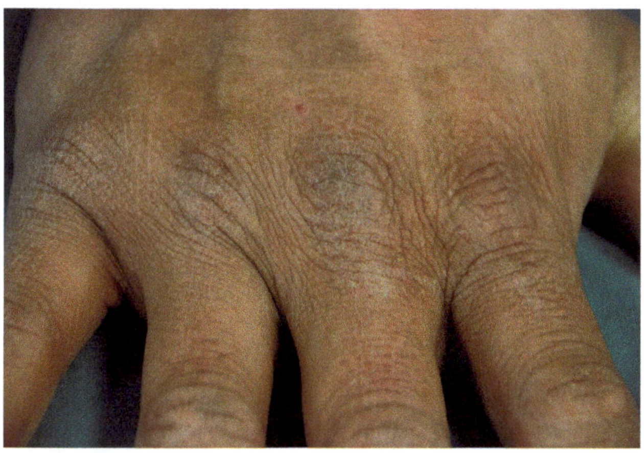

Fig. 14.5 Russell's sign

seen in 67% of patients with the purging subtype of anorexia nervosa [16]. Of note, males who suffer from AN are almost exclusively of the restricting subtype and therefore do not exhibit purging sequelae [14]. Histopathology demonstrates regenerative epidermal hyperplasia and dermal fibrosis. Cessation of manually-induced purging does not resolve the changes entirely.

14.2.12 Finger Clubbing, Fixed Drug Eruption, and Photosensitivity Dermatitis

Patients with the purging subtype of anorexia nervosa are also subject to the clinical consequences of laxatives, diuretics, and other pharmaceutical and alternative medicines. Abuse of laxatives containing senna has been said to cause clubbing of the distal digits, while phenolphthalein laxatives are associated with urticarial eruptions [17]. Thiazide diuretics have been implicated in photosensitivity reactions. Phenothiazines are associated with fixed drug eruptions (Fig. 14.6a) and/or hyperpigmentation [1]. Fixed drug reactions classically display lichenoid infiltration, dyskeratosis, and dermal melanin incontinence (Fig. 14.6b).

14.2.13 Miscellanea

Pellagra, scurvy (Fig. 14.7), acrodermatitis enteropathica, and other manifestations due to nutritional deficiencies are not uncommon in anorexia nervosa (see Chap. 3.1). Hyperpigmentation, seborrheic dermatitis, perniosis, livedo reticularis, interdigital intertrigo, paronychia, acquired striae

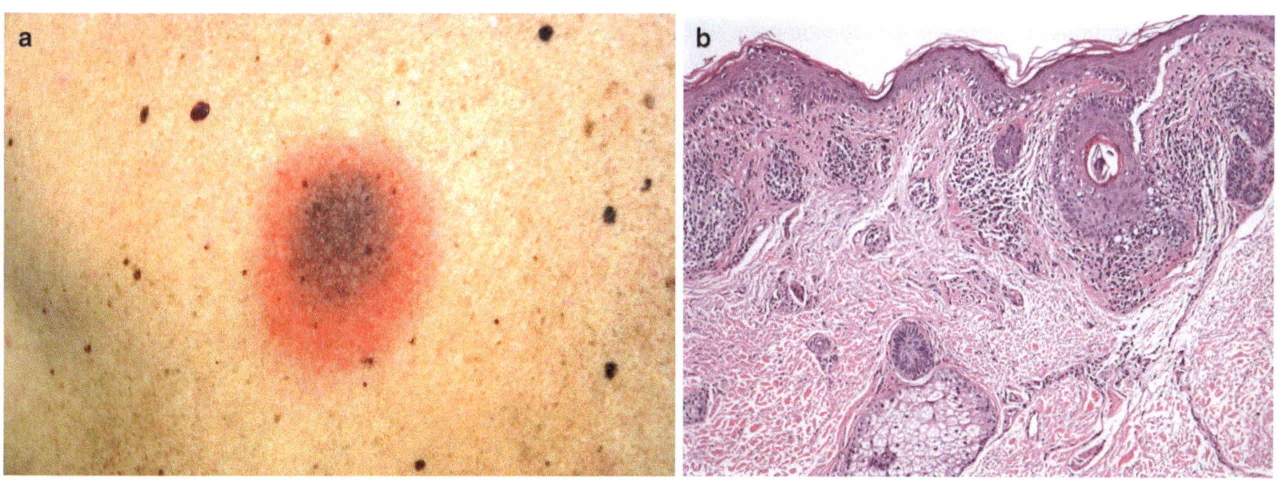

Fig. 14.6 (**a**) Fixed drug eruption. (**b**) Histopathology of fixed drug eruption

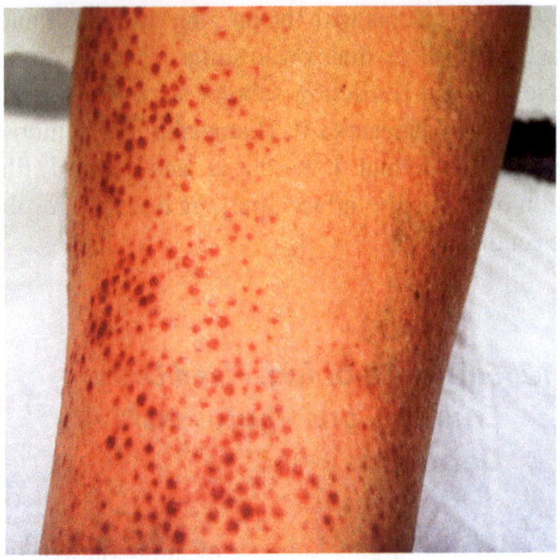

Fig. 14.7 Perifollicular hemorrhages in scurvy due to anorexia nervosa

distensae, delayed healing, prurigo pigmentosa, edema, linear erythema craquele, and self-induced dermatitis artefacta are other nonspecific dermatological signs whose concomitance, albeit in the appropriate context, may permit an early diagnosis of anorexia nervosa.

14.3 Treatment and Prognosis

Most cutaneous sequelae of anorexia nervosa will abate upon reestablishing normal body weight and nutritional status [1]. Even though skin sequelae of anorexia nervosa improve with weight gain, dermatological symptomatic treatment should be considered. Xerosis improves with moisturizing ointments and humidification of the environment Acne may be treated with topical benzoyl peroxide, retinoids, and antibacterials, but systemic treatment may also be considered. Cheilitis, angular stomatitis, and nail fragility appear to respond to topical tocopherol. Russell's sign may decrease in size following applications of ointments that contain urea.

References

1. Strumia R (2005) Dermatologic signs in patients with eating disorders. Am J Clin Dermatol 6:1–10
2. APA (2000) Diagnostic and statistical manual of mental disorders, 4th edn. Washington, DC, American Psychiatric Association, text revision
3. Hudson JI, Hiripi E, Pope HG Jr, Kessler RC (2007) The prevalence and correlates of eating disorders in the National Comorbidity Survey Replication. Biol Psychiatry 61:348–358
4. Gupta MA, Gupta AK, Haberman HF (1987) Dermatologic signs in anorexia nervosa and bulimia nervosa. Arch Dermatol 123:1386–1390
5. Glorio R, Allevato M, De Pablo A et al (2000) Prevalence of cutaneous manifestations in 200 patients with eating disorders. Int J Dermatol 39:348–353
6. Tyler I, Wiseman MC, Crawford RI, Birmingham CL (2002) Cutaneous manifestations of eating disorders. J Cutan Med Surg 6(4):345–353
7. Vogt MW, HJ FMM, Stahl S (1990) Dermatologic aspects of anorexia nervosa and bulimia nervosa. Hautarzt 41:476–484
8. Strumia R, Varotti E, Manzato E, Gualandi M (2001) Skin signs in anorexia nervosa. Dermatology 203:314–317
9. Lee S, Leung CM, Wing YK, Chiu HF, Chen CN (1991) Acne as a risk factor for anorexia nervosa in Chinese. Aust N Z J Psychiatry 25:134–137
10. Marshman GM, Hanna MJ, Ben-Tovim DI, Walker MK (1990) Cutaneous abnormalities in anorexia nervosa. Australas J Dermatol 31:9–12
11. Schulze UM, Pettke-Rank CV, Kreienkamp M et al (1999) Dermatologic findings in anorexia and bulimia nervosa of childhood and adolescence. Pediatr Dermatol 16:90–94
12. Morgan JF, Lacey JH (1999) Scratching and fasting: a study of pruritus and anorexia nervosa. Br J Dermatol 140:453–456
13. Taniguchi S, Yamamoto N, Kono T et al (1996) Generalized pruritus in anorexia nervosa. Br J Dermatol 134:510–511
14. Strumia R, Manzato E, Gualandi M (2003) Cutaneous manifestations in male anorexia nervosa: four cases. Acta Derm Venereol 83:464–465
15. Abella E, Feliu E, Granada I et al (2002) Bone marrow changes in anorexia nervosa are correlated with the amount of weight loss and not with other clinical findings. Am J Clin Pathol 118:582–588
16. Hediger C, Rost B, Itin P (2000) Cutaneous manifestations in anorexia nervosa. Schweiz Med Wochenschr 130:565–575
17. Pines A, Olchovsky D, Bregman J (1983) Finger clubbing associated with laxative abuse. South Med J 76:1071–1072

Chapter 15
Alcohol Abuse

Torello Lotti and Angelo Massimiliano D'Erme

Key Points

- Alcoholism is associated with many cutaneous stigmata.
- Most of the skin manifestations significantly associated with alcoholism are mediated by liver toxicity.
- Other cutaneous manifestations in alcoholics are due to nutritional and metabolic diseases that are capable of inducing skin symptoms.
- Alcohol can exacerbate or trigger many common skin manifestations, which may exhibit atypical or severe manifestations in alcoholics.
- Awareness of the skin manifestations of alcohol abuse can allow early detection and intervention for reducing the adverse medical implications.

Keywords Alcoholism • Liver disease • Vascular manifestations • Nutritional and metabolic diseases

15.1 Introduction

Alcoholism is a chronic, progressive, and potentially lethal disease characterized by alcohol dependence and multiorgan dysfunction. It is characterized by the loss of consumption control and by a continuous alcohol intake. Genetic, environmental, and psychosocial factors play a very important role in its development [1–4]. An alcoholic is defined as a patient who is used to drinking 80 g/day (3 oz) of alcohol, corresponding to about seven to nine drinks or bottles of beer or glasses of wine for more than 3 months. Alcohol abuse leads to several physical and social problems, and for these reasons, it represents one of the major topics in which medical interest is focused.

The World Health Organization estimates that about 76 million people throughout the world suffer from alcohol-related disorders. Problem drinkers are mostly found in young adults between the ages of 18 and 29. Conversely, the age group with the fewest alcohol problems is adults who are 65 years old or older.

Numerous studies suggest a significant relationship between work stress and the development of drinking problems [1, 2, 4, 5].

Alcohol is a water and lipid-soluble molecule, and it spreads into all tissues of the body and affects most vital functions. In fact, it can cause many physical and mental diseases and can lead ultimately to liver cirrhosis. It is also an important factor in cancer development. People with serious drinking problems have a significantly increased morbidity and mortality when compared with people of same sex and age.

15.2 Clinical and Pathological Aspects of Skin Manifestations

Cutaneous manifestations are common in alcoholics. In fact, the prevalence and severity of some skin diseases are increased in patients prone to excessive alcohol intake, even though there are no specific signs of alcoholism [4, 6, 7]. Most of them are induced by liver toxicity, by an inappropriate diet or by various organ dysfunctions.

Cutaneous manifestations in alcoholics can be divided into: (1) Skin diseases significantly associated with alcoholism and mediated by liver toxicity, (2) Nutritional and metabolic diseases with skin symptoms induced by alcoholism, and (3) Skin diseases exacerbated by alcohol.

15.2.1 Skin Diseases Significantly Associated with Alcoholism

They include *vascular manifestations* such as *flushing, spider angiomas, palmar erythema, purpura, and teleangiectasias* [8]. "*Flushing*" represents one of the most common skin

T. Lotti (✉)
Department of Dermatological Sciences, University of Florence, Via Lorenzo il Magnifico, 104, 50129 Florence, Italy
e-mail: torello.lotti@unifi.it

F. Rongioletti and B.R. Smoller (eds.), *Clinical and Pathological Aspects of Skin Diseases in Endocrine, Metabolic, Nutritional and Deposition Disease*, DOI 10.1007/978-1-60761-181-3_15, © Springer Science+Business Media, LLC 2010

manifestations of acute alcohol consumption, characterized by a transient reddening of the face and neck (Fig. 15.1), leading to the development of rosacea. Flushing accompanied by nausea, dizziness, headache, vomiting, and somnolence is a symptom of the alcohol flush reaction (Oriental flushing syndrome), especially occurring in persons of Oriental origin due to a liver deficit of aldehyde dehydrogenase that leads to acetaldehyde accumulation and vasodilatation. Topical calcineurin inhibitor use has been implicated in a flushing reaction associated with ethanol ingestion [9]. Alcoholics often suffer from erythematous conjunctivae, with thickened eyelid margins [2, 4, 6].

Spider angiomas, palmar erythema, petechiae, and teleangiectasias represent the classic cutaneous stigmata of liver cirrhosis [3, 4]. *Spider angiomas* are the most common vascular abnormalities of liver disease and alcohol abuse, due to a dilatation of superficial cutaneous arterioles (Figs. 15.2 and 15.3). They appear as slightly raised, reddish,

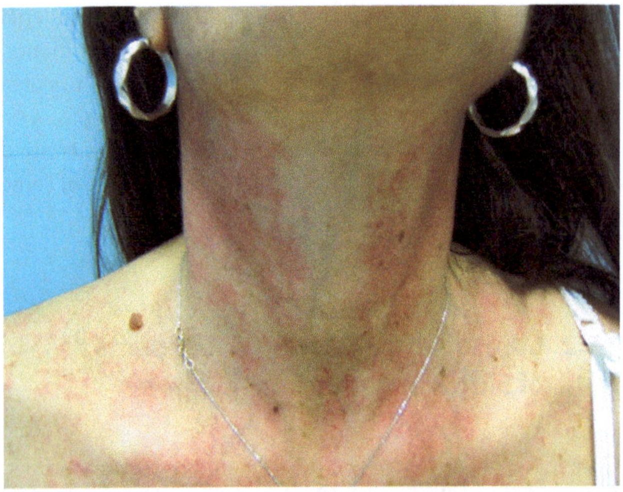

Fig. 15.1 Flushing reaction after alcohol intake

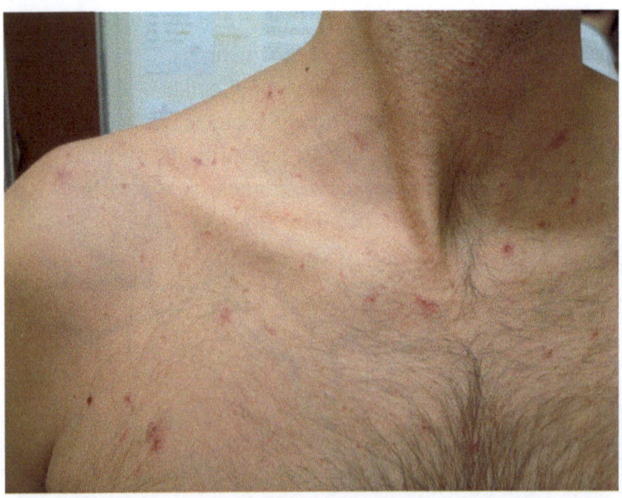

Fig. 15.2 Multiple spider angiomas in an alcoholic

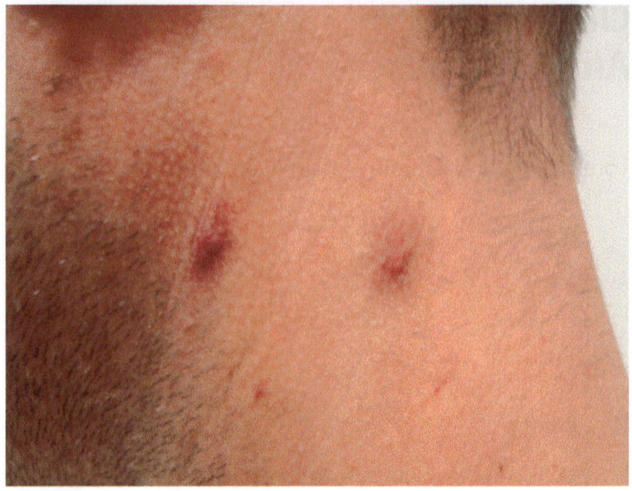

Fig. 15.3 Close-up of some spider angiomas

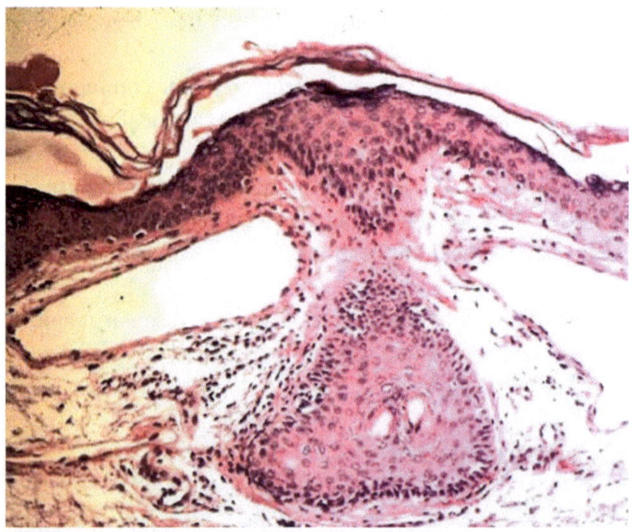

Fig. 15.4 Histopathology of spider angiomas showing a dilated dermal arteriole that communicates with dilated superficial capillaries

small spots from which fine lines radiate outward, giving them a spider-like appearance. Spider nevi can occur anywhere on the body, but preferential sites are the face, the neck, and the trunk [3, 4]. A number of more than 20 spider angiomas seems to be related to the severity of liver cirrhosis. Histologically, spider angioma consists of a vertically oriented central dilated arteriole branching into smaller vessels in the dermis (Fig. 15.4).

Palmar erythema is characterized by warm, florid, light-red patches usually on the palms of the hands and the fingertips (Fig. 15.5) [3, 4]. It has been attributed to a disruption of the body's androgen balance that causes local vasodilatation and erythema. The combination of palmar erythema, spider angiomas and Dupuytren contracture, a progressive fibrosis and thickening of palmar fascia is common in alcoholic cirrhosis [10].

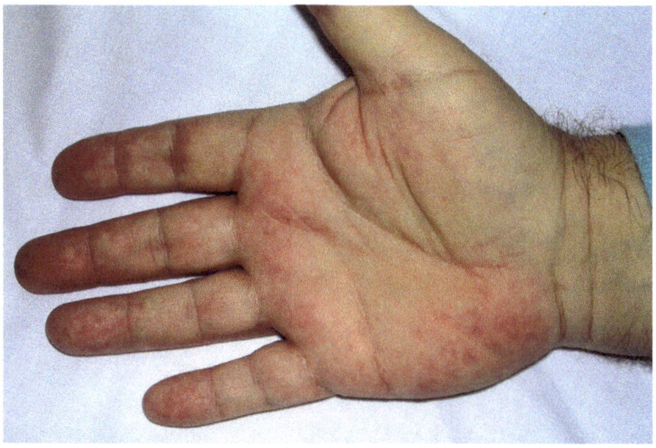

Fig. 15.5 Palmar erythema in an alcoholic with liver disease

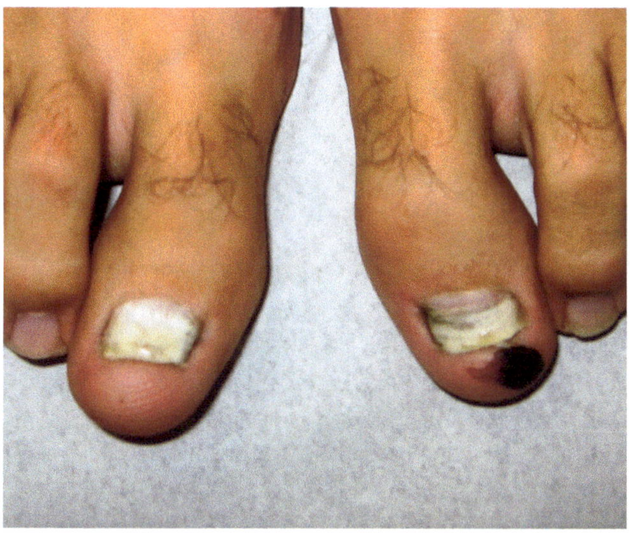

Fig. 15.6 Ecchymotic lesion and white onychomycosis in an alcoholic

Paper-money skin (or dollar-paper markings) describes a condition in which the upper trunk is covered with many randomly scattered, thin capillaries [10].

Petechiae and ecchymoses (Fig. 15.6), mainly on the lower limbs, are due to prothrombin deficiency consequent to impaired liver function. In addition, skin of the abdomen can exhibit dilated umbilical veins that are called caput medusae due to portal hypertension.

Other common skin manifestations of alcoholic liver cirrhosis are *nail changes seen in* 25% of patients and oral mucosal changes found in 54% of patients [11]. The former include clubbing, koilonychias (Fig. 15.7), leukonychia (Fig. 15.8), Terry's nails, and Muercke nails. Terry's nails present with an opaque white nail plate, with the exception of the distal part, which retains its normal color (Fig. 15.9) [10–13], while in Muercke nails we observe multiple, parallel white bands. These forms of leukonychia are due to an increase in subungual connective tissue leading to compression of

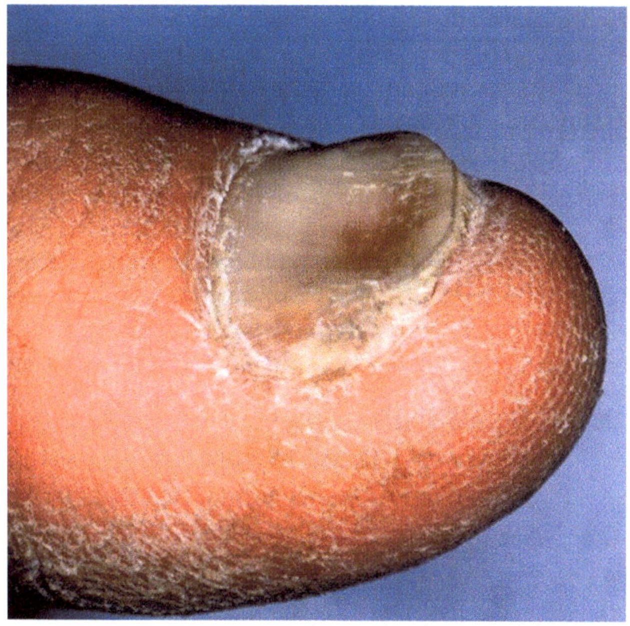

Fig. 15.7 Koilonychia (courtesy of G.E. Cannata, Imperia, Italy)

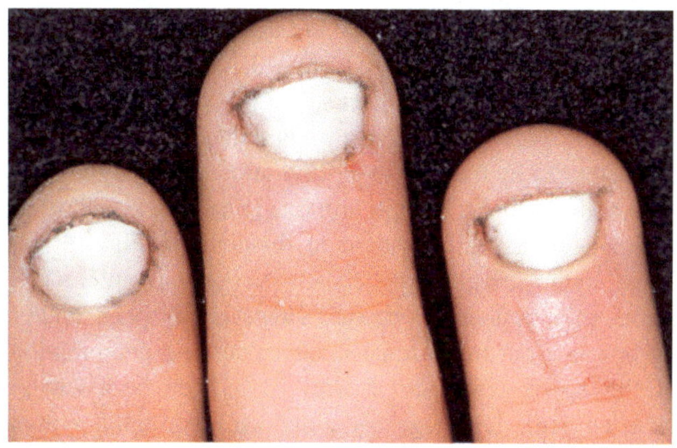

Fig. 15.8 Total leukonychia (courtesy of G.E. Cannata, Imperia, Italy)

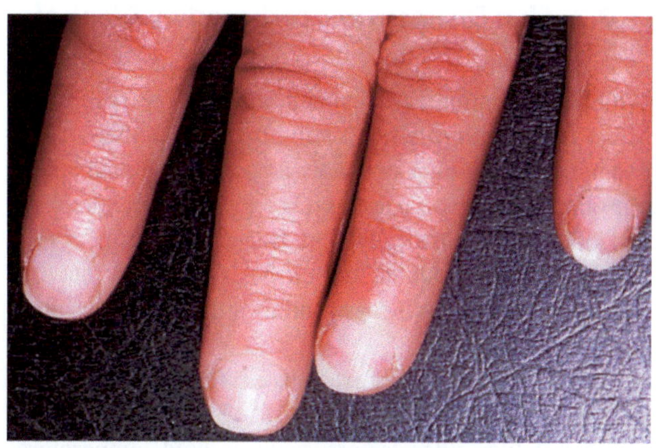

Fig. 15.9 Terry's nail (half and half nail) in a cirrhotic patient

capillaries. Alopecia of axillary, pubic, and chest hairs induced by hormonal changes is seen mostly in men.

Pruritus may precede liver cirrhosis, and it does not seem to be necessarily related to hepatic functional impairment itself [3, 4, 6]. An eczematous reaction with features of acquired zinc deficiency dermatosis in the perineum and inner thighs and histological features of spongiotic dermatitis has been considered as a separate skin manifestation of chronic alcohol excess [14].

15.2.2 Nutritional and Metabolic Diseases with Skin Symptoms Induced by Alcoholism

Porphyria cutanea tarda, characterized by blistering of the skin in areas that receive higher levels of exposure to sunlight, has been associated with alcohol intake and liver dysfunction [22, 23] (see also Chap. 10). *Oral changes* including glossitis, angular cheilitis, pellagra and pellagroid dermatoses, hyperpigmentation, and acquired manifestation of acrodermatitis enteropathica are due to nutritional dysvitaminoses [3, 4, 15] (see also Chap. 13).

Multiple Symmetrical Lipomatosis (Lipomatosis of Lanois–Bensaude, Madelung's Disease) is a metabolic condition characterized by the growth of fatty masses around the face, back of the head, neck, upper arms, abdomen, back, and upper leg in a very specific pattern or distribution (Fig. 15.10). These symmetrical fatty deposits are asymptomatic and cause only aesthetic concerns. However, dyspnea and/or dysphagia from mediastinal involvement and compression of the upper aerodigestive tract have been occasionally reported [16]. Histologically adipocytes are smaller than normal and relatively uniform in size (see also Chap. 8).

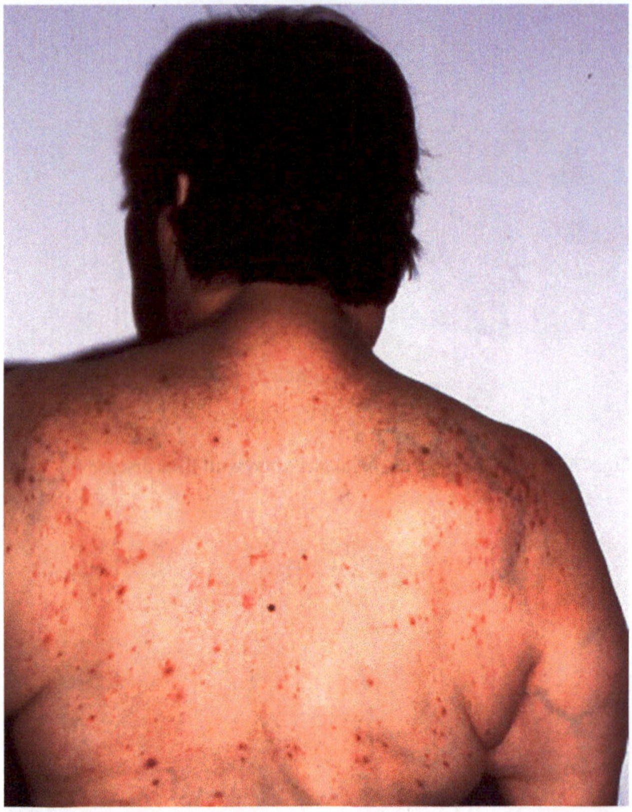

Fig. 15.10 Madelung's disease (multiple symmetrical lipomatosis) with multiple spider angiomas in an alcoholic

15.2.3 Skin Diseases Exacerbated by Alcohol

Alcohol assumption is associated with a more severe and diffuse form of *psoriasis*. It is still not clear whether alcohol assumption is causative or simply associated with the course of psoriasis and its social and psychological burden. Excessive alcohol intake is statistically more frequent in psoriatics than in the general population, and cirrhosis has been found to cause more deaths among psoriatics than among other patients [4, 17, 18].

Alcohol assumption also exacerbates *seborrheic dermatitis*, *rosacea*, and *acne vulgaris* [15].

Alcohol like other factors, such as cold temperature, sunlight, spicy food emotions, irritant cosmetics, and drugs, can worsen the progression of rosacea. In addition, patients with excessive alcohol intake had an increased level of collagen III propeptide, a marker of enhanced collagen metabolism that may play a role in the mechanism of hyperplasia of connective and sebaceous tissues such as *rhinophyma*, observed in grade IV rosacea (Fig. 15.11a, b) [4].

Alcohol consumption in some patients could aggravate acne vulgaris, even though no direct causal relationship has been demonstrated. The metabolism and pharmacokinetics of isotretinoin and its main metabolites are not influenced by ethanol during long-term isotretinoin treatment [19]. Several atopic and allergic disorders are common in people with alcohol abuse. In fact, alcohol intake may aggravate *nummular eczematous dermatitis* that is characterized by a persistent, itchy rash forming coin-shaped patches on the skin (Fig. 15.12).

Urticaria, anaphylactoid reactions, and intolerance syndromes can be induced by ethanol itself and are dose-dependent [20].

Alcohol can result in a depression of the immune system [3, 4] by inhibiting T-lymphocytes and reducing the function of neutrophils and natural killer cells; consequently, skin infections such as pityriasis versicolor, onychomycosis (Fig. 15.6), and other forms of dermatomycoses are increased in alcoholics [4, 15]. Disseminated superficial porokeratosis

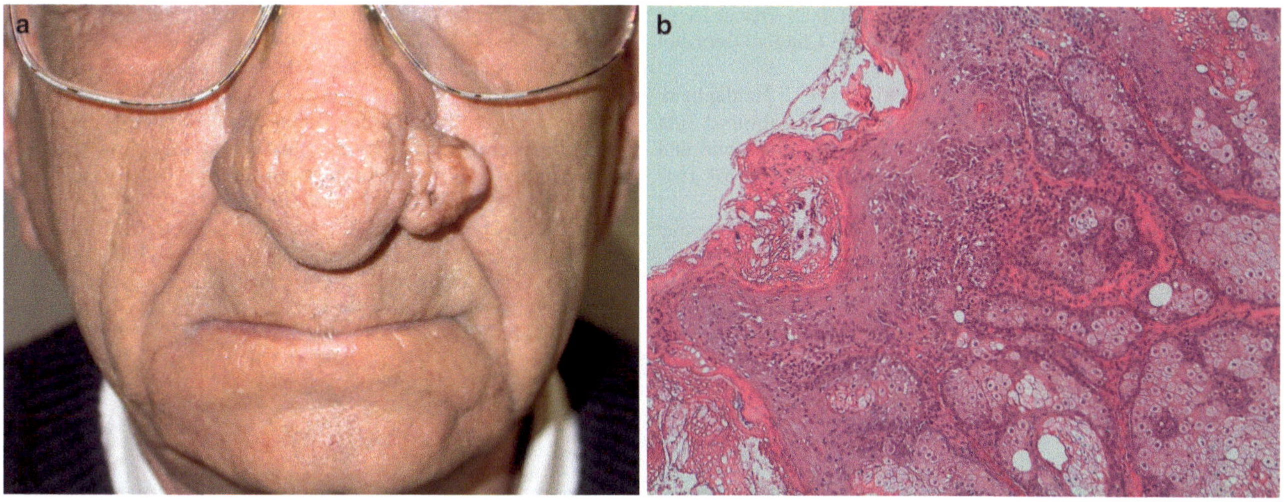

Fig. 15.11 (**a**) Rhinophyma in an alcoholic. (**b**) Rhinophyma with hyperkeratosis, sebaceous hyperplasia, fibrosis, ectatic vessels, and Demodex in the follicular ostium

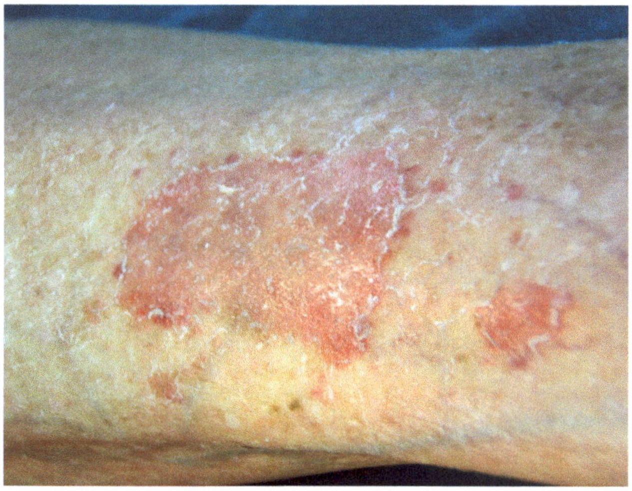

Fig. 15.12 Nummular eczema in alcoholic

has also been described in the setting of alcohol-induced immune depression [4]. Alcohol is also involved in the development of oral cancer [21].

15.3 Treatment and Prognosis

Reducing or avoiding alcohol intake and its metabolites is the most important measure in treating all the manifestations induced by alcohol abuse, including cutaneous signs.

Vascular manifestations such as spider angiomas can be treated with electrodessication or laser therapy. Surgery is the most effective treatment for multiple symmetric lipomatosis.

References

1. Morse RM, Flavin DK (1992) The definition of alcoholism. JAMA 268:1012–1014
2. Sanchez MR (1999) Alcohol, social behavior disorders, and their cutaneous manifestations. Clin Dermatol 17:479–489
3. Vogl A, Landthaler M, Vogt T (2005) Skin and alcohol (article in German). J Dtsch Dermatol Ges 3:788–790, 792–807
4. Kostović K, Lipozencić J (2004) Skin diseases in alcoholics. Acta Dermatovenerol Croat 12:181–190
5. Rosset M, Oki G (1971) Skin diseases in alcoholics. Q J Stud Alcohol 32:1017–1022
6. Wegrzynek I, Budzanowska E (2001) Alcohol and the skin. Przegl Lek 58:198–203
7. Higgins EM, du Vivier AW (1994) Alcohol abuse and treatment resistance in skin disease. J Am Acad Dermatol 30:1048
8. Wolf R, Tüzün B, Tüzün Y (1999) Alcohol ingestion and the cutaneous vasculature. Clin Dermatol 17:395–403
9. Stinco G, Piccirillo F, Sallustio M, Patrone P (2009) Facial flush reaction after alcohol ingestion during topical pimecrolimus and tacrolimus treatment. Dermatology 218:71–72
10. Hazin R, Abu-Rajab Tamimi TI, Abuzetun JY, Zein NN (2009) Recognizing and treating cutaneous signs of liver disease. Cleve Clin J Med 76:599–606
11. Rao GS (2004) Cutaneous changes in chronic alcoholics. Indian J Dermatol Venereol Leprol 70(2):79–81
12. Ruocco V, Psilogenis M, Schiavo A, Wolf R (1999) Dermatological manifestations of alcoholic cirrhosis. Clin Dermatol 17:463–468
13. Albrecht G (2000) Skin manifestations of alcoholic liver damage. Ther Umsch 57(4):232–235
14. Wahie S, Lawrence CM (2006) Cutaneous signs as a presenting manifestation of alcohol excess. Br J Dermatol 155:195–197
15. Smith K, Fenske N (2000) Cutaneous manifestations of alcohol abuse. J Am Acad Dermatol 43:1–16
16. Adamo C, Vescio G, Battaglia M et al (2001) Madelung's disease: case report and discussion of treatment options. Ann Plast Surg 46:43–45
17. Wolf R, Wolf D, Ruocco V (1999) Alcohol intake and psoriasis. Clin Dermatol 17:423–430

18. Tobin AM, Higgins EM, Norris S, Kirby B (2009) Prevalence of psoriasis in patients with alcoholic liver disease. Clin Exp Dermatol 34:698–701
19. Grønhøj Larsen F, Jakobsen P, Grønhøj Larsen C, Heidenheim M, Held E, Nielsen-Kudsk F (2009) The metabolism and pharmacokinetics of isotretinoin in patients with acne and rosacea are not influenced by ethanol. Br J Dermatol 161: 664–670
20. Sticherling M, Brasch J (1999) Alcohol: intolerance syndrome, urticarial and anaphylactoid reactions. Clin Dermatol 17: 417–422
21. Figuero Ruiz E, Carretero Peláez MA, Cerero Lapiedra R, Esparza Gómez G, Moreno López LA (2004) Effects of the consumption of alcohol in the oral cavity: relationship with oral cancer. Med Oral 9:14–23
23. Castiella A, Zapata E, de Juan MD, Múgica F, Barrio J, Otazua P, Arriola JA, Cosme A, Elosegui E, Fernández J, Zubiaurre L, Alzate LF, Utrilla E; Grupo Porfiria Guipúzcoa (2008) Porphyria cutanea tarda. An analysis of HFE gene mutations, hepatitis viruses, alcohol intake, and other risk factors in 54 patients from Guipúzcoa, Basque Country, Spain. Rev Esp Enferm Dig 100:774–778
24. Cassiman D, Vannoote J, Roelandts R, Libbrecht L, Roskams T, Van den Oord J, Fevery J, Garmyn M, Nevens F (2008) Porphyria cutanea tarda and liver disease. A retrospective analysis of 17 cases from a single centre and review of the literature. Acta Gastroenterol Belg 71:237–242

Chapter 16
Glucagonoma Syndrome and Necrolytic Migratory Erythema

Franco Rongioletti

Key Points

- Necrolytic migratory erythema is a cutaneous paraneoplastic manifestation, which is usually associated with a glucagon-secreting pancreatic tumor.
- Clues to the diagnosis are the anatomic distribution (perioral, acral, and genital), the waxing and waning course, the figurate migratory lesions with advancing scaling borders, and the distinctive histopathologic pattern with pale, vacuolated keratinocytes in the upper epidermis.
- Necrolytic migratory erythema heals once the glucagonoma has been surgically removed, but in 50% of these cases metastasis exists at the moment of the diagnosis.

Keywords Necrolytic migratory erythema • Glucagon-secreting pancreatic tumor • Glucagonoma syndrome

16.1 Introduction

Glucagonoma is a rare neuroendocrine tumor that originates from the alpha-2 cells of the pancreas. The occurrence rate for glucagonoma is estimated to be 1 in 20 million per year [1]. In 75–80% of cases, the glucagonoma starts in malignant form, and in 50% of these cases, metastasis exists at the moment of the diagnosis. The most common site for metastasis is the liver. Glucagonoma syndrome is an uncommon clinicopathologic entity, typically present near the fifth decade with an even male/female distribution, characterized by a glucagonoma associated with hyperglucagonemia, diabetes mellitus, weight loss, diarrhea, steatorrhea, anemia, hypoaminoacidemia, thromboembolic disease, psychiatric disturbances, and *necrolytic migratory erythema* (NME).

F. Rongioletti (✉)
Department of Endocrinological and Medical Sciences (DISEM)
Section of Dermatology and Department of Pathology
University of Genova, Genova, Italy
e-mail: franco.rongioletti@unige.it

16.2 Clinical and Pathological Aspects of Skin Manifestations

The cutaneous lesions are called NME owing to their similarities to both toxic epidermal necrolysis and annular erythema and present in approximately 65–70% of patients at the time of diagnosis. The eruption usually is widespread and occurs as spontaneous exacerbations and remissions (for weeks or months). It commonly manifests as itchy and painful erythematous figurate, annular or circinate migratory lesions with advancing scaling borders (Fig. 16.1), vesicles or bulla formation, and crusts (Fig. 16.2) that leave a residual hyperpigmentation. The intertriginous areas such as the groin (Fig. 16.3), perineum, buttocks, the trunk, the lower extremities (Fig. 16.4), the perioral skin, and sites of minor trauma are the preferred locations. Other dermatological manifestations of the glucagonoma syndrome are dystrophic nails, angular cheilitis (Fig. 16.5), and atrophic glossitis. Differential diagnoses include pemphigus foliaceus, acrodermatitis enteropathica, chronic mucocutaneous candidiasis, psoriasis, and severe seborrheic dermatitis [2].

Clues to the diagnosis are the anatomic distribution (perioral, acral, and genital), the waxing and waning course, and the characteristic or suggestive histopathologic features.

The most distinctive histopathologic pattern of NME is the presence of pale and sometimes vacuolated, swollen keratinocytes of the upper epidermis (Fig. 16.6). Dyskeratotic or necrotic keratinocytes are common, leading to confluent superficial epidermal necrosis with cleavage beneath the stratum corneum or within the upper third of the viable epidermis (Fig. 16.7). Angioplasia of the papillary dermis and a superficial mild perivascular lymphohistiocytic infiltrate are usually present. Subcorneal pustules can be found, sometimes associated with *Candida* superinfection (Fig. 16.8), in which case a neutrophilic infiltration is present [3, 4].

Irregular acanthosis with focal spongiosis, crust formation, confluent parakeratosis, and psoriasiform hyperplasia in the absence of vacuolated and necrotic keratinocytes have also been reported (Fig. 16.9) [5]. Eosinophils in the infiltrate and acantholysis are rare features. The results of direct

F. Rongioletti and B.R. Smoller (eds.), *Clinical and Pathological Aspects of Skin Diseases in Endocrine, Metabolic, Nutritional and Deposition Disease*, DOI 10.1007/978-1-60761-181-3_16, © Springer Science+Business Media, LLC 2010

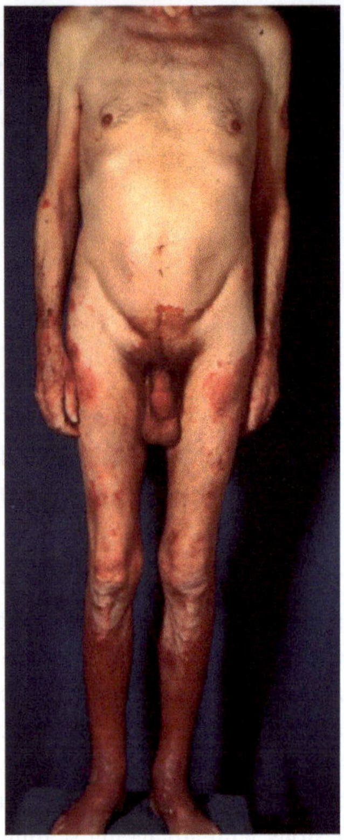

Fig. 16.1 Necrolytic migratory erythema

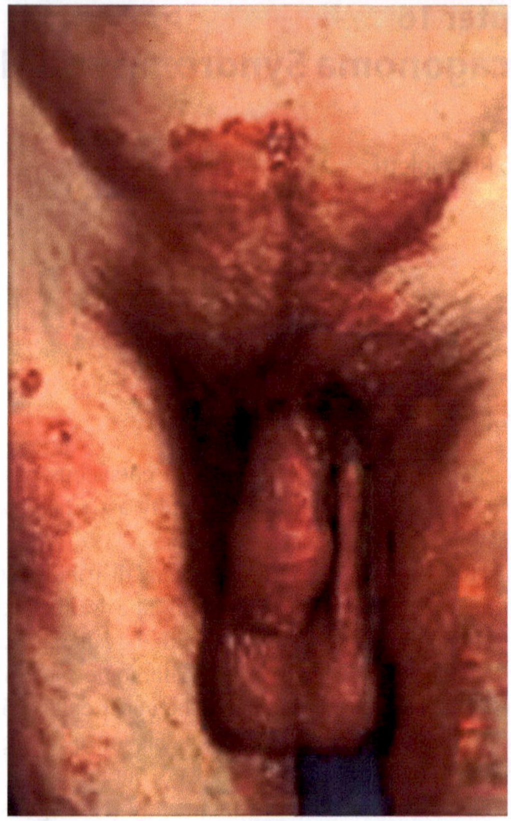

Fig. 16.3 Lesions on the groin and genital area

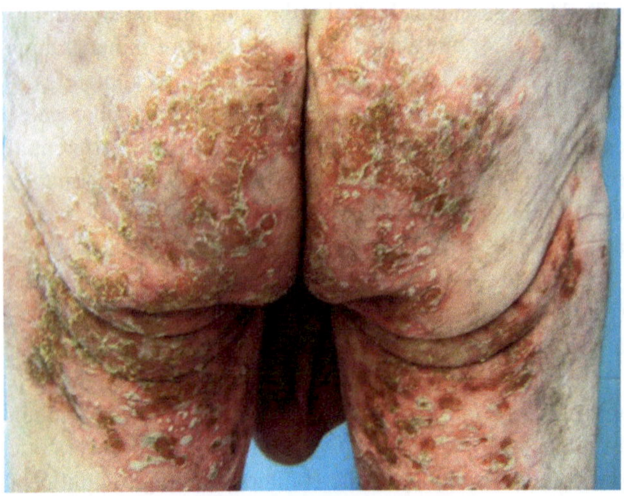

Fig. 16.2 Figurate migratory lesions with vesicopustules and advancing scaling borders

immunofluorescence studies usually are negative, but C3 deposits may occur at the dermal – epidermal junction and around blood vessels. Histological features of NME are quite similar to acrodermatitis enteropathica and pellagra.

Alhough NME is suggestive of glucagonoma, it is not specific. Pseudoglucagonoma syndrome refers to NME in the absence of a glucagon-secreting tumor. The pseudoglucagonoma syndrome may be due to liver diseases, pellagra,

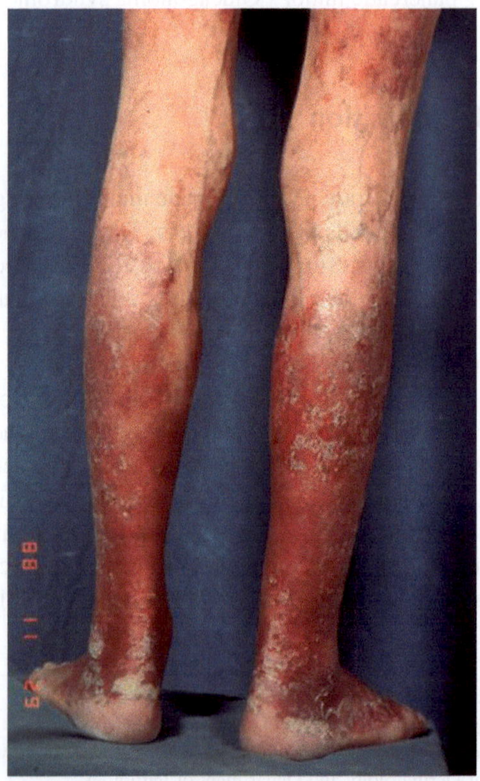

Fig. 16.4 Erythematous lesions of the legs in necrolytic migratory erythema

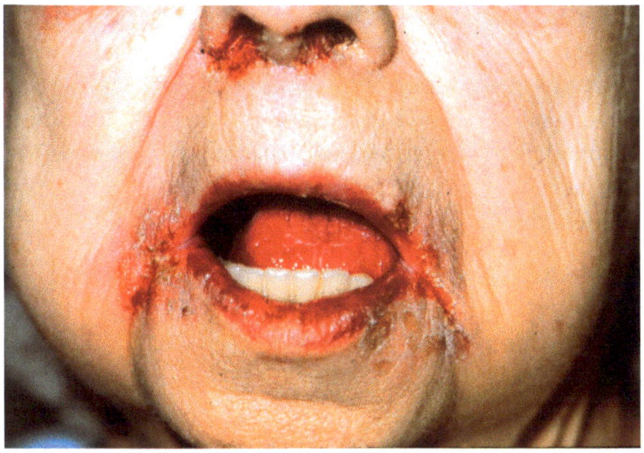

Fig. 16.5 Angular cheilitis and perinasal dermatitis in necrolytic migratory erythema

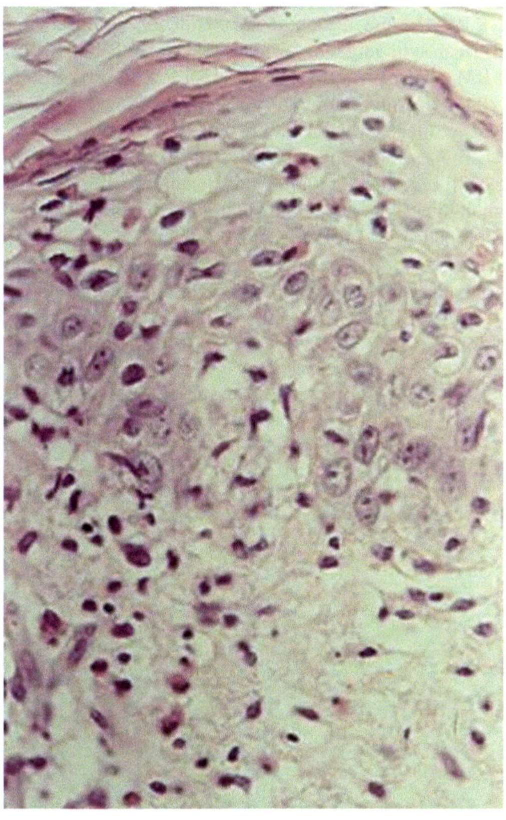

Fig. 16.6 Pale, vacuolated, swollen keratinocytes of the upper epidermis (HE stain)

acrodermatitis enteropathica, celiac sprue, chronic pancreatitis, jejunal adenocarcinoma, neuroendocrine insulin-producing tumor, myelodysplastic syndrome, inflammatory bowel disease, heroin abuse, or odontogenic abscess [6].

Although the pathogenesis of this disorder is still poorly understood, the cutaneous manifestation seems to be due to a deficiency of amino acids secondary to diversion of them to synthesis of glucagon rather than to the excess of

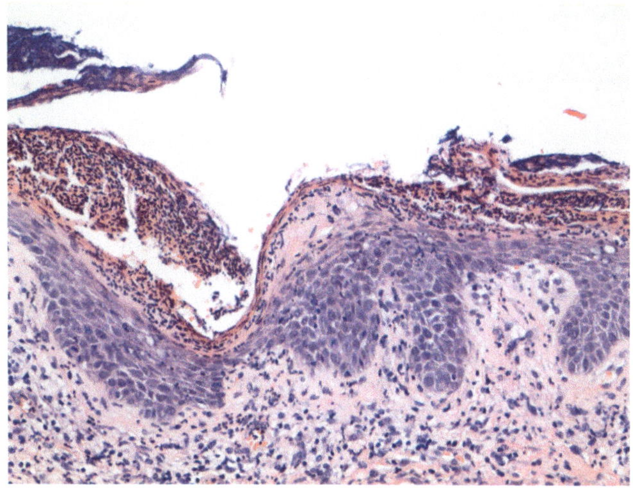

Fig. 16.7 Confluent superficial epidermal necrosis with cleavage beneath the parakeratotic and crusted stratum corneum (HE stain)

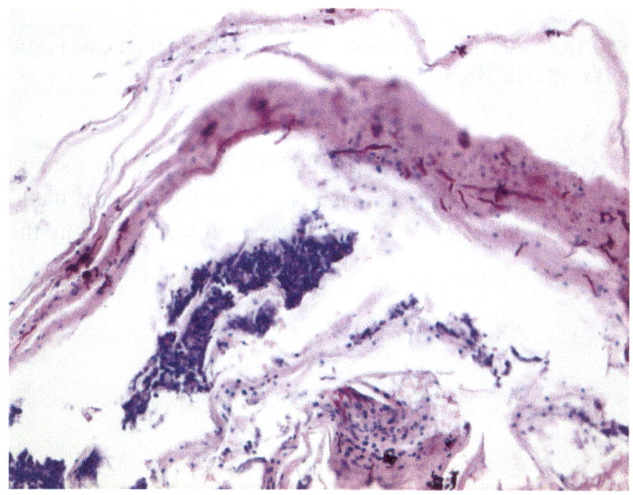

Fig. 16.8 *Candida* infection superimposed on necrolytic migratory erythema (PAS stain)

glucagon. Nonetheless, it appears that a nutritional lack of zinc and fatty acids, or hepatocellular dysfunctions might be involved.

16.3 Treatment and Prognosis

NML usually heals once the glucagonoma tumor has been surgically removed. Treatment of the skin eruption before surgery may be challenging. Topical and systemic steroids, antibiotics, radiation, ultraviolet-light therapy, vitamins including nicotinamide, methotrexate, dapsone, tar preparations, and other medications have been used singly or in combination with limited success.

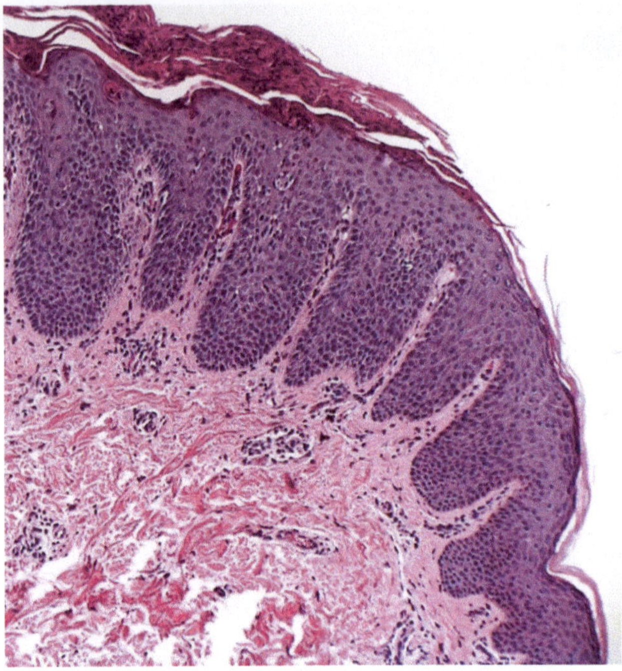

Fig. 16.9 Psoriasiform dermatitis in a patient with necrolytic migratory erythema (HE stain)

Glucagonomas are generally slow-growing but usually advanced by the time of diagnosis. Once the tumor is metastatic, cure is rarely, if ever, achieved. However, despite the presence of metastases, many patients are able to experience prolonged survival. Estimations of mean survival after diagnosis have ranged from 3 to 7 years or more. Often, the correct diagnosis is delayed for a long period, up to 12 years. It is important to recognize NME because early diagnosis and treatment may prevent metastasis of the islet-cell tumor and be lifesaving.

References

1. Remes-Troche JM, García-de-Acevedo B, Zuñiga-Varga J, Avila-Funes A, Orozco-Topete R (2004) Necrolytic migratory erythema: a cutaneous clue to glucagonoma syndrome. J Eur Acad Dermatol Venereol 18:591–595
2. Gantcheva ML, Broshtilova VK, Lalova AI (2007) Necrolytic migratory erythema: the outermost marker for glucagonoma syndrome. Arch Dermatol 143:1221–1222
3. Kovács RK, Korom I, Dobozy A, Farkas G, Ormos J, Kemény L (2006) Necrolytic migratory erythema. J Cutan Pathol 33:242–245
4. Pujol RM, Wang CY, el-Azhary RA, Su WP, Gibson LE, Schroeter AL (2004) Necrolytic migratory erythema: clinicopathologic study of 13 cases. Int J Dermatol 43:12–18
5. Vega J, Bouzari N, Romanelli P, Lanuti EL, Benedetto P, Green A, Rongioletti F, Kerdel F (2008) Clinicopathologic challenge: an intermittent inguinal rash of 3 months' duration that progressed to involve the hands and arms. Int J Dermatol 47:332–334
6. Technau K, Renkl A, Norgauer J, Ziemer M (2005) Necrolytic migratory erythema with myelodysplastic syndrome without glucagonoma. Eur J Dermatol 15:110–112

Part IV
Cutaneous Deposition Disease

Chapter 17
Amyloidoses

Franco Rongioletti

Key Points

- Amyloidoses are a heterogeneous group of diseases in which a fibrillar proteinaceous insoluble material called amyloid accumulates in various tissues and organs.
- Amyloid is not a single substance but describes various types of *protein* aggregations that share the characteristic unifying properties of congophilia and doubly refractile green color under polariscopy, distinctive fibrillar ultrastructure, and a β-pleated sheet structural conformation.
- Amyloidoses are identified according to the nature of the main amyloid precursor protein and classified into systemic amyloidoses and localized cutaneous amyloidoses.
- Systemic amyloidoses include primary, secondary, and hereditary/familial forms, while the primary localized cutaneous amyloidoses include three major forms: lichen amyloidosis and macular amyloidosis in which amyloid deposits are due to keratin, and primary nodular cutaneous amyloidosis that occurs as a result of deposition of immunoglobulin light chains produced by a local proliferation of plasma cells.
- Among the systemic amyloidoses, primary and myeloma-associated systemic amyloidosis is the most common form in which 40% of patients develop mucocutaneous disease, while secondary systemic amyloidoses and hemodialysis-associated amyloidosis present rarely with cutaneous involvement.

Keywords Amyloid • Systemic amyloidoses • Primary localized cutaneous amyloidoses • Lichen amyloidosis • Macular amyloidosis • Nodular amyloidosis

17.1 Introduction

Amyloidoses are a heterogeneous group of diseases in which a fibrillar proteinaceous insoluble material called amyloid accumulates in various tissues and organs, impairing normal function. Amyloid is not a single chemically distinct substance but describes various types of *protein* aggregations that share the unifying feature of a β-pleated sheet structural conformation through X-ray diffraction with unique staining features. Characteristic properties of amyloid include an eosinophilic amorphous hyaline appearance with the hematoxylin and eosin stain, an orange-red color with Congo red staining resulting in doubly refractile green color under polariscopy, metachromasia with crystal violet stain, thioflavine T fluorescence, and a fibrillar structure made by straight, nonbranching filaments (7–10 nm in diameter) on electron microscopy (1). All amyloid deposits, irrespective of their chemical nature and the clinical type of amyloidosis, have a common amyloid P component which is a nonfibrillar protein derived from a serum precursor, known as serum amyloid P (SAP). Amyloid can be detected by immunohistochemical stains on paraffin-embedded sections using antibodies against human component P (anti-SAP); however, the specificity of this reaction is limited as amyloid P is also present in elastic tissue. Immunohistochemical staining with antibodies directed against specific precursors is more helpful in differentiating the various types of amyloid. DNA testing is also useful in the hereditary forms.

The most recent classification identifies amyloidoses according to the nature of the main amyloid precursor protein, and up to 27 different proteins have been recognized to date to be amyloidogenic in humans. However, six are the major precursor proteins of dermatological interest: immunoglobulin light chain-derived (AL), serum amyloid A protein (SAA), ß2-microglobulin, transthyretin (ATTR), gelsolin (AGel amyloidosis), and epidermal keratinocyte keratins (amyloid-K). Clinically, amyloidoses can be classified as systemic (generalized) or localized (limited to a single organ, i.e., the skin) and acquired or hereditary (2). Systemic and localized cutaneous amyloidoses can be further subclassified as primary or secondary.

AL is seen in the setting of primary and myeloma-associated systemic amyloidosis or nodular cutaneous amyloidosis; serum amyloid A protein (SAA), an acute phase reactant synthesized by the liver, is found in secondary AA

F. Rongioletti (✉)
Department of Endocrinological and Medical Sciences (DISEM)
Section of Dermatology and Department of Pathology
University of Genova, Genova, Italy
e-mail: franco.rongioletti@unige.it

F. Rongioletti and B.R. Smoller (eds.), *Clinical and Pathological Aspects of Skin Diseases in Endocrine, Metabolic, Nutritional and Deposition Disease*, DOI 10.1007/978-1-60761-181-3_17,

Table 17.1 Main forms of amyloidoses with dermatologic interest

Amyloid protein	Precursor	Systemic (S) or localized cutaneous (LC)	Underlying disease
AL	Immunoglobulin light chain (kappa, lambda)	S LC (Nodular amyloidosis)	Primary Myeloma-associated
AA	(Apo)serum amyloid A	S	Chronic inflammation
$A\beta_2M$	β_2-microglobulin	S	Long-standing hemodialysis
ATTR	Transthyretin	S	Hereditary (familial amyloidotic polyneuropathy)
AGel	Gelsolin	S	Hereditary
A-K	Epidermal keratinocyte keratin	LC, lichen and macular type	None, sometimes MEN 2A

systemic amyloidosis caused by chronic inflammation; β_2-microglobulin is seen in the setting of amyloidosis of chronic hemodialysis; ATTR is seen in a hereditary form caused by more than 80 autosomal dominant hereditary point mutations; gelsolin amyloidosis (AGel amyloidosis) is responsible for an hereditary amyloidosis-associated form of cutis laxa; amyloid-K is found in primary localized cutaneous amyloidoses (Table 17.1).

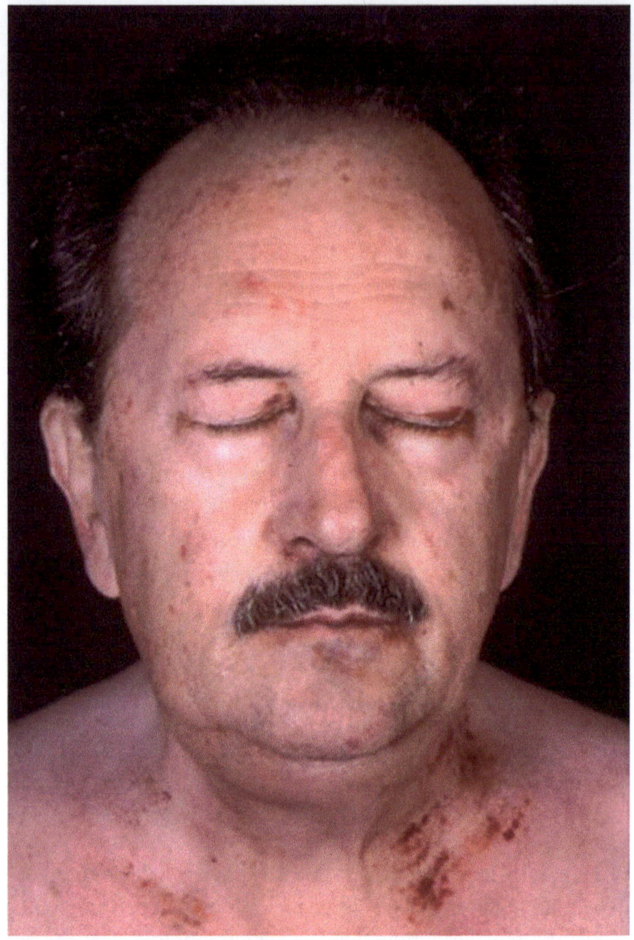

Fig. 17.1 Purpura in periorbital area (racoon sign) and around neck in primary systemic amyloidosis

17.2 Clinical and Pathological Aspects of Skin Manifestations

17.2.1 Acquired Systemic Amyloidoses with Cutaneous Involvement

They can be classified as follows: (1) primary systemic amyloidosis, usually with no evidence of preceding or coexisting paraproteinemia, or plasma-cell dyscrasia and amyloidosis associated with multiple myeloma; (2) secondary systemic amyloidosis with evidence of coexisting previous chronic inflammatory or infectious conditions where cutaneous involvement is nonspecific; (3) β_2-microglobulin hemodialysis-associated amyloidosis.

17.2.1.1 Primary and Myeloma-Associated Amyloidosis (AL Amyloidosis)

Primary and myeloma-associated amyloidosis, also known as amyloid light chain (AL) amyloidosis, is the most common form with an estimated incidence of 0.8 per 100,000 person years in western countries and 1,275–3,200 new cases per year in the USA (3).

Patients are most commonly in their sixties with a slight male predominance. No racial predilection exists. Primary systemic amyloidosis is caused by an occult underlying plasma-cell dyscrasia, and 20% of patients with primary (AL) amyloidosis also have multiple myeloma. Conversely, of all patients with multiple myeloma, 5–15% develop AL amyloid deposits. The AL amyloid is produced by plasma cells in the bone marrow and is more frequently due to lambda than kappa chains (ratio 3:1). These light chains are secreted into the serum and are unique in that they undergo partial lysosomal proteolysis within macrophages, and then, they are extracellularly deposited as insoluble amyloid filaments.

Between 29 and 40% of patients with primary systemic amyloidosis develop mucocutaneous disease (4). These mucocutaneous manifestations are sometimes the first clue to the discovery of systemic involvement. *Nonvasculitic petechiae, purpura, and ecchymoses* involving sites such as the periorbital area (*racoon sign*), lateral side of the neck, axillae, and anogenital area are typical findings (Figs. 17.1 and 17.2). Purpura may be elicited with coughing,

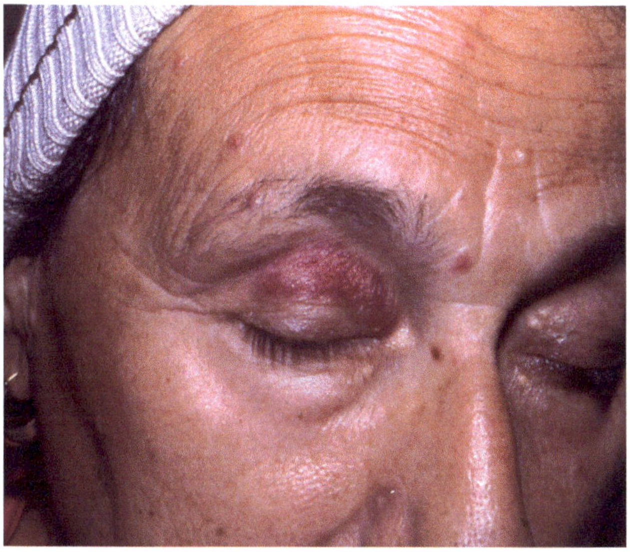

Fig. 17.2 Purpura on the lid in primary systemic amyloidosis

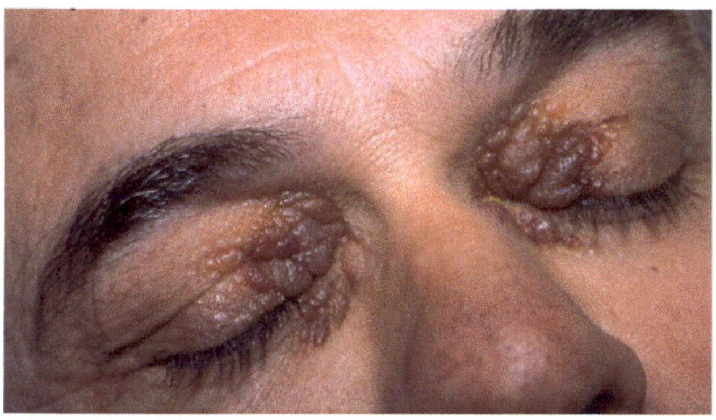

Fig. 17.3 Waxy nodules with hemorrhagic hue in myeloma-associated amyloidosis

after pinching the skin (*pinch purpura*), following proctoscopy or the Valsalva maneuver and is mainly caused by infiltration of vessel walls with amyloid. Acquired factor X deficiency, decreased vitamin K-dependent clotting factors, increased antithrombin activity, or increased fibrinolysis may also play a role. *Waxy translucent papules, plaques and nodules with an hemorrhagic hue* on the flexural folds, face (Fig. 17.3), and trunk (Fig. 17.4) are other common manifestations. Localized deposits of amyloid on the shoulder may result in the *shoulder pad sign*. Other skin signs include yellowish xanthoma-like lesions, diffuse infiltration of the extremities and trunk resulting in scleroderma-like lesions, infiltration of the scalp resembling cutis verticis gyrate with alopecia (Fig. 17.5), bullous lesions with hemorrhagic contents predominating in the axillary folds, anal and inguinal areas mimicking an autoimmune bullous disease, nail dystrophy (Fig. 17.6), cord-like thickening of the blood vessels, cutis laxa-like or pseudoxanthoma elasticum-like lesions and elastolytic lesions of the fingers whose skin

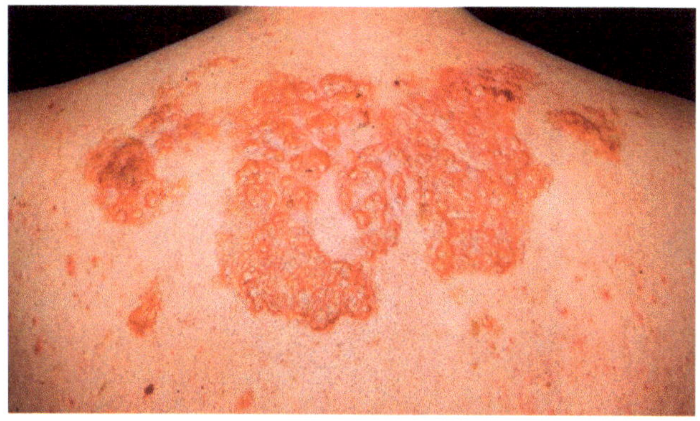

Fig. 17.4 Waxy translucent plaques in primary systemic amyloidosis (Courtesy of M. Black, London)

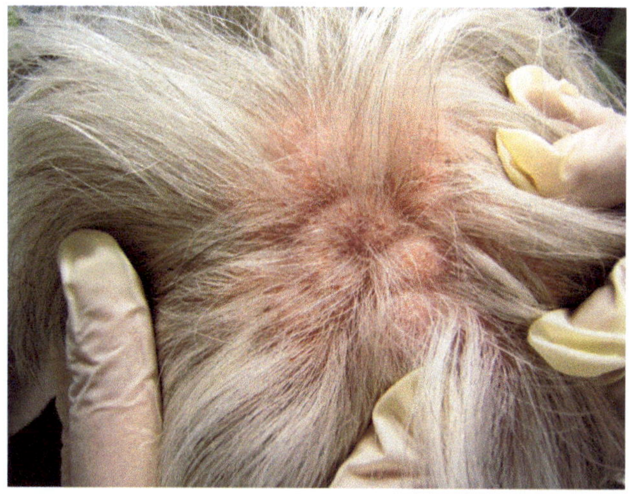

Fig. 17.5 Cutis verticis gyrata due to amyloid in primary systemic amyloidosis

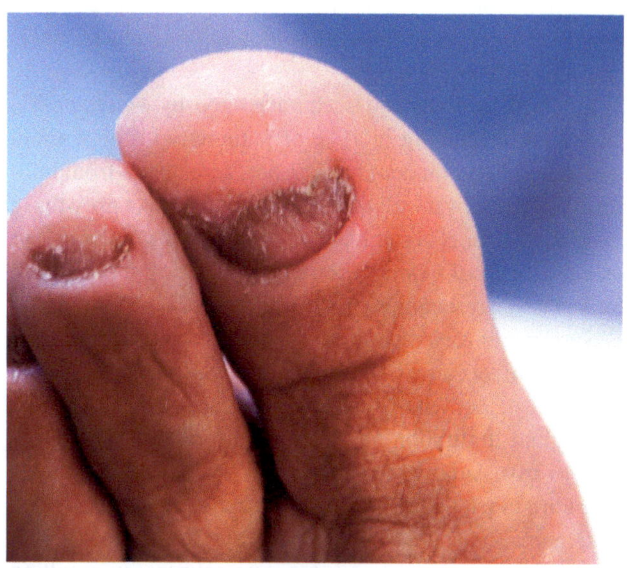

Fig. 17.6 Nail dystrophy due to amyloidosis

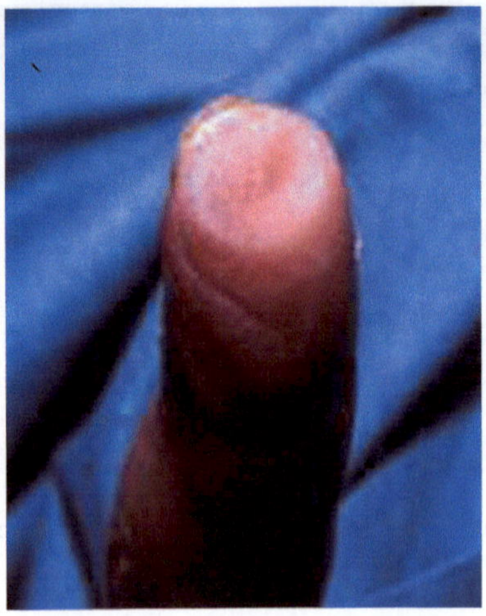

Fig. 17.7 Elastolytic lesion of the pulp of finger in myeloma-associated amyloidosis

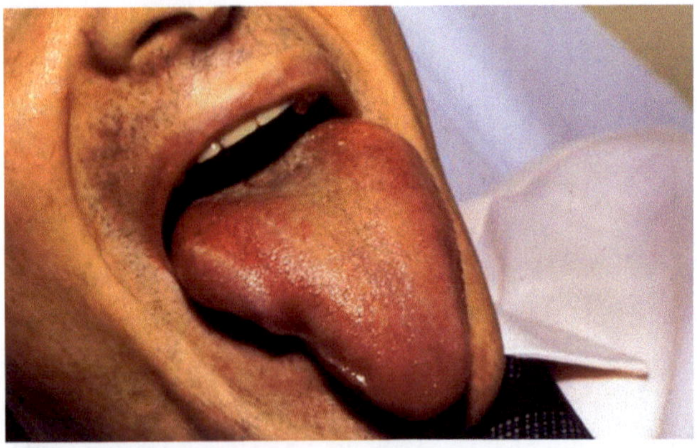

Fig. 17.8 Macroglossia in primary systemic amyloidosis

depresses with pressure and remains depressed for an abnormally long period of time (Fig. 17.7). The latter corresponds to an amyloid deposition in relation to elastic fibers (*amyloid elastosis*) (5).

Mucosal involvement is characterized by *macroglossia* (Fig. 17.8) occurring in 19% of patients with or without hardening of oral mucous membranes, xerostomia from infiltration of the salivary glands, and condyloma-like growths in the genital skin. The findings of *macroglossia*, *bilateral* or *unilateral carpal tunnel syndrome*, and *periorbital purpura* are a classic presentation of AL amyloidosis.

Systemic involvement includes cardiac disease that is the most important cause of mortality secondary to arrhythmias, ischemia or congestive heart failure; hepatomegaly due to amyloid infiltration and cardiac failure seen in 50% of patients associated with splenomegaly; kidney involvement (one-third of patients) manifested as nephrotic syndrome with proteinuria and edema; carpal tunnel syndrome seen in 25% of patients; peripheral and autonomic neuropathy resulting in postural hypotension; gastrointestinal disease with an

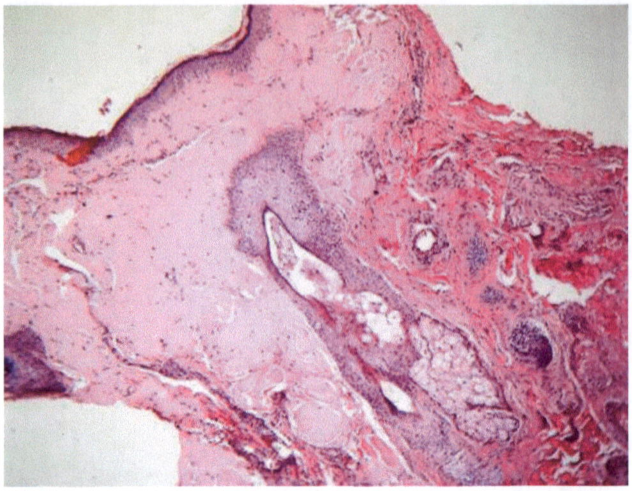

Fig. 17.9 Diffuse, eosinophilic, fissured dermal amyloid deposits in primary systemic amyloidosis (HE stain)

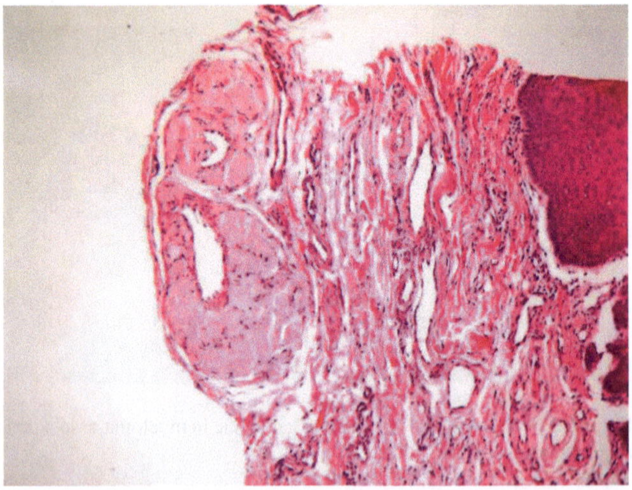

Fig. 17.10 Amyloid in the vessel walls (HE stain)

ulcerative colitis-like presentation and pseudo-obstruction of the small intestine.

Biopsy of a skin lesion, if available, has the advantage of safety and a high diagnostic yield showing diffuse or nodular, eosinophilic, often fissured amyloid deposits in the dermis and subcutis (Fig. 17.9). Amyloid is often seen within the blood vessels (Fig. 17.10), around sweat glands and pilosebaceous units leading to follicular atrophy and alopecia, and encircling the adipocytes (amyloid ring). Hemorrhages are present and the deposits are not usually associated with an inflammatory infiltrate (Fig. 17.11). Fibroblasts are often attached to the fissured edges. In the blistering form, the bulla may be both intradermal and subepidermal. Amyloid shows an apple-green birefringence with Congo red under polarized light (Fig. 17.12), a positive fluorescence with thioflavine T (Fig. 17.13), and a fibrillar structure made by straight, nonbranching filaments on electron microscopy

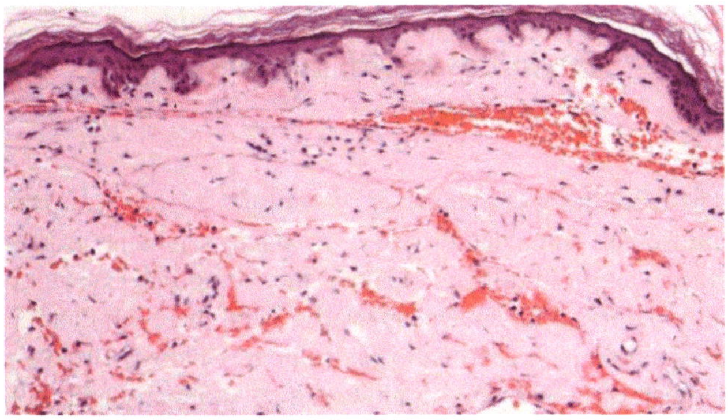

Fig. 17.11 Amyloid deposition with hemorrhages in the absence of inflammatory infiltrate (HE stain)

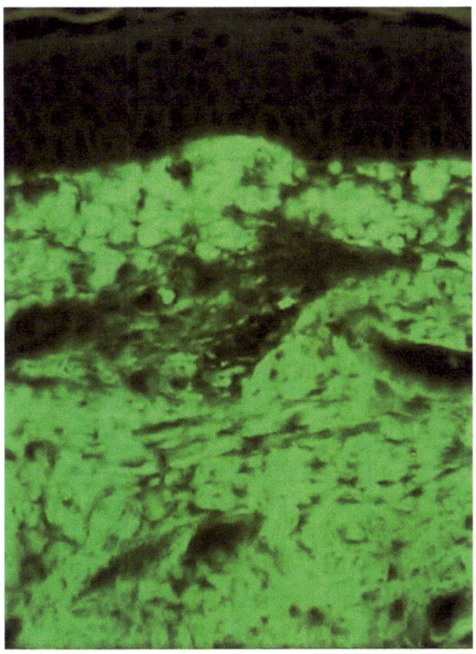

Fig. 17.12 Apple green birefringence of amyloid under polarized light (Courtesy of Martin Black, London)

(Fig. 17.14). The affinity of amyloid for Congo red after incubation with potassium permanganate does not change in patients with myeloma-associated amyloidosis. Antibodies to immunoglobulin light chains highlight amyloid deposits (Fig. 17.15). Biopsy results from clinically normal skin may be positive in as many as 50% of cases of primary systemic amyloidosis. Findings from abdominal subcutaneous aspirates and rectal biopsy are positive in almost 80% of patients. Gingival biopsies may also be useful.

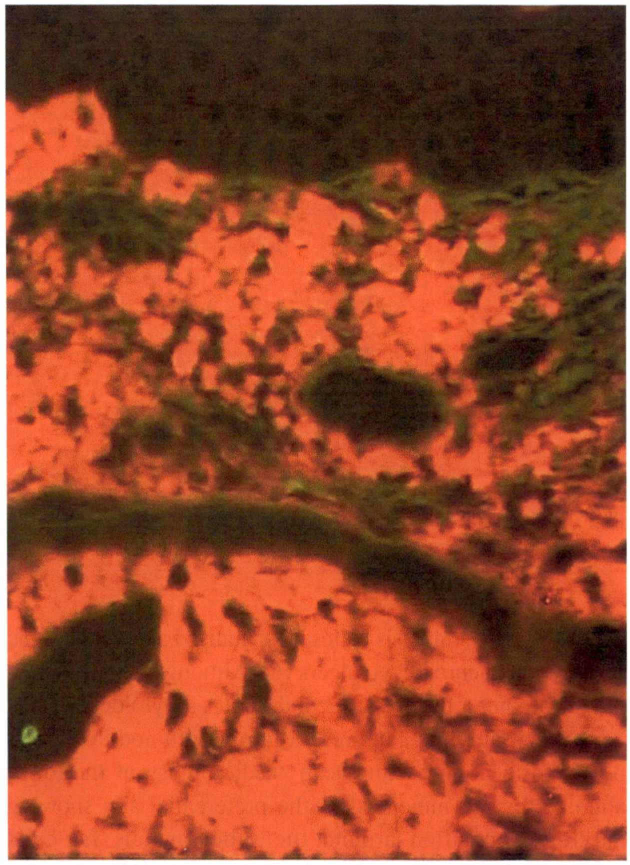

Fig. 17.13 Positive fluorescence of amyloid with thioflavine-T (Courtesy of Martin Black, London)

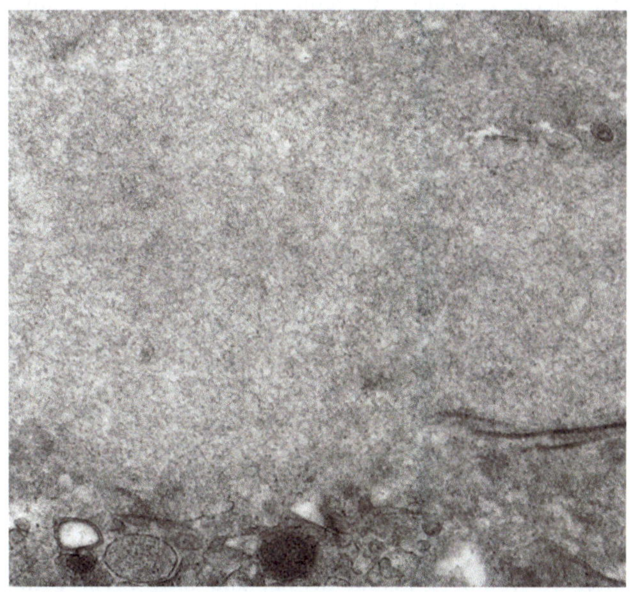

Fig. 17.14 Ultrastructural features of amyloid characterized by straight, nonbranching filaments (Courtesy of Martin Black, London)

17.2.1.2 Secondary Systemic AA Amyloidosis

AA amyloidosis is caused by serum amyloid protein A (SAA), a reactive inflammatory protein. It occurs in association with a variety of chronic inflammatory or infectious diseases such as rheumatoid arthritis, connective tissue diseases, familial Mediterranean fever, Muckle–Wells syndrome, lepromatous leprosy, hidradenitis suppurativa,

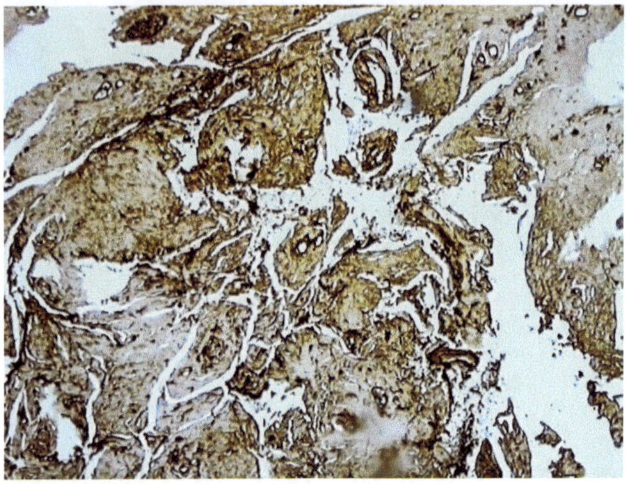

Fig. 17.15 Positive immunostaining of amyloid with antibodies to the immunoglobulin light chains

dystrophic epidermolysis bullosa, generalized and arthropathic psoriasis, and chronic leg ulcers (6). Although skin manifestations are not a feature of secondary AA amyloidosis, focal deposits of amyloid can present rarely with nodules (7) or be found in normal skin. Deep needle biopsy of the lower abdomen is recommended as the preferential site showing amyloid deposition around the subcutaneous fat cells (amyloid rings) and eccrine glands in about 66% of cases. As the amount of amyloid increases, the dermis may be diffusely infiltrated. After treatment with potassium permanganate, AA amyloid becomes nonreactive for alkaline Congo red stain while amyloid L is not affected by this treatment. The main clinical manifestations of secondary AA amyloidosis, however, are related to renal or gastrointestinal involvement.

17.2.1.3 β_2-Microglobulin Hemodialysis-Associated Amyloidosis

Dialysis-related amyloidosis is caused by the deposition of fibrillar β_2-microglobulin and is a serious complication in patients undergoing long-term dialysis (mean duration time 8–10 years). The main clinical manifestations include carpal tunnel syndrome and chronic arthralgias starting in the shoulder, or destructive arthropathies of large peripheral joints. Visceral amyloid deposition occurs late, usually after 15 years of hemodialysis, and may involve the heart or the gastrointestinal tract (with macroglossia, bowel infarction and perforation). Cutaneous signs are nonspecific and include small, shiny, lichenoid papules on the arms and trunk as well as subcutaneous masses on the buttocks (8). Dermal deposition of amyloid is similar to that of AL amyloid.

17.2.2 Hereditary/Familial Systemic Amyloidoses with Cutaneous Involvement

The hereditary amyloidoses constitute a group of rare autosomal dominant diseases in which a mutant protein forms amyloid fibrils. Among the hereditary systemic amyloidoses with cutaneous involvement, there are familial amyloidotic polyneuropathy, gelsolin amyloidosis (AGel) – Finnish type, and ApoA1 amyloidosis (Apolipoprotein A1). Familial amyloidotic polyneuropathy is caused by mutant transthyretin (Amyloid ATTR) (9). Skin changes consist of *trophic leg ulcers* and *atrophic scars* due to the accumulation of transthyretin-derived amyloid in peripheral nerves. There are Portuguese, Japanese, and Swedish subtypes. Histopathological features from clinically normal skin show amyloid in blood vessels, arrector pili muscles, elastic fibers, and cutaneous nerves. In gelsolin amyloidosis, widespread *cutis laxa* is the principal clinical manifestation associated with increased fragility and risk for intracutaneous bleeding (10). Histopathology shows cutaneous deposition of amyloid (AGel), mainly attached to basement membranes or basal laminae of various cutaneous structures, dermal nerves and blood vessel walls, and elastic fibers, which are fragmented and lost. ApoA1 autosomal dominant hereditary amyloidosis, associated with a mutation of the apolipoprotein A1 gene, exhibits a cardiac presentation with death secondary to heart failure by the sixth or seventh decade and cutaneous involvement with yellowish patches (11).

Muckle–Wells syndrome and familial Mediterranean fever are not hereditary amyloidoses *sensu strictu*, but are genetic autoinflammatory diseases characterized by recurrent fevers in which systemic reactive (AA) amyloidosis may be a severe long-term complication. Muckle–Wells syndrome is a rare autosomal dominant disease, caused by a defect in the *CIAS1* gene (now renamed *NLRP3*), which creates the protein cryopirin involved in the regulation of inflammation. It is characterized by the triad of renal amyloidosis, sensorineural deafness, and *urticarial rash* associated with periodic attacks of fever and limb pain (12). Histopathology of the hives includes vasodilatation and inflammation with neutrophils. Familial Mediterranean fever is an autosomal recessive disorder characterized by episodes of recurrent fever and serositis. Skin manifestations include mainly an erysipela-like reaction of the lower limbs with dermal neutrophilic infiltration.

17.2.3 Localized Cutaneous Amyloidoses

Localized cutaneous amyloidoses can be classified into primary and secondary forms.

17.2.3.1 Primary Localized Cutaneous Amyloidoses

Primary localized cutaneous amyloidoses (PLCA) include two major categories according to the type of amyloid: (1) Lichen, macular, and biphasic amyloidoses caused by trauma to the epidermis, producing globular amyloid deposits due to keratin (amyloid K) (13) and (2) primary nodular cutaneous amyloidosis (PNCA) that occurs as a result of deposition of amyloid L protein, produced by a local proliferation of plasma cells. Other primary cutaneous variants such as anosacral, poikiloderma-like, bullous, vitiliginous, and dyschromic have been described, though they are all quite rare (Table 17.2).

Table 17.2 Primary localized cutaneous amyloidoses

Type	Clinical appearance	Amyloid deposition
Macular	Poorly demarcated pruritic pigmented patches. Upper aspect of back	Degenerated keratinocyte intermediate filaments
Lichenoid	Pruritic lichenoid papules that may be smooth or hyperkeratotic and commonly coalesce into plaques on shins	Degenerated keratinocyte intermediate filaments
Biphasic	Coexistence of papules and pigmented patches	Degenerated keratinocyte intermediate filaments
Nodular	Single or multiple waxy nodules with or without overlying atrophic epidermis resulting in hemorrhage from slight trauma	Immunoglobulin light chains
Others	Auricular concha, penis, anosacral, poikiloderma-like, bullous, amyloidosis cutis dyschromica, vitiliginous	Usually, degenerated keratinocyte intermediate filaments

Macular and lichen amyloidoses are the most common form of PLCA (14). Lichen amyloidosis is more common in Chinese, while macular amyloidosis is more frequent in Central and South Americans, Middle Easterners, and Asians.

Lichen amyoidosis is characterized by dome-shaped, flesh-colored or pigmented, slightly hyperkeratotic papules coalescing into plaques on the shins (Fig. 17.16a, b) and, in severe cases, on the extensor surface of the arms including shoulders. Severe pruritus is a characteristic feature, and some authors have proposed that lichen amyloidosis is always a consequence of scratching an underlying pruritic condition. Macular amyloidosis consists of macular hyperpigmented areas, predominantly on the upper back (interscapular area), and less commonly on the buttocks, chest, and extremities. Lesions appear as grayish brown macules, 2–3 mm in diameter coalescing into patches (Fig. 17.17) exhibiting a reticulate or rippled pattern of pigmentation. Pruritus is not a constant feature. It is also known as frictional amyloidosis and is partially caused by the habit of vigorous rubbing of the skin with a nylon towel or brush. Notalgia paresthetica is somehow related to macular amyloidosis. Unusual variants of the macular type have been reported including periocular hyperpigmentation and nevoid hyperpigmentation (15).

In biphasic amyloidosis, the macular and lichen amyloidosis patterns coexist with fine papules superimposed upon a background of hyperpigmentation giving rise to the characteristic rippled pattern. The occasional transformation of macular amyloidosis into lichen amyloidosis has been observed. Lichen and macular amyloidoses have been described in association with connective tissue diseases (scleroderma, systemic lupus erythematosus), pachyonychia, and primary biliary cirrhosis.

Lichen and macular amyloidoses with an early onset before the age of 10 years have been described in multiple endocrine neoplasia type 2A (MEN 2A) and familial medullary thyroid

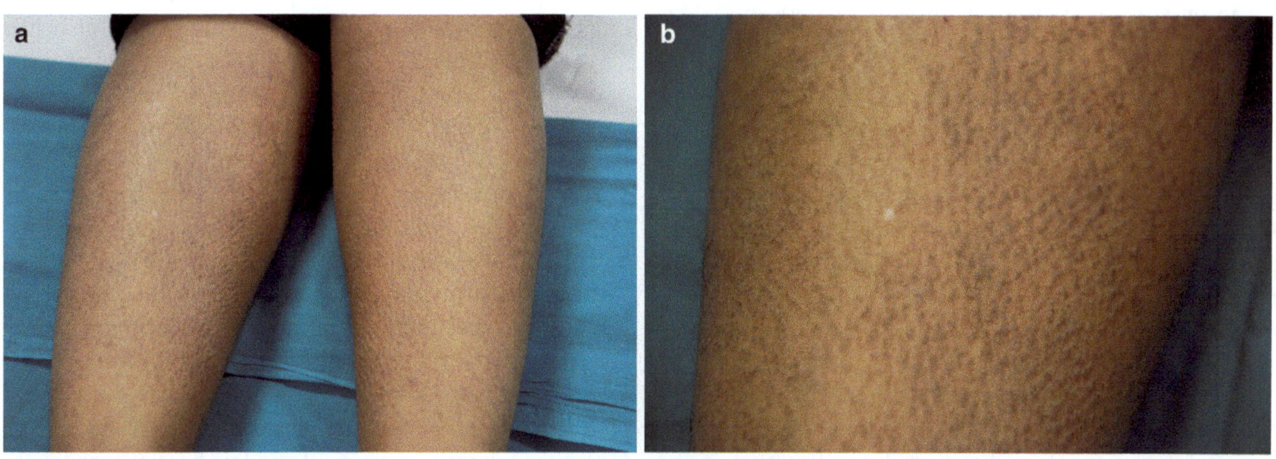

Fig. 17.16 (**a**) Lichen amyoidosis involving the shins. (**b**) Hyperkeratotic papules of lichen amyloidosis

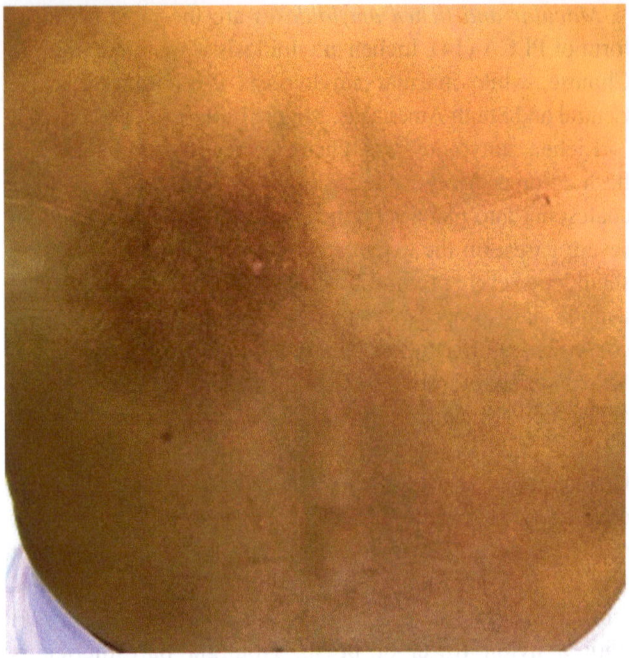

Fig. 17.17 Macular amyloidosis

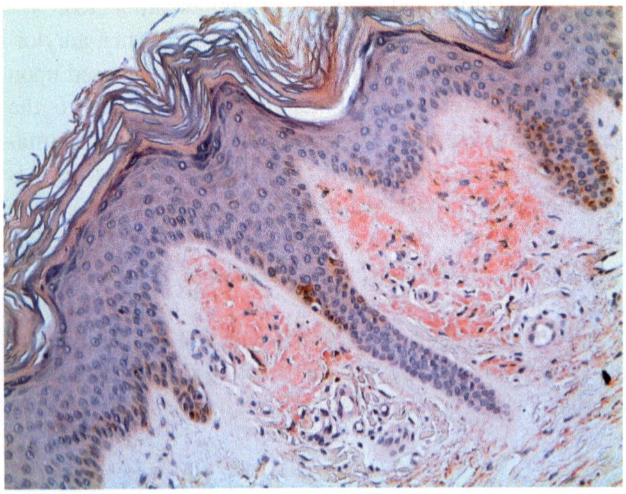

Fig. 17.18 Lichen amyloidosis with staining of amyloid by Congo red

carcinoma, which are genetic diseases caused by activating mutations of the RET proto-oncogene (16). In this setting, cutaneous manifestations are important markers for an early genetic diagnosis and an early prophylactic thyroidectomy. However, familial primary cutaneous amyloidosis with only cutaneous features of lichen amyloidosis or less frequently macular amyloidosis in the absence of multiple endocrine neoplasia type 2A (MEN 2A) may also occur as an autosomal dominant condition.

Histopathologically, the lesions of macular and lichen amyloid are similar, with the deposition of amorphous eosinophilic material in the dermal papillae that stains with Congo red (Fig. 17.18) and crystal violet (Fig. 17.19).

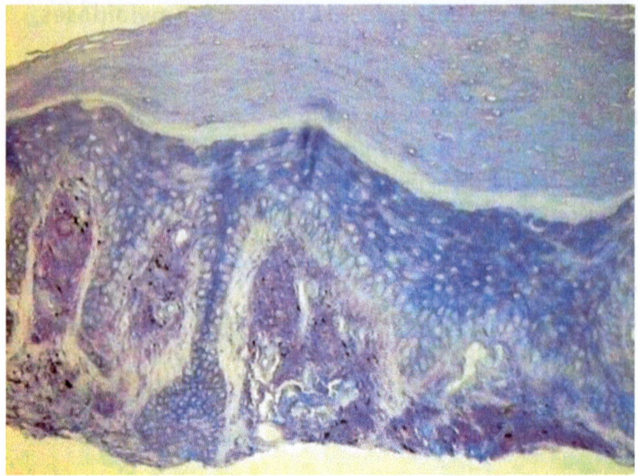

Fig. 17.19 Crystal violet stains amyloid in lichen amyloidosis (Courtesy of P. Romanelli, Miami)

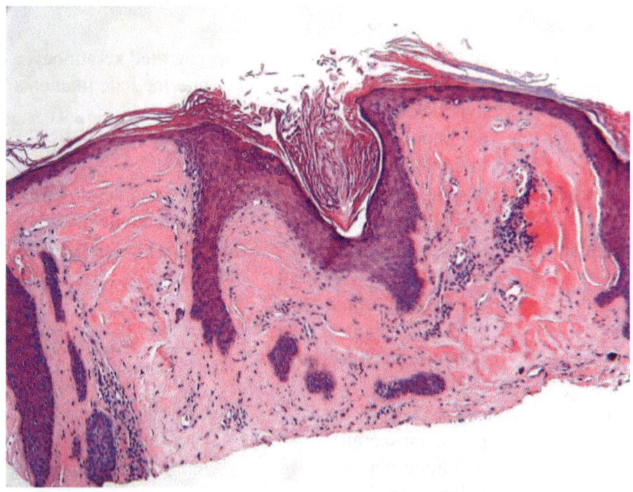

Fig. 17.20 Lichen amyloidosis with the epidermal changes of orthokeratotic hyperkeratosis, acanthosis, and hypergranulosis (HE stain)

Scattered necrotic keratinocytes, pigment incontinence, and a sparse perivascular lymphohistiocytic infiltrate are often seen in both. However, the papular lesions of lichen amyloidosis can be distinguished by the epidermal changes of orthokeratotic hyperkeratosis, acanthosis, and hypergranulosis (Fig. 17.20). In macular amyloidosis, pigmentary incontinence in papillary dermis is prominent (Fig. 17.21). The amyloid deposits stain positively with antibodies to cytokeratins. In particular, 34betaE12 and MNF116, which have in common the labeling of keratin K5, are useful (13).

Besides the three main types, some unusual cutaneous variants have been described: amyloidosis of the auricular concha (previously named collagenous papules) is considered as a topographic variant of lichen amyloidosis (Fig. 17.22) (17); amyloidosis of the glans penis mimicking condylomata (18), although the true nature of amyloid has not been totally clarified in this condition; anosacral cutaneous amyloidosis,

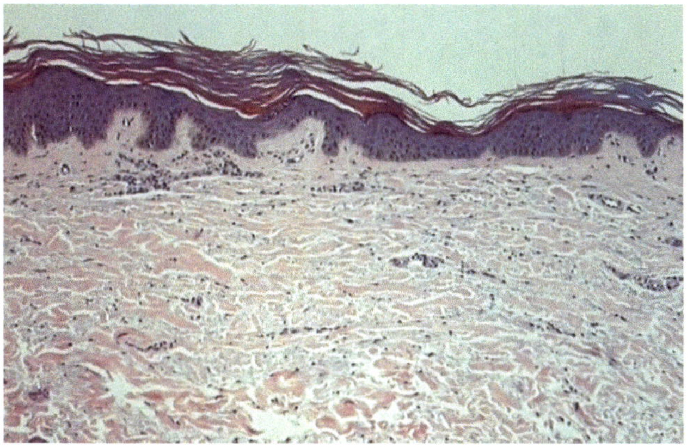

Fig. 17.21 Macular amyloidosis with pigment incontinence (HE stain) (Courtesy of P. Romanelli, Miami)

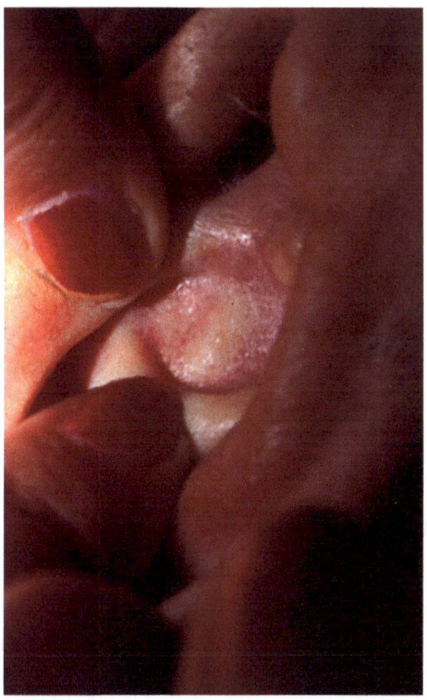

Fig. 17.22 Amyloidosis of the auricular concha

characterized by hyperpigmentation and lichenification that had mainly been reported in Japanese patients and was considered to be a senile change of the skin; bullous lesions that have been reported in the setting of lichen amyloidosis but are more commonly associated with primary systemic amyloidosis (19); amyloidosis cutis dyschromica that is characterized by generalized, asymptomatic hyperpigmentation intermingled with several hypopigmented spots without papulation, atrophy, and telangiectasia starting usually before puberty in the Middle-east countries (20); poikiloderma-like cutaneous amyloidosis, vitiliginous amyloidosis characterized by depigmented lesions with peripheral hyperpigmentation on the scalp of bald men, and tumid amyloidosis are also rare variants.

The etiology of PCLA due to amyloid K is unclear, but many risk factors have been implicated, such as ultraviolet B (UVB), Epstein–Barr virus (EBV), race, chronic trauma, genetic predisposition, and atopy.

Primary cutaneous nodular amyloidosis (PCNA), the rarest form of primary cutaneous amyloidosis, occurs as a result of deposition of amyloid L protein, produced by a local proliferation of plasma cells (21). It could be considered as a form of extramedullary plasmacytoma. Light chains may be λ or κ, or both. PCNA occurs equally in both sexes and is seen in adults, with a mean age at diagnosis of 60.8 years. Mean duration of lesions at the time of diagnosis is 13.5 years. Patients present with asymptomatic, single or multiple, firm, smooth-surfaced, waxy or rubbery, pink to tan papules, plaques, or nodules measuring up to several centimeters (Fig. 17.23). Surface telangiectasias may be seen. Clinically, the lesions may be indistinguishable from nodular deposits of amyloid occurring in primary systemic amyloidosis or myeloma-associated amyloidosis. Bullous-appearing, anetoderma-like and plantar tyloma-like lesions have been reported (22). There is a tendency for acral involvement, with the most common sites being the feet, nose, or periauricular areas. PCNA has been reported in the setting of Sjögren syndrome, and it has been suggested that this association is a distinct disease entity reflecting a particular and benign part of the polymorphic spectrum of lymphoproliferative diseases related to Sjögren syndrome (23).

Although a rate of progression of PCNA to systemic amyloidosis of 7–50% has been reported, most patients with PCNA do not do so and remain in general good health, particularly if no clinical or laboratory evidence for systemic disease exists at the time of diagnosis (24). It is, however,

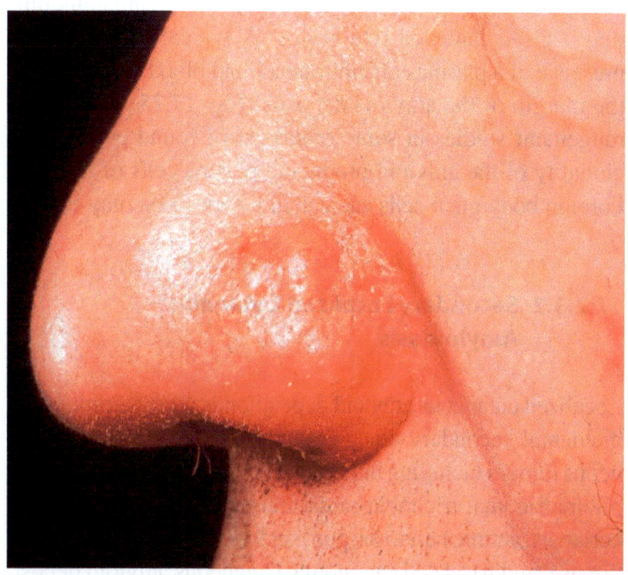

Fig. 17.23 Primary cutaneous nodular amyloidosis of the nose (Courtesy of Martin Black, London)

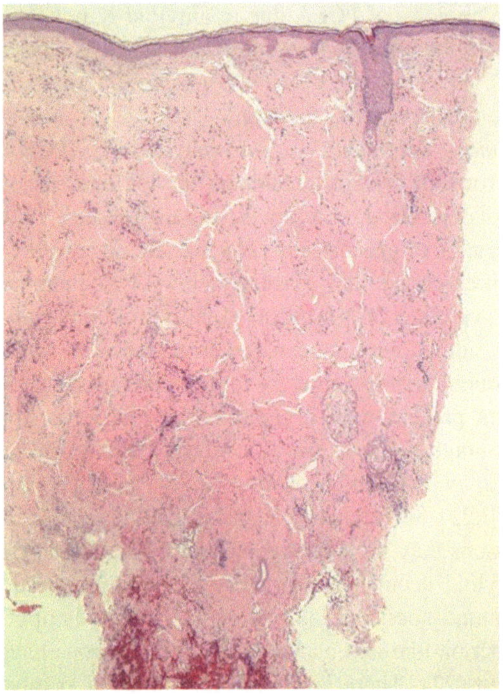

Fig. 17.24 Massive deposits of amyloid throughout the dermis in primary cutaneous nodular amyloidosis (Courtesy of Martin Black, London)

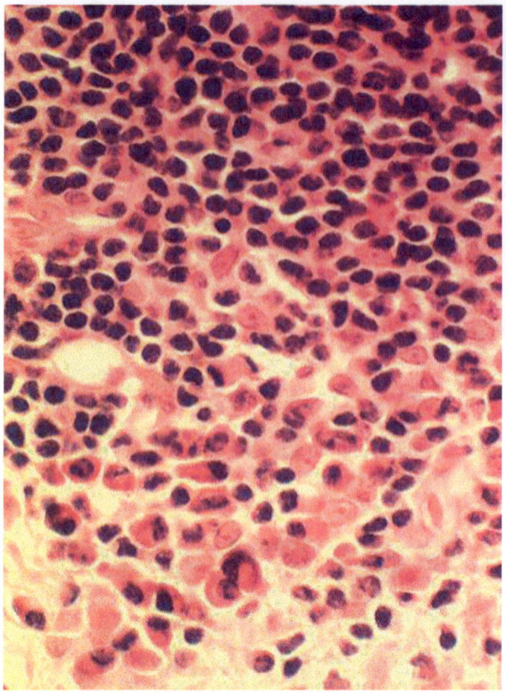

Fig. 17.25 Infiltrate of plasmocytes associated with amyloid deposit in nodular cutaneous amyloidosis

recommended that these patients are followed longterm. The use of scintigraphy with iodine 123-labelled serum amyloid P component may be useful in monitoring patients with PCNA with a monoclonal gammopathy for early occult systemic amyloidosis (25). Histopathology is similar to primary systemic amyloidosis showing massive deposits of amyloid in both the papillary and reticular dermis and sometimes the subcutis (Fig. 17.24). Amyloid may occur within vessel walls and adnexal structures. The overlying epidermis may exhibit flattened rete ridges. A typical finding is the presence of a plasma cell infiltrate around blood vessels and at the margin of the amyloid deposits (Fig. 17.25). Gene rearrangement studies in some reports have found evidence of clonality of the amyloid-producing plasma cells of the skin. Foreign body giant cells and calcium deposition may occur.

17.2.3.2 Secondary Localized Cutaneous Amyloidosis

Localized cutaneous amyloid deposition is most commonly an incidental secondary reactive process associated with cutaneous tumors including intradermal nevi, sweat gland tumors, pilomatricoma, trichoblastoma, dermatofibroma, seborrheic keratosis, actinic keratosis, porokeratosis of Mibelli, Bowen's disease, and basal cell carcinoma. Cutaneous amyloid deposition may also occur after therapy with psoralen plus ultraviolet A, or associated with mycosis fungoides and discoid lupus erythematosus (26). These amyloid deposits due to amyloid K do not have a known clinical significance. Reiterative insulin injections may cause amyloid deposition at the site of therapy.

17.3 Treatment and Prognosis

Current treatment of amyloidosis is directed to reduce the level of amyloid precursor proteins. Drugs effective in multiple myeloma such as high-dose melphalan and autologous stem-cell transplantation may be helpful in AL amyloidosis, if tolerated (27). Patients with systemic AL amyloidosis have a median survival of 1–2 years from diagnosis and <5% of all patients with AL amyloidosis survive ≥10 years from the time of diagnosis.

Treatment of secondary AA amyloidosis is difficult and relies on systemic treatment according to the underlying disease. Colchicine and other anti-inflammatory/immunosuppressive therapies and, in selected instances, anticytokine (TNF-alpha, IL-1beta) therapy or, when applicable, the eradication of an existing infectious focus (surgery, antimicrobial drugs) are useful in reducing the amyloid precursor (SAA) load (28). Prognosis is usually poor. Complications of end stage renal disease are the main cause of death, and median survival after diagnosis is 4–10 years.

In hereditary amyloidosis, there is no specific drug treatment that might specifically interfere with the progression of the disease. The possibility of suppressing the synthesis of the amyloidogenic precursor by means of liver transplantation which is the main organ synthesizing most of these proteins is actually considered as a therapeutic strategy for this group of disorders.

Most cases of PLCA remain chronic and refractory to treatment. No evidence-based therapy is recommended by controlled randomized studies. Topical glucocorticoids, intralesional glucocorticoids, cryotherapy, electrodessication and curettage, dermabrasion, narrow-band UVB, pulsed dye laser vaporization, topical and systemic retinoids, calcipotriol, and topical tacrolimus have been used with varied success (29–32). The relief of pruritus is the mainstay of treatment, but antihistamines have been found to be moderately effective.

Treatment of PCNA is difficult due to a high rate of local recurrence after all forms of treatment. Patients need to be monitored for progression to systemic amyloidosis or plasma cell dyscrasias (24). As recurrences are common, the least invasive procedure yielding cosmetically acceptable results is the best option.

References

1. Rongioletti F, Barnhill RL (2010) Deposition disorders. In: Barnhill RL, Crowson AN, Magro CM, Piepkorn MW (eds) Dermatopathology, 3rd edn. McGraw-Hill, New York, pp 362–386
2. Obici L, Perfetti V, Palladini G, Moratti R, Merlini G (2005) Clinical aspects of systemic amyloid diseases. Biochim Biophys Acta 1753:11–22
3. Black M, Upjohn E, Albert S (2008) Amyloidosis. In: Bolognia J, Jorizzo JL, Rapini R (eds) Dermatology, 2nd edn. Elsevier, St Louis, MO, pp 623–631
4. Mason AR, Rackoff EM, Pollack RB (2007) Primary systemic amyloidosis associated with multiple myeloma: a case report and review of the literature. Cutis 80:193–200
5. Bocquier B, D'Incan M, Joubert J et al (2008) Amyloid elastosis: a new case studied extensively by electron microscopy and immunohistochemistry. Br J Dermatol 158:858–860
6. Waton J, Fays-Michel S, Chandeclerc ML et al (2008) Amyloidosis: a little-known complication of chronic leg ulcer. Ann Dermatol Venereol 135:119–122
7. Katsikas GA, Maragou M, Rontogianni D, Gouma P, Koutsouvelis I, Kappou-Rigatou I (2008) Secondary cutaneous nodular AA amyloidosis in a patient with primary Sjögren syndrome and celiac disease. J Clin Rheumatol 14:27–29
8. Shimizu S, Yasui C, Yasukawa K, Nakamura H, Shimizu H, Tsuchiya K (2003) Subcutaneous nodules on the buttocks as a manifestation of dialysis-related amyloidosis: a clinicopathological entity? Br J Dermatol 149:400–404
9. Rocha N, Velho G, Horta M, Martins A, Massa A (2005) Cutaneous manifestations of familial amyloidotic polyneuropathy. J Eur Acad Dermatol Venereol 19:605–607
10. Kiuru-Enari S, Keski-Oja J, Haltia M (2005) Cutis laxa in hereditary gelsolin amyloidosis. Br J Dermatol 152:250–257
11. Hamidi Asl K, Liepnieks JJ, Nakamura M, Parker F, Benson MD (1999) A novel apolipoprotein A-1 variant, Arg173Pro, associated with cardiac and cutaneous amyloidosis. Biochem Biophys Res Commun 257:584–588
12. Haas N, Küster W, Zuberbier T, Henz BM (2004) Muckle–Wells syndrome: clinical and histological skin findings compatible with cold air urticaria in a large kindred. Br J Dermatol 151:99–104
13. Apaydin R, Gürbüz Y, Bayramgürler D, Müezzinoglu B, Bilen N (2004) Cytokeratin expression in lichen amyloidosus and macular amyloidosis. J Eur Acad Dermatol Venereol 18:305–309
14. Yoshida A, Takahashi K, Tagami H, Akasaka T (2009) Lichen amyloidosis induced on the upper back by long-term friction with a nylon towel. J Dermatol 36:56–59
15. Hung CC, Wang CM, Hong HS, Kuo TT (2003) Unusual skin manifestations of cutaneous amyloidosis. Dermatology 207:65–67
16. Jabbour SA, Davidovici BB, Wolf R (2006) Rare syndromes. Clin Dermatol 24:299–316
17. Shimauchi T, Shin JH, Tokura Y (2006) Primary cutaneous amyloidosis of the auricular concha: case report and review of published work. J Dermatol 33:128–131
18. Ritter M, Nawab RA, Tannenbaum M, Hakki SI, Morgan MB (2003) Localized amyloidosis of the glans penis mimicking condylomata: a case report and literature review. J Cutan Pathol 30:37–40
19. Khoo BP, Tay YK (2000) Lichen amyloidosus a bullous variant. Ann Acad Med 29:105–107
20. Ozcan A, Senol M, Aydin NE, Karaca S (2005) Amyloidosis cutis dyschromica: a case treated with acitretin. J Dermatol 32:474–477
21. Kalajian AH, Waldman M, Knable AL (2007) Nodular primary localized cutaneous amyloidosis after trauma: a case report and discussion of the rate of progression to systemic amyloidosis. J Am Acad Dermatol 57(Suppl):S26–S29
22. Borrowman TA, Lutz ME, Walsh JS (2003) Cutaneous nodular amyloidosis masquerading as a foot callus. J Am Acad Dermatol 49:307–310
23. Yoneyama K, Tochigi N, Oikawa A, Shinkai H, Utani A (2005) Primary localized cutaneous nodular amyloidosis in a patient with Sjögren's syndrome: a review of the literature. J Dermatol 32:120–123
24. Woollons A, Black MM (2001) Nodular localized primary cutaneous amyloidosis: a long-term follow-up study. Br J Dermatol 145:105–109
25. Rongioletti F, Romanelli P (2003) Dermal infiltrates. In: Kerdel FA, Jimenez-Acosta F (eds) Dermatology just the facts. McGraw-Hill, New York, pp 175–197
26. Powell AM, Albert S, Bhogal B, Black MM (2005) Discoid lupus erythematosus with secondary amyloidosis. Br J Dermatol 153:746–749
27. Wechalekar AD, Hawkins PN, Gillmore JD (2008) Perspectives in treatment of AL amyloidosis. Br J Haematol 140:365–377
28. Pettersson T, Konttinen YT, Maury CP (2008) Treatment strategies for amyloid A amyloidosis. Expert Opin Pharmacother 9:2117–2128
29. Castanedo-Cazares JP, Lepe V, Moncada B (2002) Lichen amyloidosis improved by 0.1% topical tacrolimus. Dermatology 205:420–421
30. Sawamura D, Sato-Matsumura KC, Shibaki A et al (2005) A case of lichen amyloidosis treated with pulsed dye laser. J Eur Acad Dermatol Venereol 19:262–263
31. Choi JY, Sippe J, Lee S (2008) Acitretin for lichen amyloidosus. Australas J Dermatol 49:109–113
32. Grimmer J, Weiss T, Weber L, Meixner D, Scharffetter-Kochanek K (2007) Successful treatment of lichen amyloidosis with combined bath PUVA photochemotherapy and oral acitretin. Clin Exp Dermatol 32:39–42

Chapter 18
Mucinoses

Franco Rongioletti

Key Points

- The cutaneous mucinoses are a heterogeneous group of disorders in which an abnormal amount of mucin accumulates in the skin.
- The etiopathogenesis of cutaneous mucinoses is unknown, although cytokines such as tumor necrosis factor α and β, interleukin-1 and transforming growth factor β and/or polyclonal and monoclonal immunoglobulins and other unidentified factors in the serum of affected patients may induce the synthesis of glycoaminoglycans.
- The cutaneous mucinoses are divided into two groups: primary cutaneous mucinoses in which the mucin deposit is the main histologic feature resulting in clinically distinctive lesions, and secondary mucinoses in which the mucin deposition is only an additional histologic epiphenomenon.
- Primary mucinoses can be divided into dermal and follicular mucinoses. The former includes lichen myxedematosus, reticular erythematous mucinosis, scleredema, dysthyroidotic mucinoses (localized (pretibial) and generalized myxedema), papular and nodular mucinosis in connective tissue diseases, self-healing juvenile cutaneous mucinosis, cutaneous focal mucinosis, digital myxoid cyst, while the latter include Pinkus' follicular mucinosis and urticaria-like follicular mucinosis.
- Associated disorders include paraproteinemia (scleromyxedema, scleredema), diabetes mellitus (scleredema), hyperthyroidism (pretibial myxedema), hypothyroidism (generalized myxedema) and lupus erythematosus, and dermatomyositis or scleroderma (papular and nodular mucinosis in connective tissue diseases).

Keywords Mucin • Dermal mucinoses • Follicular mucinoses • Lichen myxedematosus • Dysthyroidotic mucinoses • Scleredema

F. Rongioletti (✉)
Department of Endocrinological and Medical Sciences (DISEM)
Section of Dermatology and Department of Pathology
University of Genova, Genova, Italy
e-mail: franco.rongioletti@unige.it

18.1 Introduction

The cutaneous mucinoses are a heterogeneous group of disorders in which an abnormal amount of mucin accumulates in the skin (1). Mucin or protein–hyaluronic acid complex is a normal component of the dermal connective tissue produced in small amounts by fibroblasts. It is a jelly-like, amorphous mixture of acid glycosaminoglycans (formerly called acid mucopolysaccharides) that are repeating polysaccharides forming a complex carbohydrate. The acid glycosaminoglycans may be fixed on both sides of a protein core (proteoglycan monomer) as in the case of dermatan-sulfate or chondroitin-6-sulfate and chondroitin-4-sulfate, or they may be free as in the case of hyaluronic acid, which is the most important component of dermal mucin. Mucin is capable of absorbing 1,000 times its own weight of water playing a major role in maintaining the salt and water balance of the dermis. However, in disease conditions, mucin is increased and since it holds water (hygroscopic), the dermal connective tissue is edematous. A light blue staining between the separated collagen bundles or empty spaces is a good clue for mucin deposition. In such a case, special stains such as Alcian blue at pH 2.5 (negative at 0.4) and colloidal iron should be used to highlight these changes. Furthermore, mucin is hyaluronidase sensitive and periodic acid-Schiff (PAS) negative.

It is not clear why mucin production is increased in pathological states. Although the cause is probably multifactorial, it has been suggested that cytokines and/or immunoglobulins and unidentified factors in the serum of affected patients can induce the synthesis of glycoaminoglycans. Cytokines that may play an important role in the process include tumor necrosis factor α and β, interleukin-1, and transforming growth factor β. A decrease in the catabolic process of mucin degradation could be also involved. In Chinese Shar-Pei dogs, known for their distinctive features of deep wrinkles, mucin accumulation in the skin is a typical condition considered to be a consequence of a genetic defect in the metabolism of hyaluronic acid.

F. Rongioletti and B.R. Smoller (eds.), *Clinical and Pathological Aspects of Skin Diseases in Endocrine, Metabolic, Nutritional and Deposition Disease*, DOI 10.1007/978-1-60761-181-3_18, © Springer Science+Business Media, LLC 2010

The cutaneous mucinoses, which may be dermal or follicular according to the site of mucin deposition, are divided into two groups: primary (idiopathic) cutaneous mucinoses in which the mucin deposit is the main histologic feature resulting in clinically distinctive lesions and secondary mucinoses in which histologic mucin deposition is only an additional finding and secondary phenomenon.

18.2 Clinical and Pathological Aspects of Skin Manifestations

18.2.1 Lichen Myxedematosus (Papular Mucinosis)

Lichen myxedematosus (LM) is a chronic, idiopathic disorder characterized by lichenoid papules, nodules, and/or plaques due to dermal mucin deposition and a variable degree of fibrosis in the absence of thyroid disease (2). It includes two clinicopathologic subsets: a generalized papular and sclerodermoid form (also called scleromyxedema of Arndt–Gottron) with a monoclonal gammopathy and systemic, even lethal, manifestations and a localized papular form which does not run a disabling course. Occasionally, patients with LM have overlapping or atypical features and fall between scleromyxedema and localized LM.

In scleromyxedema, there is a widespread symmetric eruption of 2–3 mm, firm, waxy, closely spaced papules on an indurated, sclerodermoid background involving the hands (Fig. 18.1), forearms, head and neck region, upper trunk (Fig. 18.2), and thighs. Papules are often arranged in a strikingly linear array and the skin exhibits a brownish discoloration. The glabella is typically involved with deep longitudinal furrowing (Fig. 18.3), as well as the ears (Fig. 18.4). As the condition progresses, skin stiffening, sclerodactyly, and decreased motility of the mouth and joints occur. On the proximal interphalangeal joints, a central depression surrounded by an elevated rim (due to the skin thickening) is referred to as the "doughnut sign."

Scleromyxedema is almost always associated with a monoclonal gammopathy, usually of IgG-type with lambda light chains. Although a mild plasmacytosis may be found in the bone marrow, scleromyxedema progresses to multiple myeloma in less than 10% of cases. The significance of the monoclonal gammopathy in patients with scleromyxedema is still debated. Paraprotein levels do not correlate with either the extent or the progression of the disease. However, while serum from patients with scleromyxedema enhanced fibroblast proliferation in vitro, an immunoglobulin purified from the paraprotein-containing serum failed to do so (2),

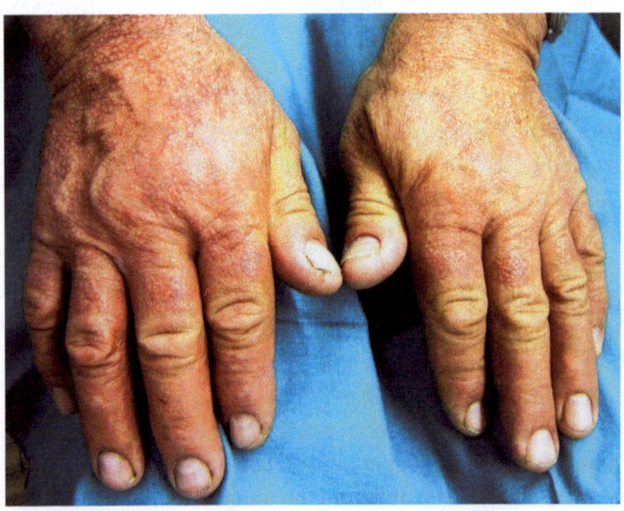

Fig. 18.1 Scleromyxedema on the hands with doughnut sign

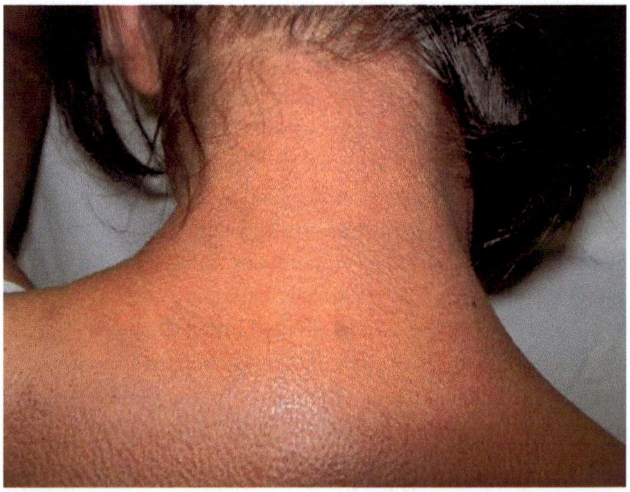

Fig. 18.2 Scleromyxedema on the trunk

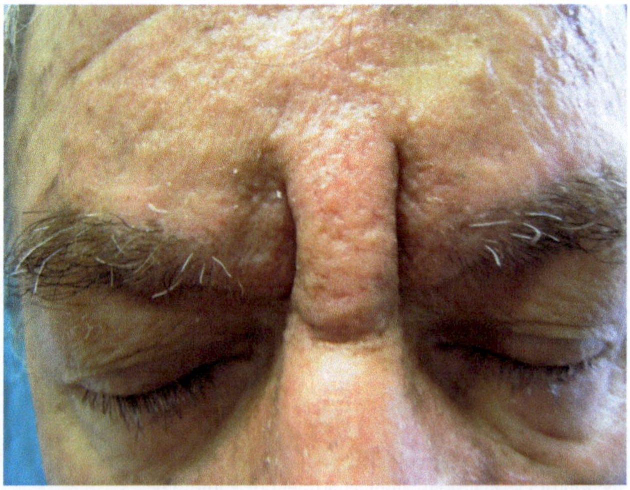

Fig. 18.3 Scleromyxedema on the glabella with deep longitudinal furrows

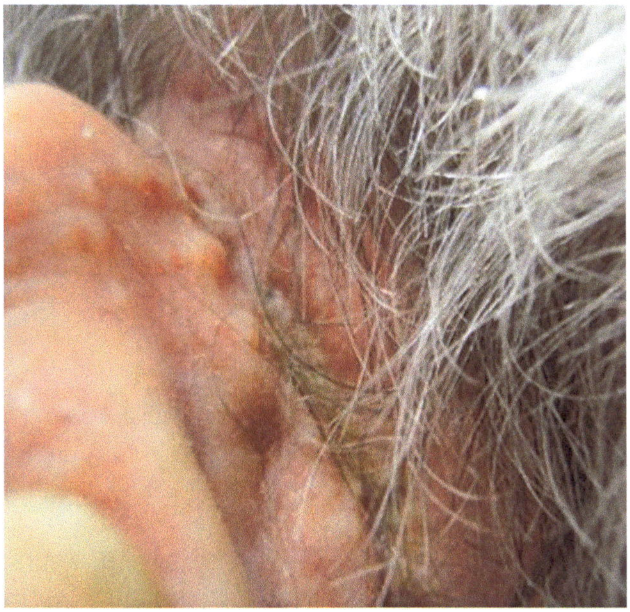

Fig. 18.4 Scleromyxedema behind the ear

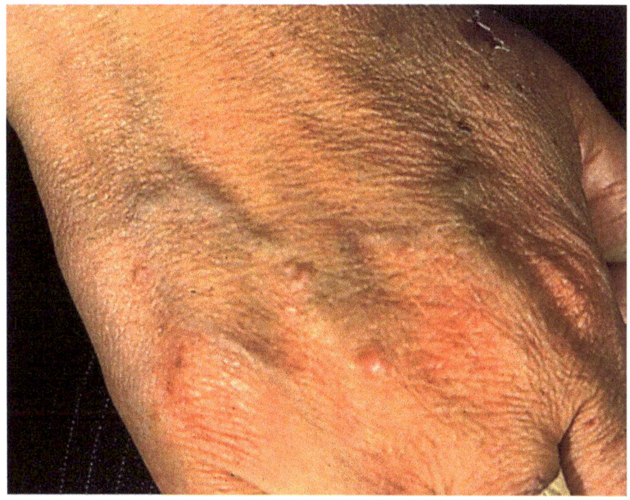

Fig. 18.5 Acral persistent papular mucinosis

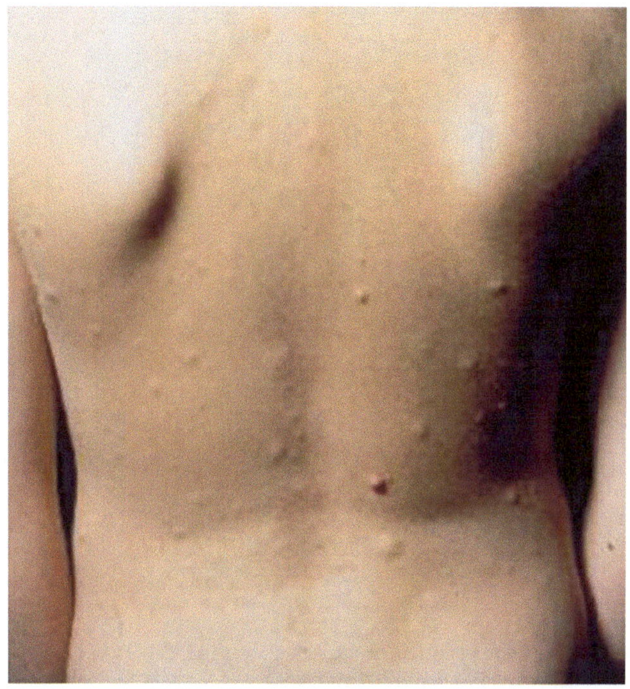

Fig. 18.6 Cutaneous mucinosis of infancy

suggesting a pathogenetic role for circulating factors other than the paraprotein. Clinical remission of scleromyxedema following autologous stem cell transplantation points to the bone marrow as a source of these circulating factors.

Patients with scleromyxedema can have a number of internal manifestations – muscular, neurologic, rheumatologic, pulmonary, renal, and cardiovascular. Dysphagia, proximal muscle weakness due to myositis, disturbances of the central nervous system leading to unexplained coma, peripheral neuropathy, arthropathies, carpal tunnel syndrome, restrictive or obstructive lung disease, and a scleroderma-like renal disease may accompany or follow the cutaneous manifestations.

In localized LM, the patients exhibit small, firm, waxy papules (or nodules and plaques produced by the confluence of papules) confined to only a few sites (usually the upper and lower limbs and trunk) without sclerotic features, paraproteinemia, systemic involvement or thyroid disease. Localized LM is subdivided into four subtypes: a discrete papular form involving the limbs and trunk; acral persistent papular mucinosis (APPM) in which flesh-colored papules develop exclusively on the back of the hands and extensor surface of the distal forearms (Fig. 18.5); cutaneous mucinosis of infancy (Fig. 18.6), and a pure nodular form with a mild or absent papular component. Moreover, localized LM may be observed in association with HIV infection, exposure to toxic oil or L-tryptophan, and hepatitis C virus infection. Familial forms of papular mucinosis have also been reported. Whether they are a distinct entity or a familial form of localized LM is, however, still unclear (4).

Histologically, scleromyxedema is characterized by a triad of microscopic features that includes a diffuse deposit of mucin in the upper and mid-reticular dermis, an increase in collagen deposition and a marked proliferation of irregularly arranged fibroblasts (Fig. 18.7a, b). Mucin may fill the walls of myocardial blood vessels as well as the interstitium of the kidney, pancreas, adrenal glands, and nerves. In the localized forms the changes are less characteristic. Mucin accumulates in the upper and mid reticular dermis, fibroblast proliferation is variable, and fibrosis is not marked and may even be absent (4). In APPM, mucin accumulates focally in the upper reticular dermis (sparing a subepidermal zone) and fibroblasts are not increased in number (Fig. 18.8a, b).

Histologic examination of the skin helps to distinguish localized LM from several papular eruptions that have a

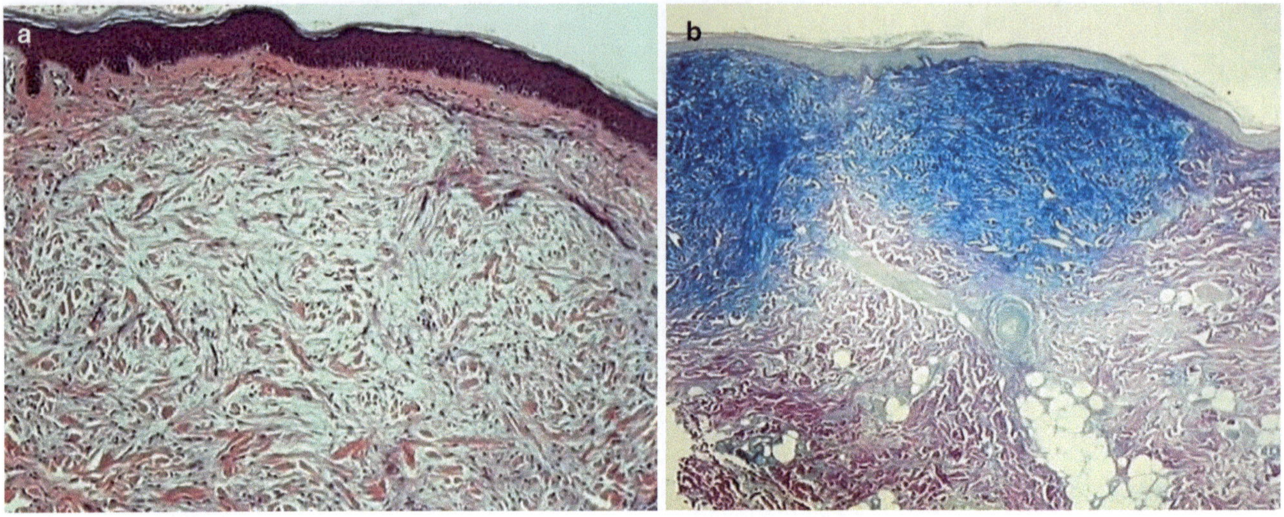

Fig. 18.7 Scleromyxedema. (**a**) Microscopic triad of mucin deposition, fibroblast proliferation, and fibrosis (HE stain). (**b**) Mucin in scleromyxedema (colloidal iron stain)

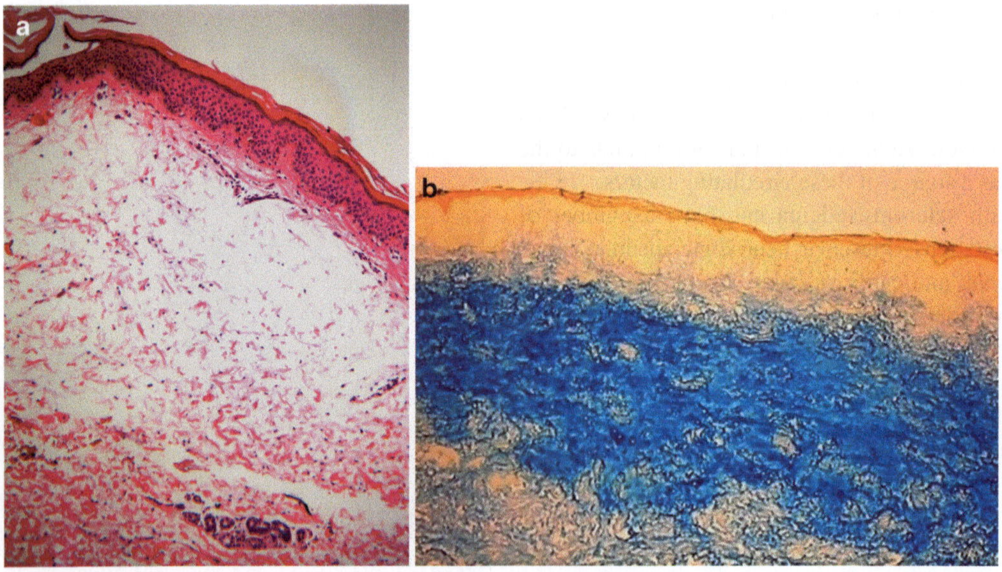

Fig. 18.8 Acral persistent papular mucinosis (APPM). (**a**) Focal mucin deposition with grenz zone and no fibroblast proliferation (HE stain). (**b**) Mucin in APPM (Colloidal iron stain)

similar appearance, such as granuloma annulare, lichen amyloidosus, lichen planus and other lichenoid eruptions, and eruptive collagenoma. Scleromyxedema should be distinguished mainly from systemic scleroderma, scleredema, and nephrogenic systemic fibrosis. The presence of papules, especially in linear arrays, is a very helpful clinical sign in scleromyxedema. Nephrogenic systemic fibrosis, seen in patients with serious renal dysfunction and a positive history of exposure to Gadolinium-containing contrast agent, differs from scleromyxedema as it lacks face involvement and paraproteinemia; moreover, a deeper fibrotic involvement of the dermis and of the septa in the subcutis with mucinous deposits and an increase of CD34+ stromal spindle cells that coexpress procollagen-I and CD45RO are more typical of the former.

18.2.2 Reticular Erythematous Mucinosis

Reticular erythematous mucinosis (REM) (syn. Plaque-like cutaneous mucinosis) occurs most often in middle-aged women (1). On the mid back or chest, reddish macules and papules merge into reticulated, net-like patterns or plaque-like lesions (Fig. 18.9). Sun exposure usually worsens the eruption, but it has occasionally been reported to be beneficial.

In general, REM is not associated with systemic diseases or abnormal laboratory tests. Oral contraceptives, menses, pregnancy, heat, X-ray therapy, and perspiration may promote or exacerbate REM. Familial cases have been reported (5).

Histologically, the epidermis is normal. Interstitial deposits of mucin are seen in the upper dermis, along with a perivascular and, at times, perifollicular T-cell infiltrate (Fig. 18.10a, b). Vascular dilation is present. Usually, direct immunofluorescence is negative, but rarely granular deposits of IgM, IgA and C3 have been seen at the dermo–epidermal junction (6).

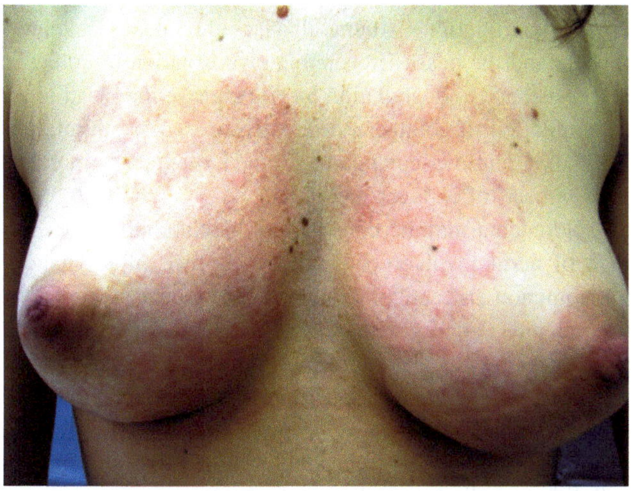

Fig. 18.9 REM. Clinical features

The main differential diagnosis is with lupus erythematosus. In biopsy specimens of cutaneous lupus erythematosus, there is involvement of the epidermis by an interface dermatitis, and deposits of IgG and C3 are found at the dermo–epidermal junction. Lupus erythematosus tumidus can be difficult to distinguish microscopically from REM, but clinically it presents as scattered smooth-topped papules and plaques, sometimes in an annular pattern. Jessner's lymphocytic infiltration usually lacks mucin deposits.

18.2.3 Scleredema

Scleredema (Buschke, diabeticorum) is a symmetrical diffuse induration of the upper part of the body caused by a thickened dermis and deposition of mucin (Fig. 18.11) (1). Classically, there are three types of scleredema, although a simpler division into those with and those without diabetes has been suggested. The *first type* affects mostly middle-aged women, but also children. It is preceded by fever, malaise, and an infection (usually streptococcal) of the upper or lower respiratory tract. The skin of the cervicofacial region suddenly hardens with extension to the trunk and proximal upper limbs. The *second type* shares the same clinical features as the first but has a more subtle onset, without a preceding illness; it persists for years. This type is more frequently associated with a monoclonal gammopathy. The *third type* occurs mainly in obese middle-aged men with insulin-dependent diabetes

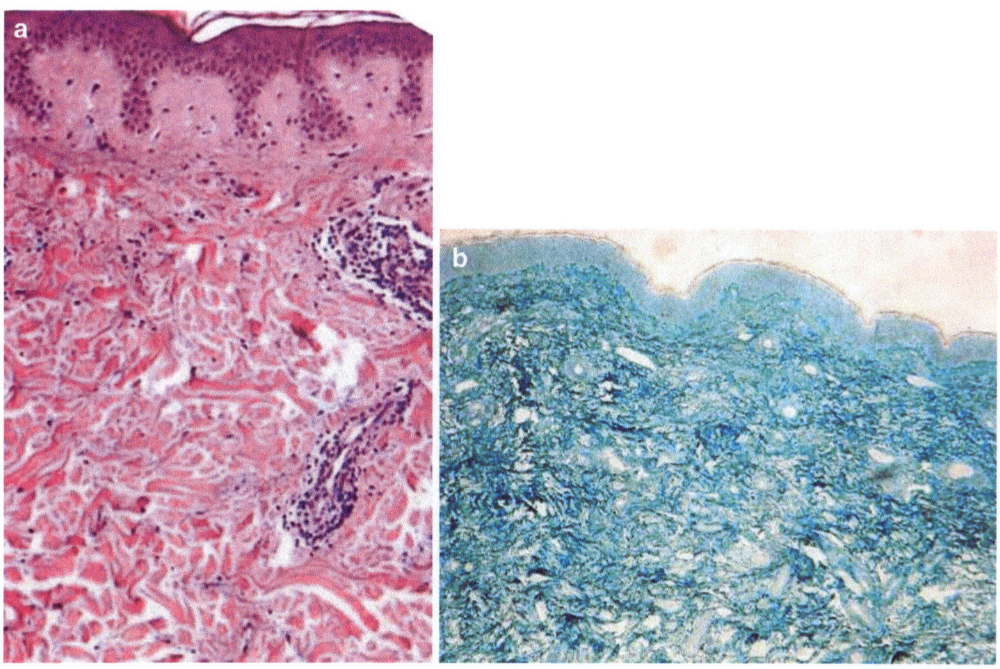

Fig. 18.10 REM. (**a**) Interstitial dermal mucin with perivascular lymphocytic infiltrate. Note the uninvolved epidermis (HE stain). (**b**) Mucin deposition in REM (Alcian blue stain)

(*scleredema diabeticorum*) (7). The onset is subtle and the involvement persistent. Erythema and induration of the posterior neck and the back are commonly observed as is a *peau d'orange* appearance of the skin. Unusual cases with limited site involvement have been reported (8).

Systemic manifestations (in all three forms) include serositis, dysarthria, dysphagia, myositis, parotitis, and ocular and cardiac abnormalities. Reported associations include hyperparathyroidism, rheumatoid arthritis, Sjögren's syndrome, malignant insulinoma, myeloma, gall bladder carcinoma, and HIV infection. Except for limitation of movement, scleredema usually causes little morbidity. Type 1 may clear in 6 months to 2 years, whereas the other types last longer. Type 3 scleredema is occasionally fatal due to systemic involvement.

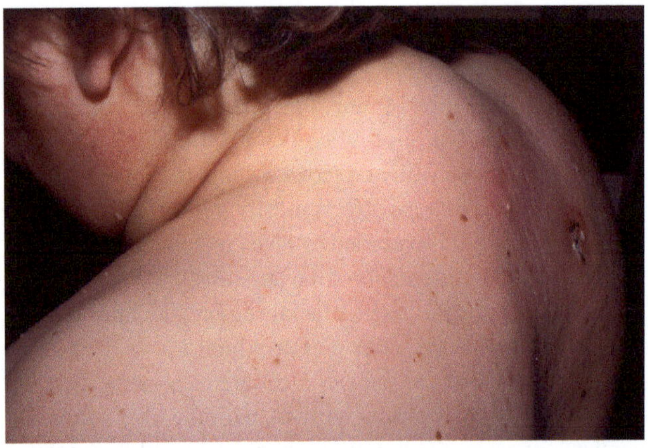

Fig. 18.11 Scleredema. Clinical features

Histologically, the principal alteration in scleredema is the thickening of the reticular dermis, with large collagen bundles separated from each other by clear spaces filled with mucin, resulting in fenestration of the dermis (Fig. 18.12 a, b). There is no increase in the number of fibroblasts, but the elastic fibers are reduced in number. At times, the mucin deposition can be slight. There is often a sparse perivascular lymphocytic infiltrate. Direct immunofluorescence is usually negative, but IgG and C3 have been found at the dermo–epidermal junction. Mucin also accumulates in skeletal muscle and the heart. Irreversible glycosylation of collagen and resistance to degradation by collagenase may lead to an accumulation of collagen. Alternatively, excess stimulation by insulin, microvascular damage, and hypoxia may increase the synthesis of collagen and mucin.

Scleredema may be confused with scleroderma, but the lack of acral involvement and the absence of Raynaud's phenomenon and cuticular and mat telangiectasias points to scleredema. Patients with scleromyxedema also have firm papules (often in a linear array) in addition to dermal induration. Histologically, there is little overlap beyond increased dermal mucin. Occasionally, because of associated erythema, patients with type 3 scleredema are misdiagnosed as having cellulitis (usually by nondermatologists).

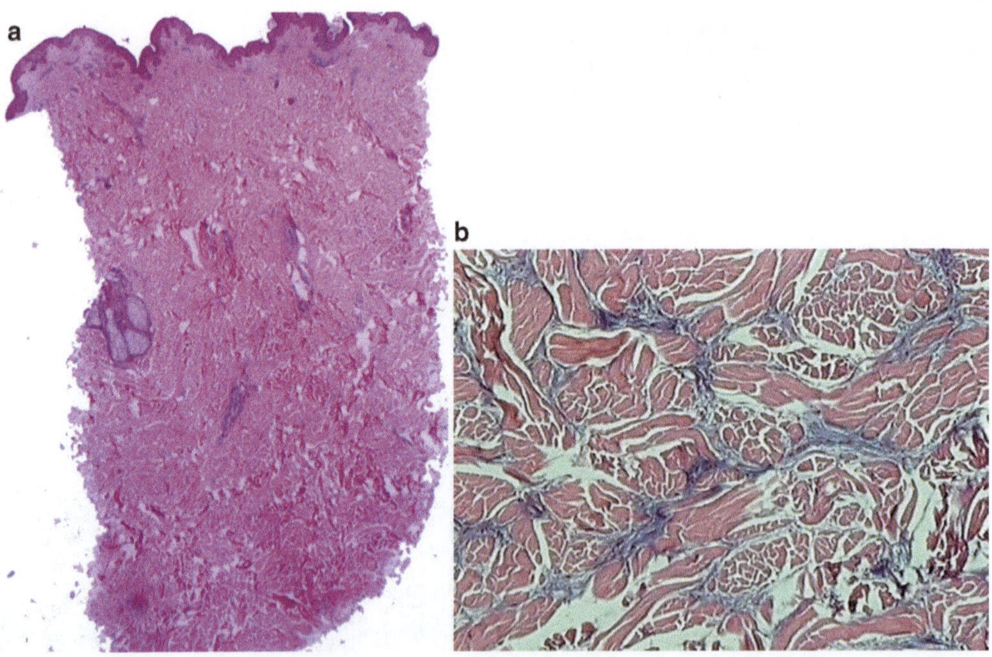

Fig. 18.12 Scleredema. (**a**) Thickening of the reticular dermis with large collagen bundles. (**b**) Fenestration of the collagen bundles separated by mucin deposition (HE stain)

18.2.4 *Mucinoses Associated with Altered Thyroid Function*

18.2.4.1 Localized (Pretibial) Myxedema

Pretibial mixoedema is one of the signs of Graves' disease (along with goiter, exophthalmus, thyroid acropathy, and high circulating levels of long-acting thyroid-stimulating hormone) and usually tends to occur at a later stage of the disease or after the patient becomes euthyroid post treatment (9). It is found in 1–5% of patients with Graves' disease, but in up to 25% of patients with exophthalmus (4). Less commonly, it has been described with Hashimoto's thyroiditis. There are four main clinical variants of pretibial myxedema: diffuse, nonpitting edema (43%); plaque (27%); nodular (18%); and elephantiasis (5%) (Fig. 18.13) (10). The lesions can vary in color and may exhibit a characteristic *peau d'orange* (orange peel) appearance and texture due to prominent hair follicles. The elephantiasic form is the most symptomatic and debilitating, consisting of nodular, polypoid, or fungating lesions with marked lymphedema (Fig. 18.14). The typical sites of involvement are the lateral or anterior aspect of the legs and dorsa of the feet, but the toes, the thighs, the shoulders, the hands and the forehead can be involved as well. Overlying hyperhidrosis or hypertrichosis may be associated. Apart from appearance, associated morbidity is usually minimal. Entrapment of peroneal nerves by mucinous connective tissue may cause foot drop or faulty dorsiflexion.

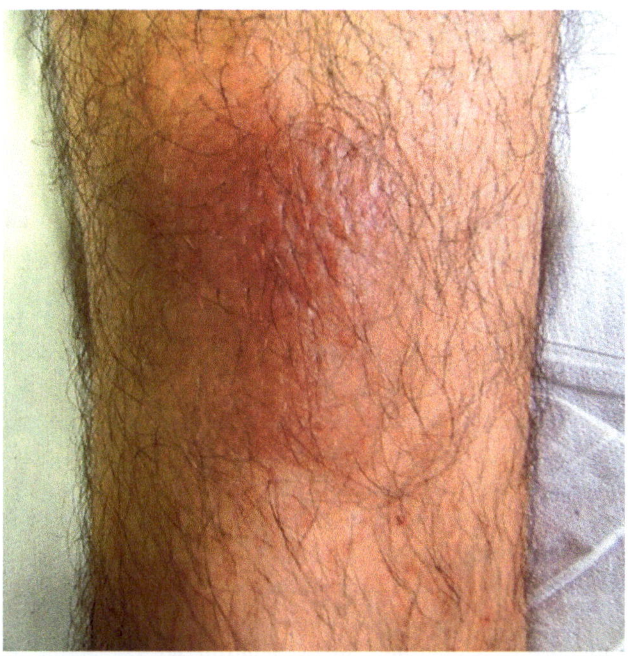

Fig. 18.13 Pretibial myxedema. Plaque-type with orange peel appearance

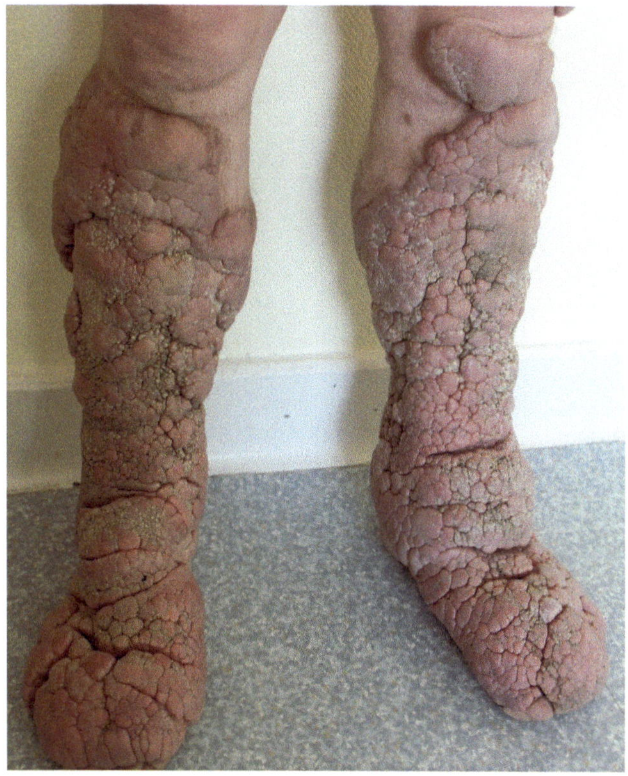

Fig. 18.14 Pretibial myxedema. Elephantiasic form (courtesy of B. Cribier, Strasbourg, France)

Histopathology reveals hyperkeratosis with follicular plugging, acanthosis and sometimes papillomatosis. The reticular dermis, particularly the mid to the lower part, shows separation of collagen bundles by large quantities of mucin (Fig. 18.15a, b). An increase in mast cells may be found but fibroblasts are normal. Elastic fibers are reduced in number.

A serum factor (unrelated to long-acting thyroid stimulating hormone) could incite fibroblasts to produce mucin. Fibroblasts from the dermis of the lower extremities have been found to be more sensitive to this factor than are fibroblasts from other areas of the body. An insulin-like growth factor, trauma, and lymphatic obstruction due to mucin may play a role.

In addition to lichen simplex chronicus and hypertrophic lichen planus in which mucin is lacking, pretibial myxedema should be differentiated from obesity-associated lymphedematous mucinosis seen in patients without thyroid disease.

18.2.4.2 Generalized Myxedema

Generalized myxedema is a manifestation of severe hypothyroidism in which mucin is deposited in the dermis leading

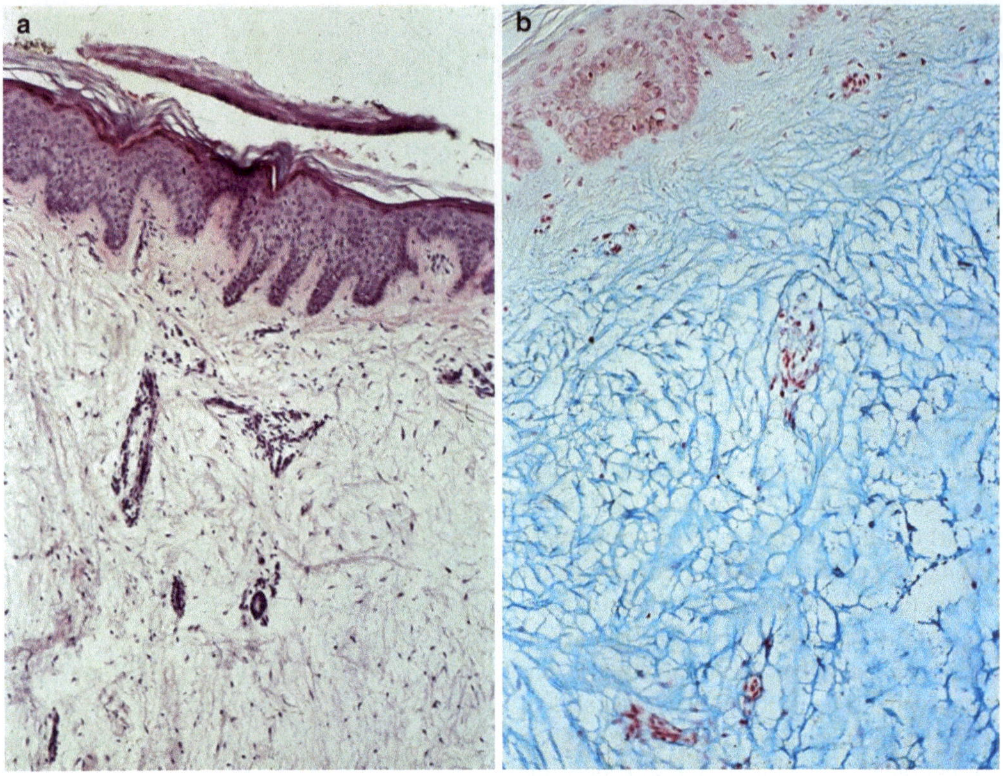

Fig. 18.15 (**a**) Pretibial myxedema. (HE stain). (**b**) Mucin in pretibial myxedema (Alcian blue stain)

to waxiness of the skin. Generalized myxedema is due to a quantitative or functional deficiency of thyroxine. Impaired degradation, rather than increased synthesis, of mucin has been suggested. Hypothyroidism may be congenital (cretinism) or of juvenile or adult onset.

Adult hypothyroidism is the most common form of the disease. It can be seen in women of 40–60 years of age as the result of autoimmune disease (usually Hashimoto's thyroiditis), therapy of hyperthyroidism (usually Graves' disease) or, rarely, pituitary or hypothalamic failure.

The initial symptoms are subtle and include mental and physical sluggishness, weight gain, constipation, leg cramps, loss of appetite, and cold intolerance. The face has a dull expression. The eyelids, lips, tongue, and hands are puffy, the nose is broad, and the speech becomes hoarse and slurred. The skin is pale, cool, waxy, and dry; an absence of sweating can lead to acquired ichthyosis or eczema craquelé. A yellowish discoloration of the palms and soles due to carotenemia may appear. Hair and nails are dry and brittle, and a diffuse nonscarring alopecia is common. Purpura involving the extremities, blue telangiectatic fingertips, delayed wound healing, and xanthomas may be seen.

Histologically, mucin deposits, mainly perivascular and perifollicular, display collagen bundles and may extend to the subcutaneous fat and nerves. Fibroblasts are not increased in number, but elastic fibers are reduced. Mucin deposits in the brain probably cause the psychiatric symptoms.

18.2.5 Papular and Nodular Mucinosis in Connective Tissue Diseases

Primary mucinoses presenting with papular, nodular, or plaque-like lesions may be associated with or antedate a connective tissue disease such as lupus erythematosus (cutaneous lupus mucinosis) (11) or, less frequently, dermatomyositis and scleroderma (Fig. 18.16) (12, 13). Cutaneous lupus mucinosis occurs in 1.5% of patients with lupus erythematosus. Only in Japan has a male predominance been observed. Pedriatic cases have also been reported (14). The clinical course may be related or not related to the underlying disease activity. Usually, patients with lupus erythematosus who develop papular and nodular mucinosis have a systemic disease, in about 75% of cases with renal and articular involvement. Cutaneous (discoid) and subacute cutaneous lupus erythematosus may also be associated. Histologically, mucin abounds in the upper and mid dermis, sometimes in association with a slight to moderately dense perivascular lymphocytic infiltrate. Mucin may involve the subcutis as well. The epidermal changes of

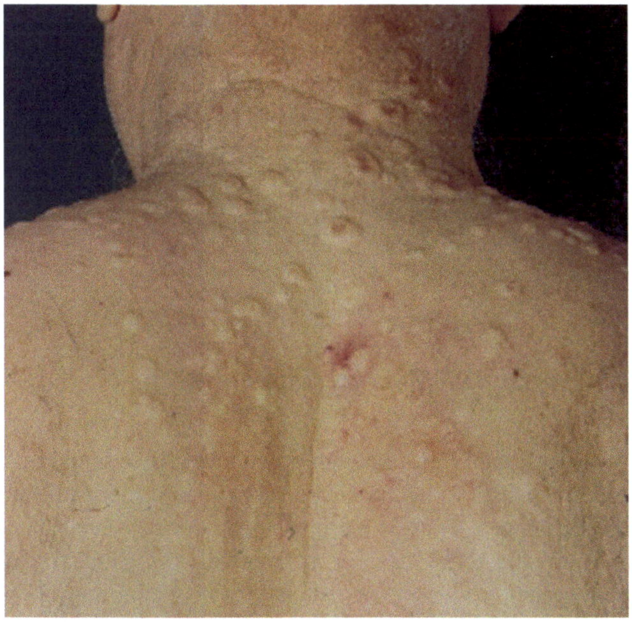

Fig. 18.16 Papular and nodular mucinosis associated with connective tissue disease

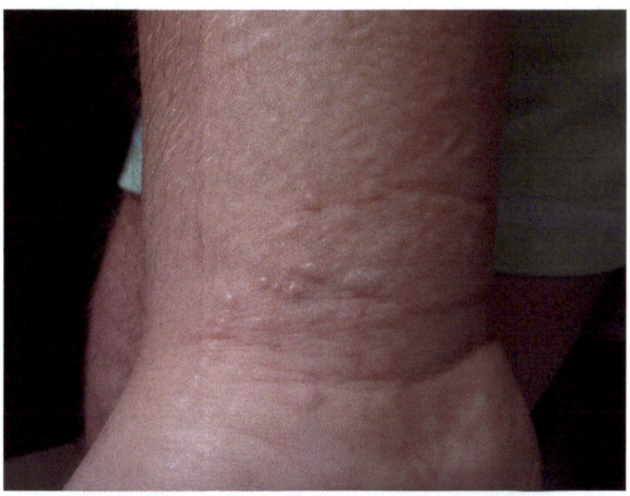

Fig. 18.17 Self-healing juvenile cutaneous mucinosis with papular lesions

lupus erythematosus are absent, but a positive lupus band is seen on direct immunofluorescence.

18.2.6 Self-healing Cutaneous Mucinosis

Self-healing cutaneous mucinosis is a rare disorder, usually involving the juvenile population, characterized by the following criteria: an acute eruption of multiple papules (Fig. 18.17), sometimes gathering in linear infiltrated plaques, on the face, neck, scalp, abdomen, and thighs; mucinous subcutaneous nodules on the face with periorbital swelling and on periarticular areas (Fig. 18.18); systemic symptoms such as fever, arthralgias, weakness, and muscle tenderness in the absence of paraproteinemia, bone marrow plasmocytosis, and thyroid dysfunction; spontaneous resolution in a period ranging from a few weeks to many months (from 2 to 8) (15). It has been also described in adults (16). Histologically, papular lesions show mucin deposition with mild inflammation and a small increase in fibroblasts while nodules show deep mucinous areas associated with bands of fibrosis and fibroblastic proliferation (Fig. 18.19).

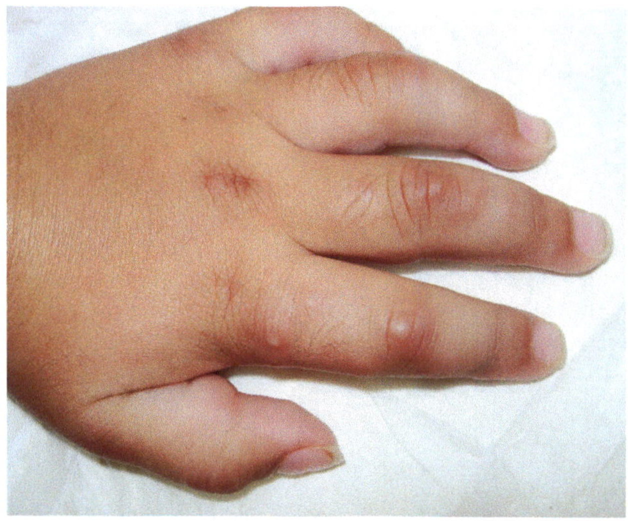

Fig. 18.18 Self-healing juvenile cutaneous mucinosis with hand nodules

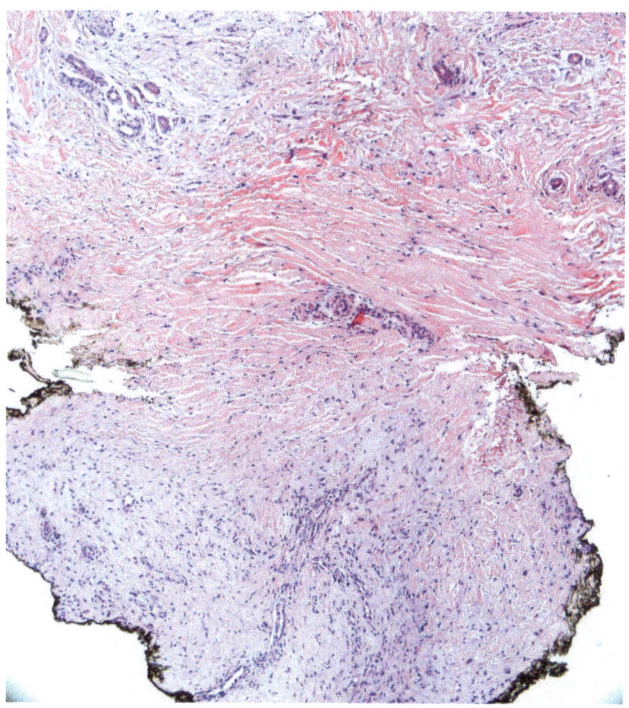

Fig. 18.19 Self-healing juvenile cutaneous mucinosis. Histopathology of a nodular lesion (HE stain)

18.2.7 Cutaneous Focal Mucinosis

The lesion is a benign, symptomless, skin-colored papule or nodule, which is less than 1 cm in diameter; it can occur anywhere on the body (Fig. 18.20) (17), except over the joints of the hands and feet. Oral involvement is not infrequent. The diagnosis is a histologic one. Mucin is dispersed throughout the upper and mid dermis sparing the subcutaneous fat (Fig. 18.21). Cleft-like spaces, but no cysts, are seen. Spindle-shaped or stellate fibroblasts are present. Moreover, a minor population of dermal dendrocytes that are partially factor XIIIa positive and partially CD34 positive is found. The elastic and reticulum fibers are absent, but capillaries are normal in number.

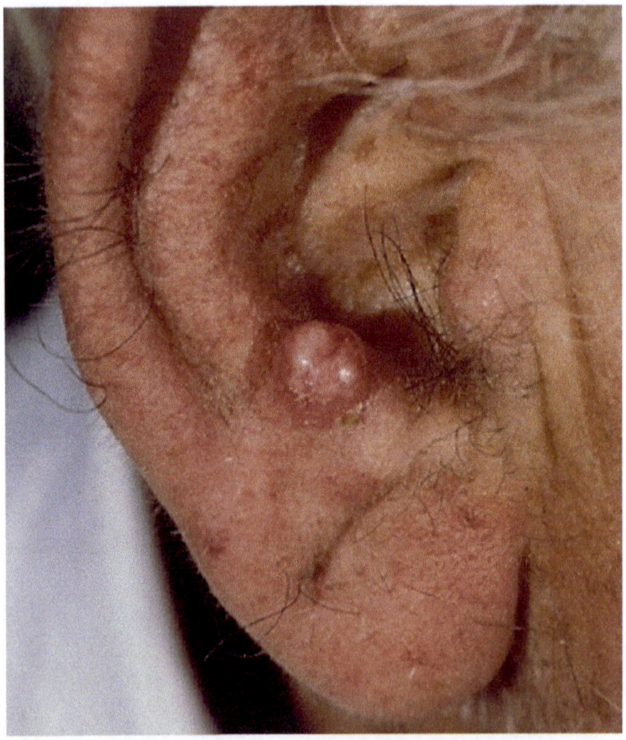

Fig. 18.20 Cutaneous focal mucinosis involving an ear

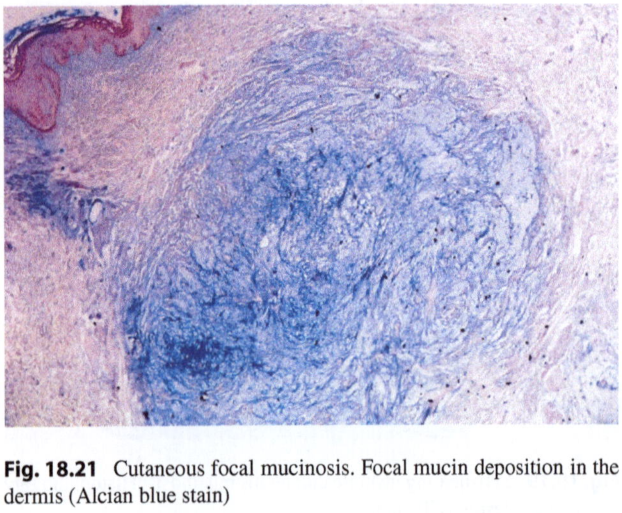

Fig. 18.21 Cutaneous focal mucinosis. Focal mucin deposition in the dermis (Alcian blue stain)

Cutaneous focal mucinosis results from a "muciparous" reaction of the connective tissue to nonspecific stimuli and should be distinguished from an angiomyxoma, which represents a true neoplasm.

18.2.8 Digital Mucous (Myxoid) Cyst

A dome-shaped elevation with or without visible semitransparent contents forms on the dorsal skin on or near a distal interphalangeal joint of the finger (Fig. 18.22). Subungual and multiple forms have been reported (17). Clinical and radiographic evidence of osteoarthritis is common (18). Grooving of the nail may associate or even precede the cyst itself by up to 6 months. Antecedent trauma has been documented in a small minority of cases (19). There are two variety of lesions: the cyst derived from synovial cells (ganglion), which is located over the joints, and that derived from dermal-based fibroblasts, which is located between the interphalangeal joints. Puncture or biopsy results in the drainage of viscous, stringy mucin from the cyst. Histopathological features show a large deposit of mucin containing stellate fibroblasts, some vascular spaces, and

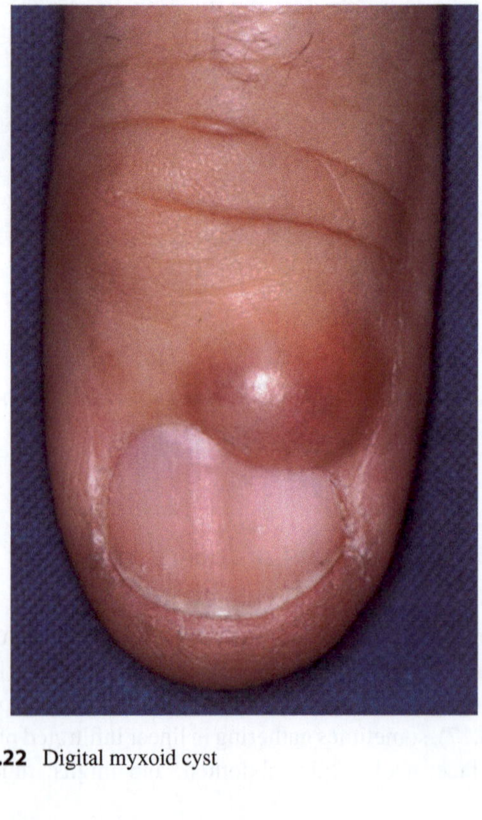

Fig. 18.22 Digital myxoid cyst

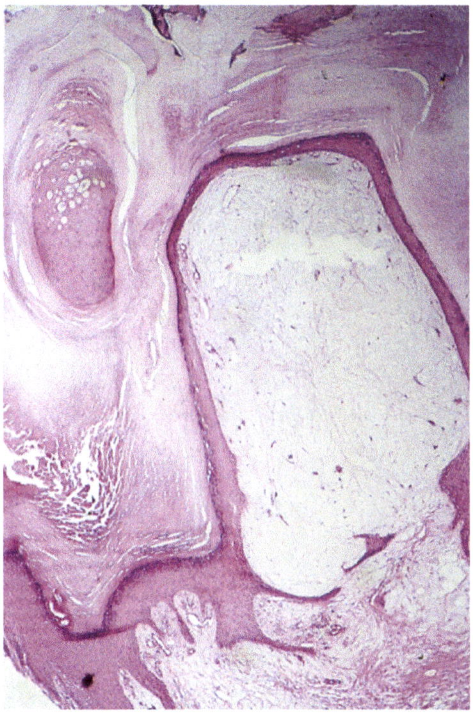

Fig. 18.23 Histopathology of digital myxoid cyst

multiple clefts (Fig. 18.23). The overlying epidermis is laterally acanthotic and centrally more atrophic. Transepidermal elimination of mucoid material may be seen.

18.2.9 Oral Mucous Cyst

Oral mucous cyst (mucocele)is a benign, single, dome-shaped, translucent, blue-whitish, mucin-containing cystic lesion of the oral cavity. They are located on the inner surface of the lower lip or on the floor of the mouth and wax and wane over several months (Fig. 18.24). The mucin deposits are made by sialomucin (neutral glycosaminoglycans) and not by acid glycosaminoglycans and are both PAS positive and Alcian blue positive.

18.2.10 Primary Follicular Mucinoses

Mucin accumulates in the follicular epithelium in two primary (idiopathic) distinctive clinical disorders: Pinkus' follicular mucinosis (20) and urticaria-like follicular mucinosis (21). Otherwise, follicular mucinosis is a histologic epiphenomenon most often seen in cutaneous T-cell lymphomas and other skin diseases

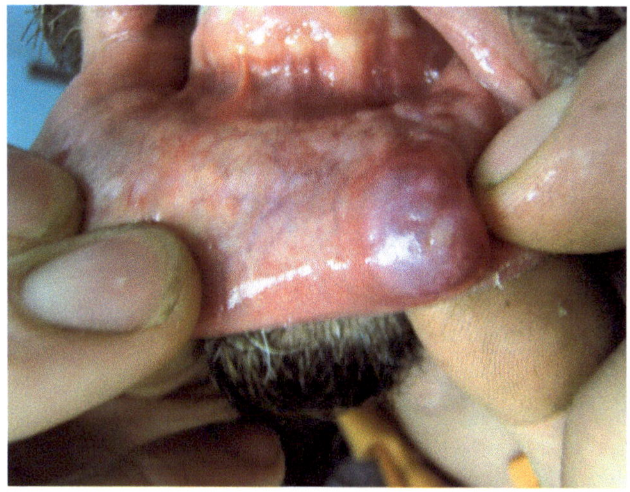

Fig. 18.24 Oral mucous cyst

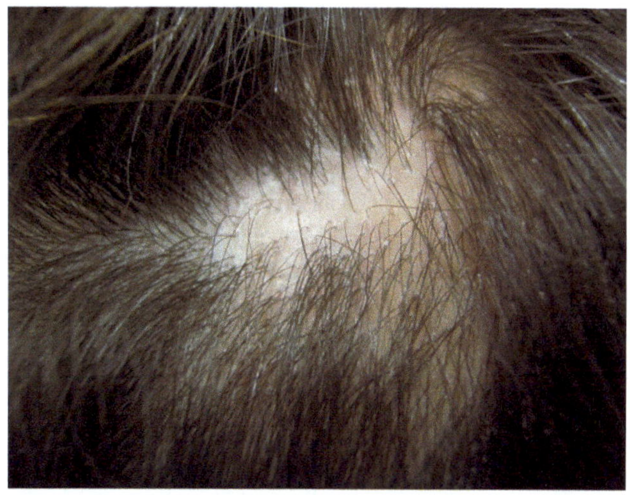

Fig. 18.25 Follicular mucinosis of the scalp

18.2.10.1 Pinkus' Follicular Mucinosis (Alopecia Mucinosa)

This uncommon inflammatory disorder, apparently not linked with lymphoma, has a predilection for children and for adults in the third and fourth decades of life. It is far from clear why dermal-type mucin is deposited selectively within an epithelial structure. Although follicular keratinocytes have been considered to be the source of the mucin, an etiologic role for cell-mediated immune mechanisms has been proposed. A reaction to persistent antigens such as *Staphylococcus aureus* has also been suggested. Clinically, it presents as an acute or subacute eruption characterized by one or several plaques of grouped follicular papules; lesions are limited to the face and scalp and are associated with alopecia (Fig. 18.25). Nodules, annular plaques, folliculitis, follicular spines, and acneiform eruptions (22) have also been described.

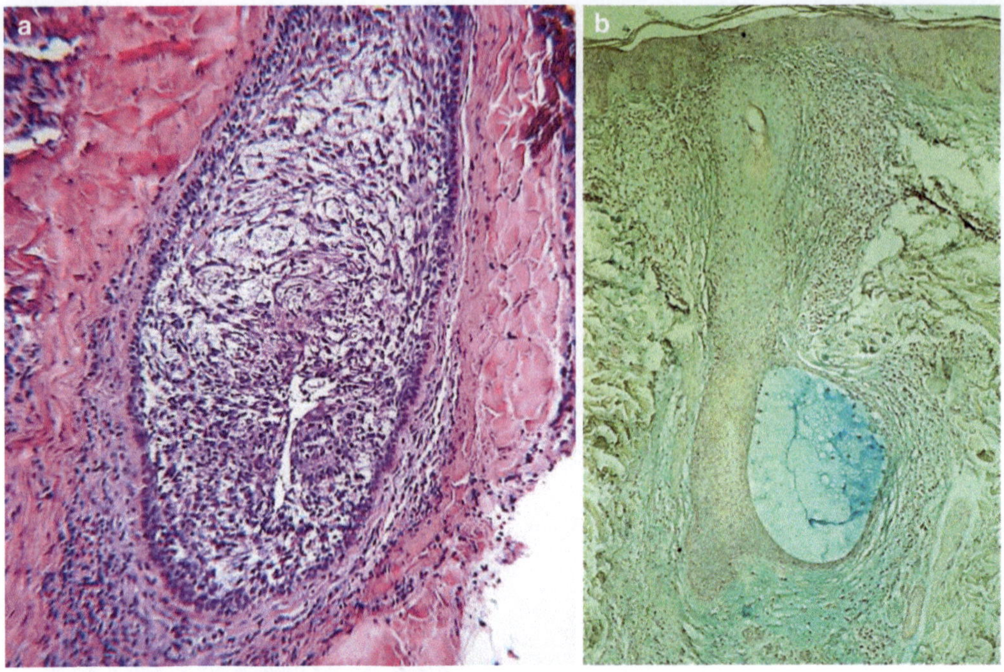

Fig. 18.26 (**a**) Follicular mucinosis (HE stain). (**b**) Mucin in the follicle (Alcian blue stain)

A second type that is characterized by a more generalized chronic form in a slightly older age group with larger and more numerous plaques on the extremities, trunk, and face is probably best regarded as a follicular mucinosis associated with a cutaneous T-cell lymphoma rather than a primary condition. Histologically, mucin accumulates within the follicular epithelium and sebaceous glands causing keratinocytes to disconnect (Fig. 18.26a, b). In more advanced lesions, the follicles are converted into cystic spaces containing mucin, inflammatory cells, and altered keratinocytes. A perifollicular infiltrate of lymphocytes, histiocytes, and eosinophils is seen. The differentiation between Pinkus' follicular mucinosis and mycosis fungoides-associated follicular mucinosis is very difficult and there is no single reliable criterion. Although the existence of a primary follicular mucinosis has been questioned as it has been considered as an "indolent" localized form of cutaneous T-cell lymphoma, clues in favor of a primary form are the young age of the patient, a solitary lesion on the face or neck, and the absence of histologic features of epidermotropism and atypical lymphocytes (23). Clonal T-cell rearrangement is not always useful to differentiate the two types. In these cases, a clinical follow-up is mandatory.

18.2.10.2 Urticaria-Like Follicular Mucinosis

This is a very rare disorder that occurs primarily in middle-aged men (21). Pruritic, urticarial papules or plaques appear on the head and neck within an erythematous "seborrheic" background. As lesions resolve, red macules persist for a few weeks. Hair-bearing regions may be involved, but neither follicular plugging nor alopecia is seen. Urticaria-like follicular mucinosis waxes and wanes irregularly over a period that can vary from a few months to 15 years. There are no associated systemic manifestations. Response to natural sunlight has been inconsistent, but it has been beneficial in a small number of cases.

As in primary follicular mucinosis, mucin accumulates inside the hair follicles. An infiltrate with lymphocytes and eosinophils is seen around blood vessels and hair follicles. In only a single patient were vascular C3 deposits seen by direct immunofluorescence.

18.3 Prognosis and Treatment of Cutaneous Mucinoses

Scleromyxedema is a disease with an unpredictable but usually progressive and disabling course, and the therapy is often disappointing. In the USA, melphalan has been the therapy of choice for long time, targeting the plasma cell dyscrasia. This alkylating agent can result in some clinical improvement, but it has also been implicated in 30% of the deaths secondary to its induction of hematologic malignancies and septic complications. Other chemotherapeutic agents have been tried, such as cyclophosphamide, methotrexate, chlorambucil or 2-chlorodesoxyadenosine, but with no better results and similar side effects. Systemic corticosteroids are also often used with limited or good, but temporary, results. Interferon alpha has led to paradoxical effects, both improving and worsening LM. Actually, high-dose intravenous immunoglobulins (24), autologous stem cell transplantation, and thalidomide may represent promising therapies. On the other hand, spontaneous improvement and clinical resolution, even after 15 years, have been described. The use of potentially toxic drugs should be limited to patients who are disfigured, disabled, or very ill. Dysarthria and a flu-like illness may herald coma, and the patient should be promptly admitted to hospital for close observation.

Localized LM is a benign condition and does not require therapy, and a wait-and-see approach is recommended. Topical corticosteroids and calcineurin inhibitors (25) may be of some benefit. However, spontaneous resolution may occur, even in the setting of HIV-associated cases.

The therapy of choice for REM is antimalarials (e.g. hydroxychloroquine) which are usually effective in clearing the lesions in 2–4 weeks. Calcineurin inhibitors may be also effective (26). Broad-spectrum sunscreens should also be used. The lesions may clear spontaneously, even after 15 years.

Therapy is unnecessary for type 1 scleredema because it is self-limited in duration. Regression of scleredema associated with diabetes or monoclonal gammopathy is more uncommon and no specific treatment is available. Control of the hyperglycemia does not have any influence on the skin. PUVA, pulse therapy with cyclophosphamide, oral corticosteroids, cyclosporine, factor XIII infusion, electron-beam, and UV-A1 therapy (27) have all been reported to be of benefit. Chemotherapeutic treatment of associated multiple myeloma also improved the lesions of scleredema. Aggressive therapies, however, should be limited to those cases associated with myeloma or with systemic, disabling manifestations.

Localized (pretibial) myxedema can be treated with corticosteroids applied under occlusive dressings or delivered by intralesional injection. Usually, skin grafting is followed by relapses. Plasmapheresis, gradient pneumatic compression, and octreotide with and without surgical shave removal have been of some benefit (28). Therapy for the associated hyperthyroidism does not improve the cutaneous lesions and, often, localized myxedema develops after treatment has been instituted. Localized myxedema may clear spontaneously (an average 3.5 years).

In generalized myxedema, symptoms subside with thyroxine administration and recur if it is discontinued. Even areas of hair loss regrow with proper treatment. If untreated, patients can die as a result of "myxedema coma."

Therapy of papular and nodular mucinosis in lupus erythematosus is the same as for lupus erythematosus. Only a few patients respond to antimalarials, the remainder requiring systemic corticosteroids. However, the course of papulonodular mucinosis is not always related to the severity of the associated connective tissue diseases.

Cutaneous focal mucinosis and myxoid cyst can be excised. Relapsing is not uncommon in the latter and many dermatologists tend to favor more conservative treatments such as multiple needling or aspiration followed by steroid injection or cryotherapy. Surgical excision is also the treatment of choice for oral mucous cyst.

There is no specific treatment for Pinkus' follicular mucinosis. A wait-and-see approach is recommended as many cases of Pinkus' follicular mucinosis resolve spontaneously in 2–24 months. Topical, intralesional and systemic corticosteroids, dapsone, antimalarials, indomethacin, minocycline, oral isotretinoin, interferon alfa-2b, and UVA1 phototherapy have produced some beneficial effects. Urticaria-like follicular mucinosis has a good prognosis and antimalarials and dapsone were reportedly beneficial (21).

References

1. Rongioletti F, Rebora A (2008) Mucinoses. In Bolognia J, Jorizzo JL, Rapini R. (eds). Dermatology, 2nd edn. Elsevier, St Louis, MO, pp 611–621
2. Rongioletti F (2006) Lichen myxedematosus (papular mucinosis): new concepts and perspectives for an old disease. Semin Cutan Med Surg 25:100–104
3. Scheidegger EP, Itin P, Kempf W (2005) Familial occurrence of axillary papular mucinosis. Eur J Dermatol 15:70–72
4. Rongioletti F, Rebora A (2001) Cutaneous mucinoses: microscopic criteria for diagnosis. Am J Dermatopathol 23:257–267
5. Caputo R, Marzano AV, Tourlaki A, Marchini M (2006) Reticular erythematous mucinosis occurring in a brother and sister. Dermatology 212:385–387
6. Gasior-Chrzan B, Husebekk A (2004) Reticular erythematous mucinosis syndrome: report of a case with positive immunofluorescence. J Eur Acad Dermatol Venereol 18:375–378
7. Lewerenz V, Ruzicka T (2007) Scleredema adultorum associated with type 2 diabetes mellitus: a report of three cases. J Eur Acad Dermatol Venereol 21:560–561
8. Ioannidou DI, Krasagakis K, Stefanidou MP et al (2005) Scleredema adultorum of Buschke presenting as periorbital edema: a diagnostic challenge. J Am Acad Dermatol 52(Suppl):41–44
9. Doshi DN, Blyumin ML, Kimball AB (2008) Cutaneous manifestations of thyroid disease. Clin Dermatol 26:283–287
10. Fatourechi V (2005) Pretibial myxedema: pathophysiology and treatment options. Am J Clin Dermatol 6:295–309
11. Ortiz VG, Krishnan RS, Chen LL, Hsu S (2004) Papulonodular mucinosis in systemic lupus erythematosus. Dermatol Online J 10:16
12. Rongioletti F, Rampini P, Parodi A, Rebora A (1999) Papular mucinosis associated with generalized morphoea. Br J Dermatol 141:905–908
13. Tan E, Tan S, Ng SH (2003) Cutaneous mucinosis in dermatomyositis associated with a malignant tumor. J Am Acad Dermatol 48:S41–S42
14. Bachmeyer C, Chesneau AM, Loirat C, Asensi D, Babinet JM, Blum L (2007) Papulonodular mucinosis in a child with systemic lupus erythematosus. Pediatr Dermatol 24:585–586
15. Nagaraj LV, Fangman W, White WL, Woosley JT, Prose N, Selim MA, Morrell DS (2006) Self-healing juvenile cutaneous mucinosis: cases highlighting subcutaneous/fascial involvement. J Am Acad Dermatol 55:1036–1043

16. Yokoyama E, Muto M (2006) Adult variant of self-healing papular mucinosis in a patient with rheumatoid arthritis: predominant proliferation of dermal dendritic cells expressing CD34 or factor XIIIa in association with dermal deposition of mucin. J Dermatol 33:30–35
17. Takemura N, Fujii N, Tanaka T (2005) Cutaneous focal mucinosis: a case report. J Dermatol 32:1051–1054
18. Lin YC, Wu YH, Scher RK (2008) Nail changes and association of osteoarthritis in digital myxoid cyst. Dermatol Surg 34:364–369
19. Connolly M, de Berker DA (2006) Multiple myxoid cysts secondary to occupation. Clin Exp Dermatol 31:404–406
20. Arca E, Köse O, Taştan HB, Gür AR, Safali M (2004) Follicular mucinosis responding to isotretinoin treatment. J Dermatolog Treat 15:391–395
21. Harthi FA, Kudwah A, Ailan A et al (2003) Urticaria-like follicular mucinosis responding to dapsone. Acta Derm Venereol 83:389–390
22. Passaro EM, Silveira MT, Valente NY (2004) Acneiform follicular mucinosis. Clin Exp Dermatol 29:396–398
23. Rongioletti F, De Lucchi S, Meyes D et al (2010) Follicular mucinosis: a clinicopathologic, histochemical, immunohistochemical and molecular study comparing the primary benign form and the mycosis fungoides-associated follicular mucinosis. J Cutan Pathol 37:15–19
24. Blum M, Wigley FM, Hummers LK (2008) Scleromyxedema: a case series highlighting long-term outcomes of treatment with intravenous immunoglobulin (IVIG). Medicine (Baltimore) 87:10–20
25. Rongioletti F, Zaccaria E, Cozzani E, Parodi A (2008) Treatment of localized lichen myxedematosus of discrete type with tacrolimus ointment. J Am Acad Dermatol 58:530–532
26. Rubegni P, Sbano P, Risulo M, Poggiali S, Fimiani M (2004) A case of reticular erythematous mucinosis treated with topical tacrolimus. Br J Dermatol 150:173–174
27. Kroft EB, de Jong EM (2008) Scleredema diabeticorum case series: successful treatment with UV-A1. Arch Dermatol 144:947–948
28. Felton J, Derrick EK, Prince ML (2003) Successful combined surgical and octreotide treatment of severe pretibial myxoedema reviewed after 9 years. Br J Dermatol 148:825–826

Chapter 19
Lipoid Proteinosis

Franco Rongioletti

Key Points

- Lipoid proteinosis is rare autosomal recessive disorder starting in early infancy and characterized by deposition of hyaline material in the skin, mucous membranes, and multiple organs.
- Typical clinical symptoms are hoarseness, vesicles leaving pitted scars, beaded papules on the eyelid margins, diffuse thickening of the skin with verrucous change on frictional areas, and infiltration of the oral mucosa.
- Mutations within the extracellular matrix protein gene (ECM-1) are the underlying defect.

Keywords Urbach-Wiethe disease • Hyalinosis cutis et mucosae • Hoarseness • Moniliform blepharosis

19.1 Introduction

"Hyaline" is not a single substance. Traditionally, this term included a variety of skin deposits that appeared eosinophilic and somewhat glassy by the refraction of light. Lipoid proteinosis (LiP) (OMIM 247100), also known as Urbach-Wiethe disease or hyalinosis cutis et mucosae, is a rare autosomal recessive or sporadic (new mutation) disorder in which an amorphous hyaline material is primarily deposited in the skin, the oropharyngeal mucosa, the larynx, and the brain. Its prevalence is high in South Africa, suggesting a probable founder effect (descendents of German and Dutch immigrants) [1]. Only about 300 cases have been reported in the literature, with only a few case series [2]. LiP is caused by loss of function mutations in the extracellular matrix protein 1 gene, ECM1, on chromosome 1q21 [3]. At least, 26 different inherited mutations in ECM1 have been reported, and exons 6 and 7 are the most common sites for ECM 1 gene mutations. It has been suggested that individuals with mutations in exon 7 have a slightly milder phenotype than those with exon 6 mutations.

F. Rongioletti (✉)
Department of Endocrinological and Medical Sciences (DISEM)
Section of Dermatology and Department of Pathology
University of Genova, Genova, Italy
e-mail: franco.rongioletti@unige.it

19.2 Clinical and Pathological Aspects of Skin Manifestations

LiP is clinically heterogeneous with affected individuals displaying differing degrees of skin scarring and infiltration, variable signs of hoarseness and respiratory distress, and in some cases neurological abnormalities such as temporal lobe epilepsy [4]. There is no sex predilection. The initial symptom of LiP is a weak cry after birth or hoarseness in early infancy, caused by infiltration of the vocal cords. Skin lesions usually develop during the first few years of life or may appear later and are characterized by inflammatory vesicles, bullae, and hemorrhagic crusts that resolve leaving pox-like and acneiform scars on the face and extremities. In the later stages, waxy, yellow papules and plaques with generalized skin thickening develop on the face (Fig. 19.1) and flexures. The classic and pathognonomic sign is the beaded papules on the eyelid margins (moniliform blepharosis) (Fig. 19.2), sometimes involving the nose (Fig. 19.3). Hyperkeratotic, verrucous lesions may appear in regions exposed to mechanical friction, such as the hands (Fig. 19.4), feet, elbows, and knees. Scalp involvement may lead to patchy or diffuse alopecia. Infiltration of the oral mucosa leads to a cobblestone appearance of the lips and tongue (Fig. 19.5). The tongue is short with a thickened frenulum that limits lingual movements and causes speech difficulties. Extracutaneous features may include epilepsy and neuropsychiatric abnormalities, dyspnea, intestinal bleeding, dental anomalies, and recurrent inflammation of the parotid and submandibular glands. A typical radiographic finding is bilateral, comma-shaped intracranial calcifications in the temporal lobes or hippocampus. No diagnostic laboratory abnormalities are found. Polymerase chain amplification and direct nucleotide sequencing of the ECM1 gene can confirm the diagnosis.

F. Rongioletti and B.R. Smoller (eds.), *Clinical and Pathological Aspects of Skin Diseases in Endocrine, Metabolic, Nutritional and Deposition Disease*, DOI 10.1007/978-1-60761-181-3_19, © Springer Science+Business Media, LLC 2010

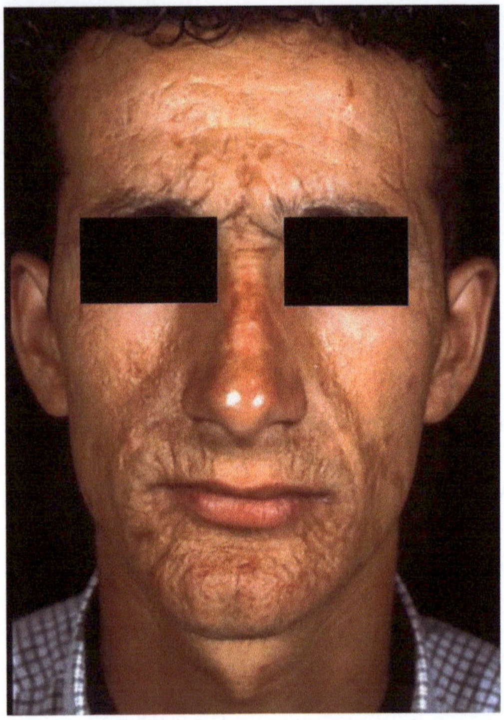

Fig. 19.1 Yellowish plaques with skin thickening and residual scars (Courtesy of A. Amantea and P. Donati, Rome, Italy)

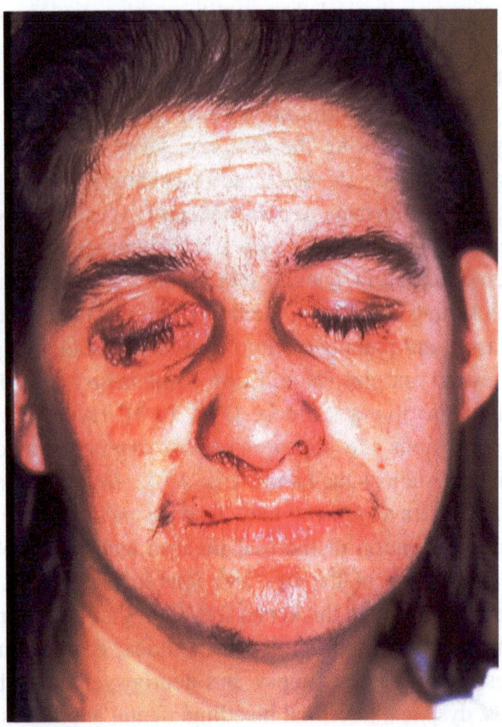

Fig. 19.2 Beaded papules on the eyelid margins (moniliform blepharosis)

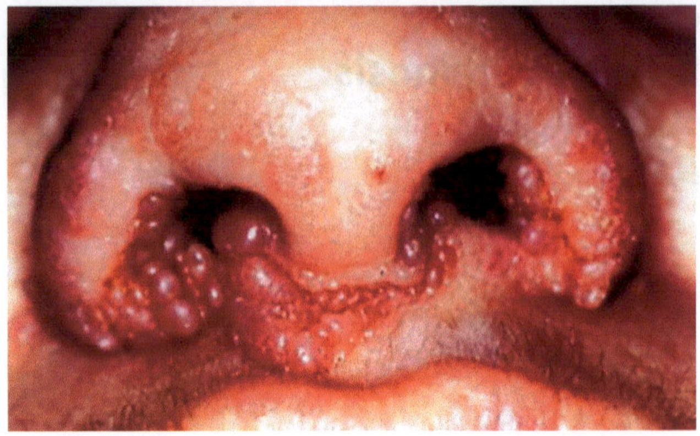

Fig. 19.3 Beaded papules on the nose (Courtesy of G.E. Cannata, Imperia, Italy)

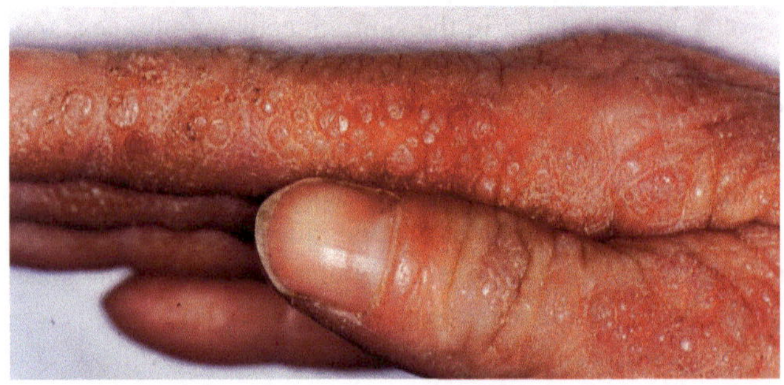

Fig. 19.4 Verrucous lesions on the hands (Courtesy of G.E. Cannata, Imperia, Italy)

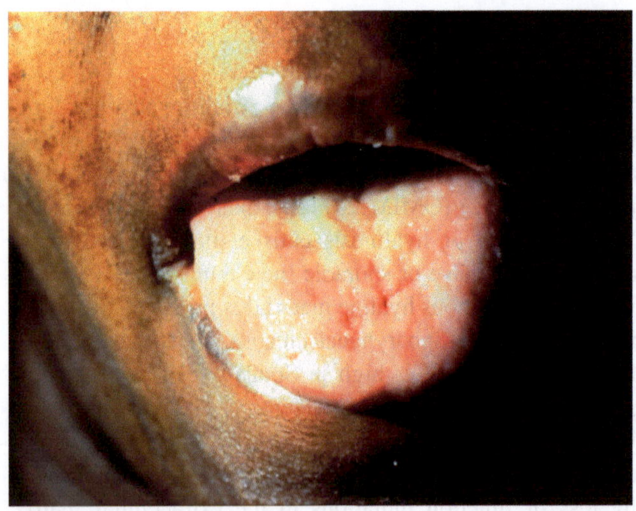

Fig. 19.5 Infiltration of the oral mucosa leads to a cobblestone appearance of the tongue

Histopathology of a typical lesion reveals widespread deposition of homogeneous, pale-staining, hyaline-like material in the dermis under a hyperkeratotic, acanthotic, and papillomatous epidermis (Fig. 19.6a). Initially, the deposits are located concentrically around capillaries and eccrine sweat glands (Fig.19.6b, c) (onion-skin pattern) and less frequently around hair follicles and arrector pili muscles. Later, vertically oriented hyaline deposits fill the dermis (Fig. 19.6d) [5].

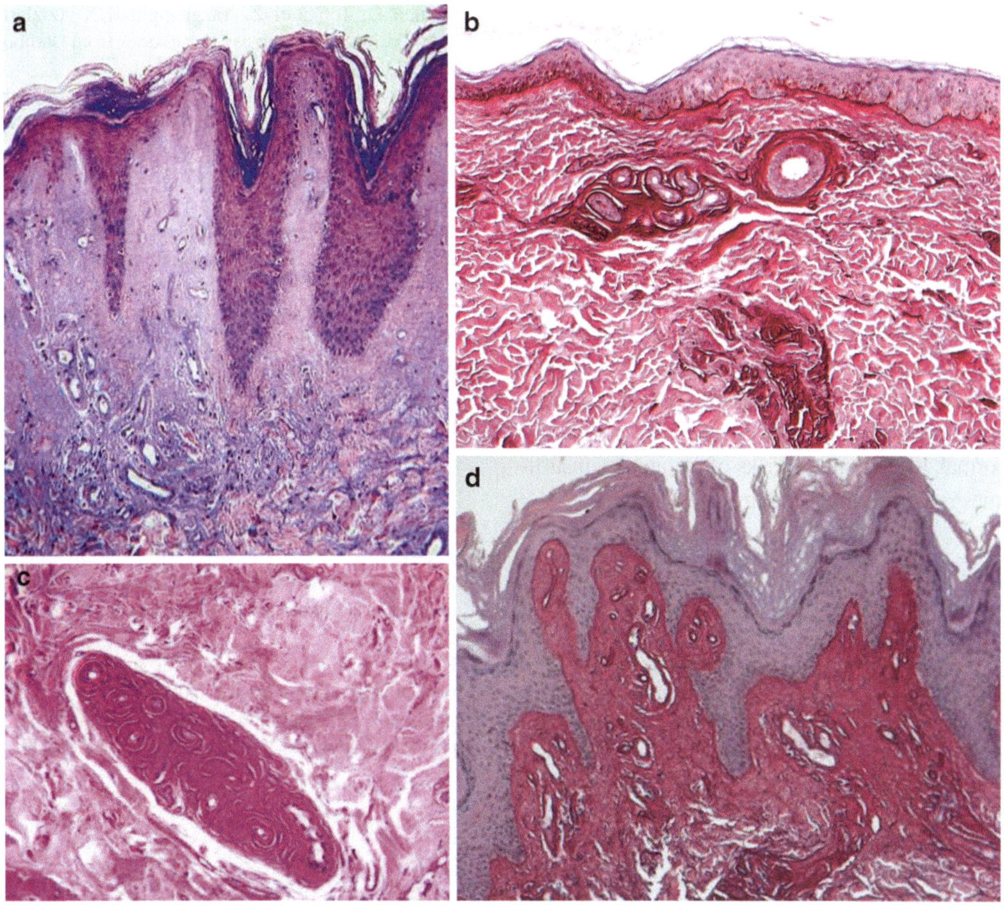

Fig. 19.6 (**a**) Homogeneous, hyaline-like material in the dermis under a hyperkeratotic, acanthotic, and papillomatous epidermis (HE stain). (**b**) Hyaline deposits located concentrically around capillaries and eccrine sweat glands (PAS stain). (**c**) Deep deposit around the eccrine coil (PAS stain) (**d**) Vertically oriented hyaline deposit fills the dermis (PAS stain) (Courtesy of A. Amantea and P. Donati, Rome, Italy)

The dermal deposits contain type IV collagen, laminin, neutral mucopolysaccharides, hyaluronic acid, and ceramide or more complex lipids. The material is periodic acid–Schiff (PAS)-positive, but diastase-resistant; furthermore, it stains positively with colloidal iron and Alcian blue at pH 2.5 and only weakly positive or negative with Congo Red and Thioflavin T. Small lipid droplets may be demonstrated with the scarlet red stain. Calcified foci and vascular and lymphatic anomalies have also been described [6, 7]. Electron microscopy demonstrates concentric rings of excess basement membrane surrounding blood vessels and adnexal structures, with irregular reduplication of lamina densa at the dermal–epidermal junction. In addition, abnormal lysosomes with curved tubular profiles in dermal eccrine glands and histiocytes, similar to those seen in Farber disease, and dermal fibroblasts with characteristic cytoplasmic vacuole formation have also been demonstrated in some patients, suggesting an abnormality in a degradation pathway of glycolipids or sphingolipids. On the contrary, histopathology of an initial vesicle reveals only the presence of an intraepidermal blister, sometimes with nondyskeratotic acantholysis [8]. In fact, ECM1 is critical to the intercellular adhesion of a keratinocyte and plays an important role in the binding of keratin intermediate filaments to the desmosomal region. Immunolabeling of affected tissue with polyclonal antibodies against the ECM1 protein may provide a faster, more efficient way of detecting mutations.

The differential diagnosis includes other deposition disorders such as erythropoietic protoporphyria, lichen amyloidosis, colloid milium, and lichen myxedematosus. Final distinction relies on clinicopathologic correlations. Histologically, in erythropoietic protoporphiria, the perivascular hyalin deposits are more focal and superficial and do not involve the adnexa. Demonstration of pathogenetic mutations in the ECM1 gene in LiP now provides a definitive means of establishing a diagnosis through molecular gene analysis.

19.3 Treatment and Prognosis

There is no specific treatment for LiP [4]. Although different therapeutic modalities such as systemic steroids, dimethyl sulphoxide, etretinate, penicillamine, and intralesional heparin injections have been proposed in an anecdotic way, they are rarely effective [9]. CO_2 laser treatment of vocal cords and eyelid papules is helpful for some patients [10]. Identification of mutations in ECM1 in LP now provides a basis for the development of more rational forms of treatment, including trials of recombinant ECM1 protein and the development of somatic gene therapy for skin or respiratory mucosa [9]. The disease typically follows a slowly progressive, yet often benign, course. Life expectancy of patients is normal, aside from the risks of respiratory insufficiency, sometimes requiring tracheostomy, and seizures.

References

1. Van Hougenhouck-Tulleken W, Chan I, Hamada T, Thornton H, Jenkins T, McLean WH, McGrath JA, Ramsay M (2004) Clinical and molecular characterization of lipoid proteinosis in Namaqualand, South Africa. Br J Dermatol 151:413–423
2. Baykal C, Topkarci Z, Yazganoglu KD, Azizlerli G, Baykan B (2007) Lipoid proteinosis: a case series from Istanbul. Int J Dermatol 46:1011–1016
3. Chan I, Liu L, Hamada T, Sethuraman G, McGrath JA (2007) The molecular basis of lipoid proteinosis: mutations in extracellular matrix protein 1. Exp Dermatol 16:881–890
4. Hamada T (2002) Lipoid proteinosis. Clin Exp Dermatol 27:624–629
5. Rongioletti F, Granese J, Junkins-Hopkins JM (2010) Deposition disorders and miscellaneous alterations of dermal connective tissue. In: Busam KJ (ed) Dermatopathology. A volume in the series Foundations in Diagnostic Pathology, 1st edn. Saunders Elsevier, New York, pp 250–265
6. Mirancea N, Hausser I, Beck R, Metze D, Fusenig NE, Breitkreutz D (2006) Vascular anomalies in lipoid proteinosis (hyalinosis cutis et mucosae): basement membrane components and ultrastructure. J Dermatol Sci 42:231–239
7. Uchida T, Hayashi H, Inaoki M, Miyamoto T, Fujimoto W (2007) A failure of mucocutaneous lymphangiogenesis may underlie the clinical features of lipoid proteinosis. Br J Dermatol 156: 152–157
8. Ko C, Barr RJ (2003) Vesicular lesions in a patient with lipoid proteinosis: a probable acantholytic dermatosis. Am J Dermatopathol 25:335–337
9. Kaya TI, Kokturk A, Tursen U et al (2002) D-penicillamine treatment for lipoid proteinosis. Pediatr Dermatol 19:359–362
10. Kroukamp G, Lehmann K (2007) Treatment of laryngeal lipoid proteinosis using CO_2 laser. S Afr Med J 97:90–92

Chapter 20
Colloid Milium

Franco Rongioletti

Key Points

- Colloid milium is a rare, degenerative skin condition characterized by deposition of amorphous hyaline-like material in the dermis.
- Colloid milium and colloid degeneration include at least four distinct clinicopathological conditions: classic adult-type colloid milium, juvenile colloid milium, nodular colloid degeneration (paracolloid), and pigmented colloid milium (hydroquinone related).
- There are usually no systemic implications, with the exception of a rare ligneous conjunctivitis or periodontitis in the juvenile type.
- Special stains, immunohistochemical studies, and electron microscopy have allowed the distinction from similar conditions such as amyloidosis.

Keywords Adult-type colloid milium • Juvenile colloid milium • Nodular colloid degeneration (paracolloid)

20.1 Introduction

Colloid milium is a rare, degenerative skin condition characterized by deposition of amorphous hyaline-like material in the dermis [1]. Various terms have been used for this disorder, including colloid pseudomilium, miliary colloidoma, nodular colloid degeneration, hyaloma, and elastosis colloidalis conglomerata [2].

20.2 Clinical and Pathological Aspects of Skin Manifestations

Colloid milium is classified into two main clinical forms: adult colloid milium (ACM) and juvenile colloid milium (JCM). A third controversial variant is reported under the name of nodular colloid degeneration or paracolloid of the skin. A fourth variant known as pigmented colloid milium is associated with hydroquinone use [1].

ACM, the most common form, affects fair-skinned, middle-aged patients (30–60 years of age) who have actinically damaged skin. ACM shows a predilection for males (4:1). It is characterized by multiple, small (1–5 mm), dome-shaped, amber- or flesh-colored translucent papules occurring on sun-exposed regions including the face (Figs. 20.1 and 20.2), neck, décolleté (Fig. 20.3), and dorsal aspects of the hands and back. A gelatinous material can often be expressed after puncture of the lesions. The underlying skin may be thickened and furrowed. Stroking may induce purpura. Patients are usually asymptomatic but may experience transient itching. Unusual sites of involvement such as the eyelid margin may mimic lipoid proteinosis [3]. Anecdotal association with multiple myeloma [4] and beta thalassemia [5] has been reported. The condition has been linked to long-term, unprotected sun exposure, which appears to cause degeneration of elastin. In fact, UV-induced colloid milium has been documented in patients with outdoor occupations, such as farmers and taxi drivers who can exhibit unilateral left-sided involvement [6]. Prolonged exposure to UVA wavelengths for cosmetic purposes may also induce lesions [7]. However, excessive UV exposure is not the only etiologic factor, as ACM has been described on the penis and even in the oral mucosa [8, 9]. Long-term exposure to petroleum derivatives is another triggering factor, and phenols have been suggested as causative agents. A verrucous variant associated with occupational lubricating oil-exposure has been reported (Fig. 20.4) [10].

Clinical differential diagnoses of ACM may include milium, syringomas, steatocystoma multiplex, lipoid proteinosis, retention cysts, sarcoidosis, molluscum contagiosum, papular mucinosis, and senile sebaceous hyperplasia.

JCM is transmitted in both autosomal recessive and autosomal dominant modes and presents before puberty [1]. The lesions are clinically indistinguishable from ACM but can occur in normal skin. More commonly, however, they follow a severe sunburn or excess sun exposure and occur on the face. Familial cases have also been reported.

F. Rongioletti (✉)
Department of Endocrinological and Medical Sciences (DISEM)
Section of Dermatology and Department of Pathology
University of Genova, Genova, Italy
e-mail: franco.rongioletti@unige.it

F. Rongioletti and B.R. Smoller (eds.), *Clinical and Pathological Aspects of Skin Diseases in Endocrine, Metabolic, Nutritional and Deposition Disease*, DOI 10.1007/978-1-60761-181-3_20, © Springer Science+Business Media, LLC 2010

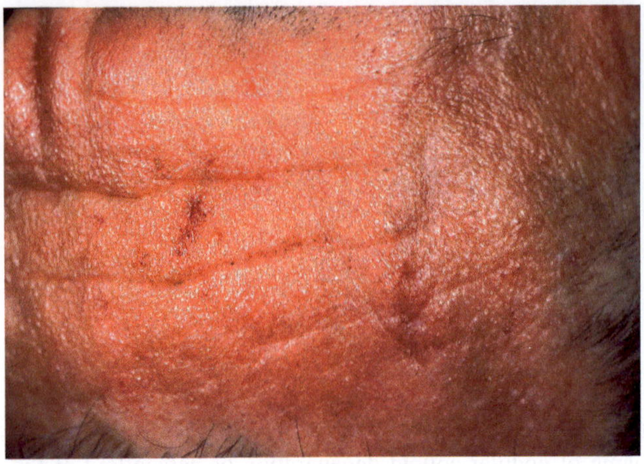

Fig. 20.1 Adult colloid milium on the forehead

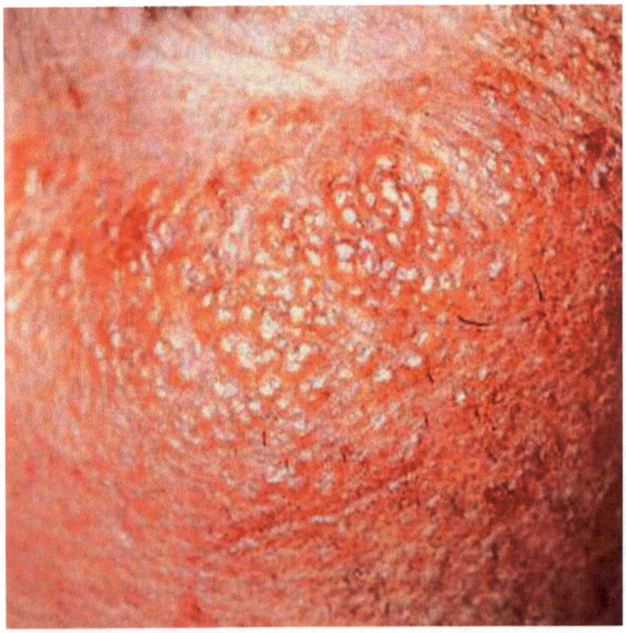

Fig. 20.2 Papules of adult colloid milium on the face

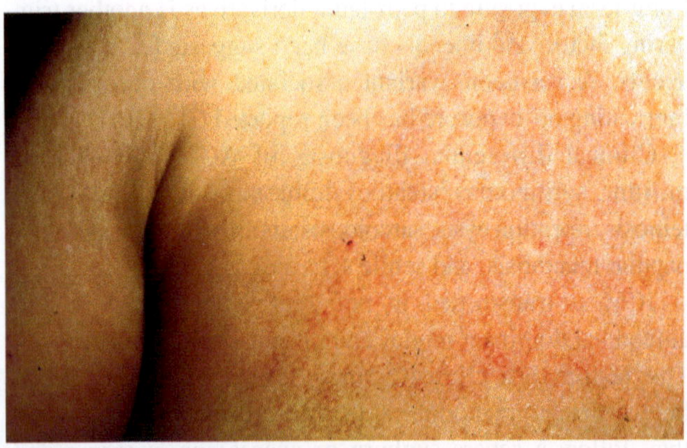

Fig. 20.3 Papules of adult colloid milium on the chest

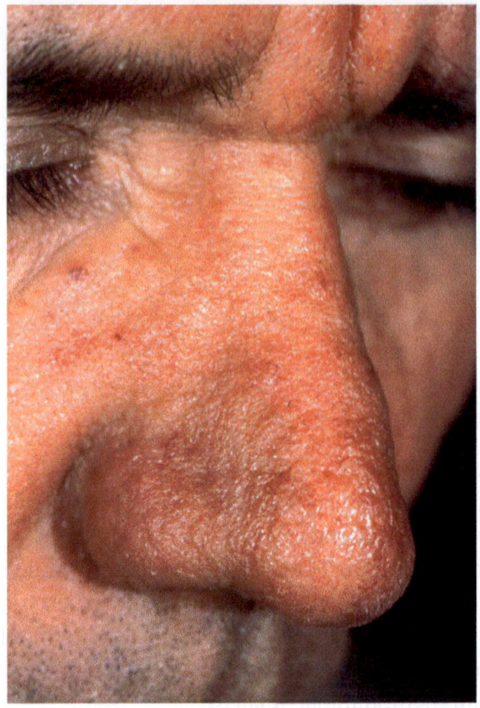

Fig. 20.4 Colloid milium associated with occupational lubricating oil-exposure (courtesy of L. Muscardin, Rome, Italy)

JCM may be associated with ligneous conjunctivitis or ligneous periodontitis due to hyalin-like infiltration of the tissue. The cause is unclear, but it may involve a hereditary predisposition to sun-induced keratinocyte damage.

Pigmented colloid milium is a disorder associated with exogenous ochronosis secondary to the use of hydroquinone-containing creams and sun exposure [11]. It has a distinct clinical presentation with the development of glistening black, caviar-like papules darker than the patient's normal skin on the face. Between the papules, atrophy may be present.

Nodular colloid degeneration or paracolloid of the skin probably represents a heterogeneous group [12, 13], including also cases of nodular amyloidosis. It usually appears in adulthood as a single pink or yellowish-brown nodule or multiple nodules up to 5 cm in size, usually on the face and occasionally on the trunk or scalp. They may be angiectatic with a slightly "lumpy" surface and sometimes itching. Sun exposure is not believed to play a role because in some patients, the lesions are restricted to the chest. However, the paucity of the reports does not allow one to draw any firm conclusions.

The histologic composition of ACM reveals homogenous, pale-pink, fissured masses in the papillary dermis (Fig. 20.5) [1, 5, 14]. Fibroblasts may be seen lining the fissures of the colloid and dispersed throughout the deposit. Solar elastosis is generally present, but an elastic tissue stain is largely negative in the main body of colloid. Inflammation is lacking, but occasionally, a few lymphocytes and mast cells can be seen (Fig. 20.6). A narrow *grenz* zone separates the colloid from the overlying atrophic epidermis and often contains elastic fibers. Dilated blood vessels may surround the colloid. The colloid material has been shown to derive from elastic fibers, although this finding does not exclude the possibility that it can also be produced by ultraviolet-damaged fibroblasts. In the verrucous variant, irregular acanthosis and papillomatosis are found (Fig. 20.7) [10].

Histopathology of JCM reveals subepidermal, eosinophilic, fissured colloid masses abutting the epidermis without a *grenz* zone (Fig. 20.8a, b). Colloid-like material appears to be derived from apoptotic keratinocytes, some of which appear as "dropping off" into the dermis [15]. Histiocytes, melanophages, and mast cells have been noted within the colloid islands. Dilated blood vessels may also be seen within the reticular dermis. Rete ridges may be elongated at the periphery of the lesion.

In pigmented CM, in addition to the acellular hyaline material, the histology shows ochronotic collagen fibers [16].

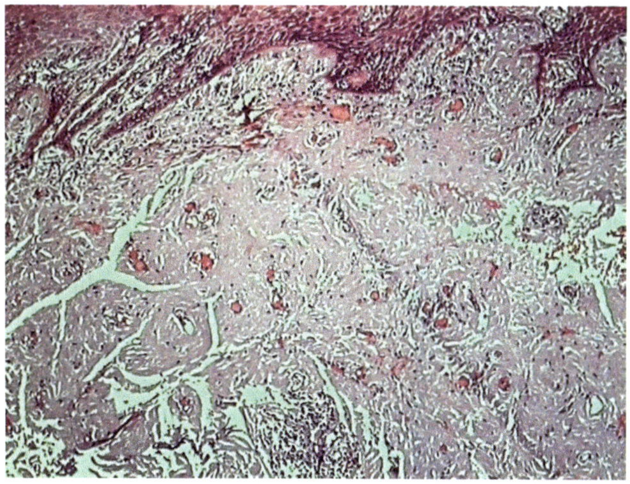

Fig. 20.6 Amorphous material of adult colloid milium with occasional inflammatory infiltrate (HE stain)

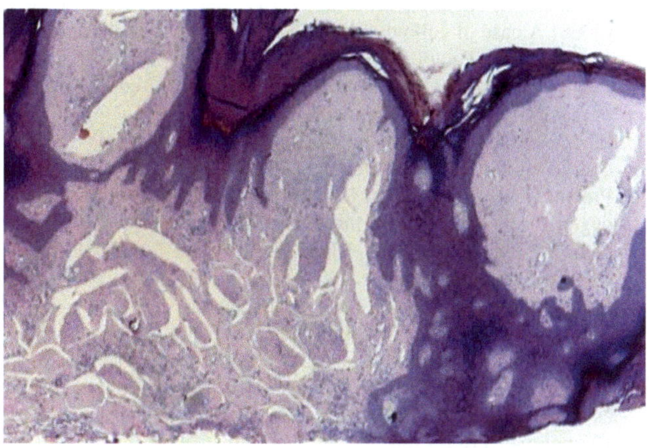

Fig. 20.5 Histopathology of adult colloid milium (HE stain)

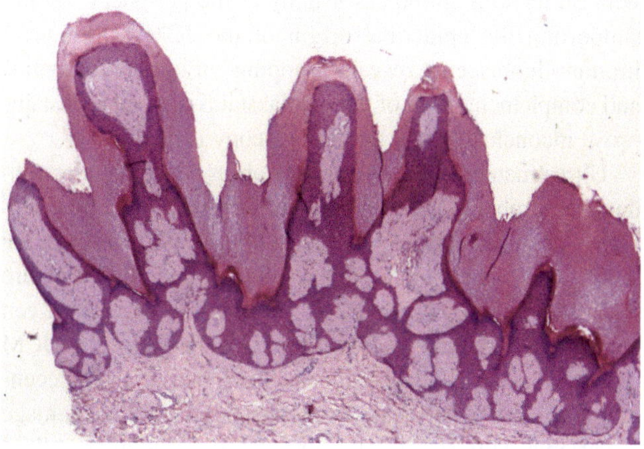

Fig. 20.7 Verrucous variant of adult colloid milium with irregular acanthosis and papillomatosis (HE stain) (courtesy of L. Muscardin, Rome, Italy)

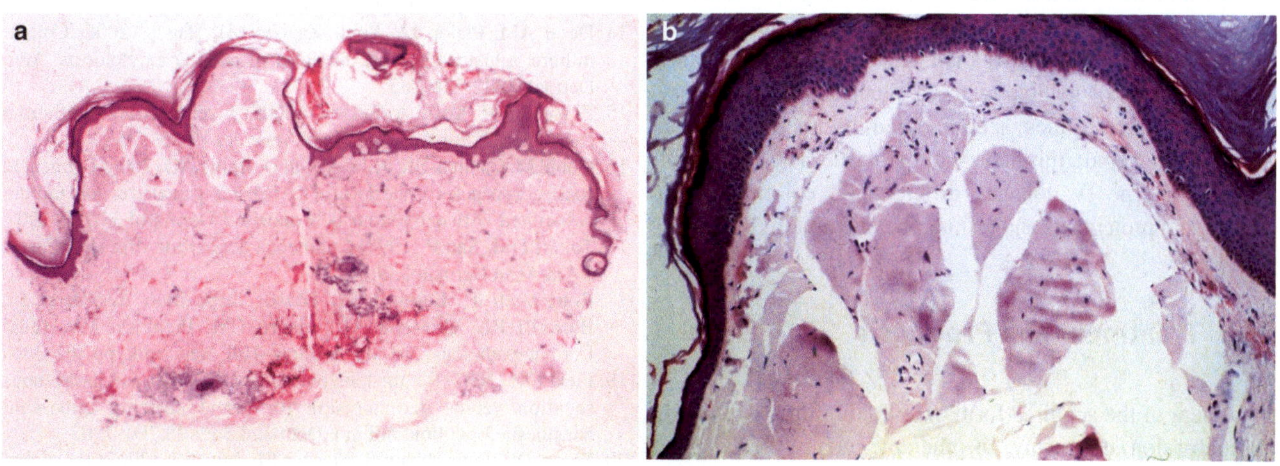

Fig. 20.8 Juvenile colloid milium. (**a**) Subepidermal, eosinophilic, fissured colloid masses abutting the epidermis (courtesy of James W. Patterson, Charlottesville, VA, USA). (**b**) Close-up of colloid masses (courtesy of James W. Patterson, Charlottesville, VA, USA)

In the nodular form, the hyaline-like deposit extends more deeply than in colloid milium throughout the reticular dermis and reveals clefting. The epidermis is usually flattened. Although the material has been reported to stain identically to ACM, some cases are probably due to amyloid deposition and other cases lack definite characteristics of either amyloid or colloid milium [12, 13].

The colloid in both the adult and the juvenile types stains positive with PAS both before and after diastase digestion and negative with alcian blue at pH 2.5 [17].The material is only weakly positive or negative with Congo red or Thioflavine T. The disparity in the results of Congo red stain could be due to the different technical procedures performed [5]. Methyl violet and crystal violet stains give variable staining patterns. The colloid in the adult form can be stained immunohistochemically for amyloid P protein, which is present in normal elastic fibers, and it fails to stain with antikeratin antibodies. JCM, in contrast, stains positively with antikeratin antibodies usually at the periphery, further supporting the epidermal origin of the JCM [18]. Direct immunofluorescence reveals "trapping" of immunoglobulins and complement. If all of the special stains and immunostains prove inconclusive, electron microscopy is helpful.

Ultrastructurally, the colloid appears as a medium electron-dense amorphous, granular material with short, branching filaments up to 2.0 nm in diameter [17]. These filaments are much shorter and smaller than those of amyloid, which are 6- to 10-nm straight filaments. Transitional stages between actinic elastosis and colloid are seen. The lesions of JCM consist of an amyloid-like substance originating from degenerated epidermal keratinocytes. Basement membrane damage is variable. Ultrastructurally, the colloid in nodular colloid degeneration appears similar to that seen in ACM.

The major histologic differential diagnosis is amyloidosis. In cutaneous primary amyloidosis, amyloid deposition occurs within the dermis, particularly around vessel walls and sometimes with extension into subcutis surrounding individual fat cells. Hemorrhage between the hyaline deposits is quite common. Lichen amyloidosis is characterized by small and sparse deposits of hyaline material situated in the papillary dermis and sometimes accompanied by melanophages. The overlying epidermis may be hyperplastic. The absence of laminin or type IV collagen differentiates colloid milium from lipoid proteinosis and primary cutaneous amyloidosis [17]. Topical tretinoin, systemic ascorbic acid, and exfoliative agents have been tried.

20.3 Treatment and Prognosis

Treatment of the acquired form of colloid milium is limited. Dermabrasion, diathermy, cryotherapy, intense pulsed light laser, and ablative and fractional laser resurfacing were reported to be effective [19, 20]. Sunscreens are also recommended

Most cases of ACM persist with no spontaneous resolution. Lesions reach their peak within 3 years, after which very few new papules occur. Genetic counseling is advisable for the rare juvenile form.

References

1. Pourrabbani S, Marra DE, Iwasaki J, Fincher EF, Moy RL (2007) Colloid milium: a review and update. J Drugs Dermatol 6:293–296
2. Dummer R, Laetsch B, Stutz S, Schärer L (2006) Elastosis colloidalis conglomerata (adult colloid milium, paracolloid of the skin): a maximal manifestation of actinic elastosis? Eur J Dermatol 16:163–166
3. Muzzaffar W, Dar NR, Malik AM (2002) Colloid milium of the upper eyelid margins: a rare presentation. Ophthalmology 109:1944–1946
4. Sanjuán EB, Planas G, Piquero J, Pérez R, Reyes O, Bretaña A (1994) Colloid milium associated with multiple myeloma. Int J Dermatol 33:793–795
5. Giordano G, Ricci R, Froio E, Izzi G, Barone A, Boccaletti V (2008) A case of colloid milium in patient with beta thalassaemia major. J Cutan Pathol 35:566–569
6. Lewis AT, Le EH, Quan LT et al (2002) Unilateral colloid milium of the arm. J Am Acad Dermatol 46:S5–S7
7. Innocenzi D, Barduagni F, Cerio R, Wolter M (1993) UV-induced colloid milium. Clin Exp Dermatol 18:347–350
8. Preston PW, Orpin SD, Muc R, Zaki I (2006) Penile colloid degeneration. Clin Exp Dermatol 31:674–676
9. Ojha J, Bhattacharyya I, Islam NM, Wong F (2008) Cohen DM.Colloid milium of the oral cavity: a rare presentation. Oral Surg Oral Med Oral Pathol Oral Radiol Endod 105:34–38
10. Muscardin LM, Bellocci M, Balus L (2000) Papuloverrucous colloid milium: an occupational variant. Br J Dermatol 143(4):884–887
11. Oskay T, Erdem C, Anadolu R et al (2003) Juvenile colloid milium associated with conjunctival and gingival involvement. J Am Acad Dermatol 49:1185–1188
12. Patterson JW, Wilkin JK, Schatzki PF (1985) Nodular colloid degeneration: distinctive histochemical and ultrastructural features. Cutis 36:355–358
13. Dupre A, Bonafe JF, Pieraggi MT, Perrot H (1979) Paracolloid of the skin. J Cutan Pathol 6:304–309
14. Desai AM, Pielop JA, Smith-Zagone MJ, Hsu S (2006) Colloid milium: a histopathologic mimicker of nodular amyloidosis. Arch Dermatol 142:784–785
15. Ekmekci TR, Koslu A, Sakiz D (2005) Juvenile colloid milium: a case report. J Eur Acad Dermatol Venereol 19:355–356
16. Gönül M, Cakmak SK, Kiliç A, Gül U, Heper AO (2006) Pigmented coalescing papules on the dorsa of the hands: pigmented colloid milium associated with exogenous ochronosis. J Dermatol 33:287–290
17. Touart DM, Sau P (1998) Cutaneous deposition diseases. Part I. J Am Acad Dermatol 39:149
18. Rongioletti F, Barnhill RL (2010) Deposition disorders. In: Barnhill RL, Crowson AN, Magro CM, Piepkorn MW (eds) Dermatopathology, 3rd edn. McGraw-Hill, New York, pp 362–386
19. Field LM (2002) Re: the long pulsed Er:YAG laser and intravenous sedation versus dermabrasion (or laser) utilizing tumescent anesthesia for colloid milium. Dermatol Surg 28:780–790
20. Marra DE, Pourrabbani S, Fincher EF, Moy RL (2007) Fractional photothermolysis for the treatment of adult colloid milium. Arch Dermatol 143:572–574

Chapter 21
Calcification and Ossification

Maxime Battistella and Bernard Cribier

Key Points

- Cutaneous calcification or ossification is the result of a disruption of the normal calcium regulatory pathway in the skin by local or systemic events.
- Calcifying disorders of the skin can be divided into four groups: dystrophic calcinosis secondary to localized or diffuse tissue alterations; metastatic calcinosis, including calciphylaxis, due to impaired calcium-phosphate metabolism; idiopathic calcinosis, and iatrogenic calcinosis.
- Cutaneous ossifications are characterized by heterotopic lamellar bone deposits in the skin and can be divided into two main groups: primary osteomas (localized or diffuse) and secondary ossifications.
- Treatment of localized forms of cutaneous calcinosis or ossification is mainly surgical while treatment of the diffuse forms remains disappointing. Drugs modifying the calcium metabolism are used with variable results. Therapy of the underlying or associated problems such as connective tissue disease or hyperparathyroidism is mandatory to prevent further calcification and tissue damage.

Keywords Dystrophic calcinosis • Metastatic calcinosis • Calciphylaxis • Idiopathic calcinosis • Iatrogenic calcinosis • Osteomas • Secondary ossifications

21.1 Introduction

Cutaneous calcification or cutaneous calcinosis consists in deposits of hydroxyapatite and calcium phosphate crystals in the skin. Two intertwined mechanisms are implicated in the development of cutaneous calcinosis in humans: (1) abnormal plasmatic rates of calcium, phosphate, or vitamin D, which are regulated by a complex hormonal, enzymatic, and environmental network (Fig. 21.1) and (2) various local tissue alterations allowing initiation of crystal formation in the skin.

Ossification is a more complex phenomenon. The initial phase also requires hydroxyapatite crystallization but, unlike calcification, hydroxyapatite crystals are tightly packed and precisely organized in a lamellar haversian bone pattern. Cutaneous ossification is a dynamic process, with continuous bone formation and destruction by osteoblasts and osteoclasts.

21.2 Clinical and Pathological Aspects of Skin Manifestations

21.2.1 Cutaneous Calcinosis

Clinically, cutaneous calcinosis consists of firm, yellow-whitish, infiltrated papules, nodules, or plaques. Hydroxyapatite deposits in the skin are radio-opaque and can be fortuitously discovered on X-rays. They can also be discovered by chance on histopathological sections when they are relatively small and not clinically suspected. Not infrequently, cutaneous calcinosis can be spontaneously eliminated through the epidermis. A chalky, whitish, more or less liquid material extrudes from the lesions. Most lesions develop gradually and are asymptomatic, although they may occasionally be tender. The distribution of the lesions varies according to the causal disorder. Radiographic examination may demonstrate the extent of tissue calcification. On histopathological grounds, calcium presents with monomorphous basophilic purple-blue deposits of various size and shape, stained deep blue to violet in H&E stained tissue sections (Fig. 21.2), black with the von Kossa stain, and red with Alizarin red. A foreign-body granulomatous reaction and/or peripheral dermal fibrosis are frequently associated.

Cutaneous calcinoses are classified according to their predominant pathogenic mechanism (1). (1) dystrophic calcinosis secondary to localized or diffuse tissue alterations; (2) metastatic calcinosis due to impaired calcium-phosphate

B. Cribier (✉)
Clinique Dermatologique, Université de Strasbourg/Faculté de Médecine, Hôpitaux Universitaires de Strasbourg, 1 place de l'Hôpital, 67091 Strasbourg, France
e-mail: bernard.cribier@chru-strasbourg.fr

F. Rongioletti and B.R. Smoller (eds.), *Clinical and Pathological Aspects of Skin Diseases in Endocrine, Metabolic, Nutritional and Deposition Disease*, DOI 10.1007/978-1-60761-181-3_21, © Springer Science+Business Media, LLC 2010

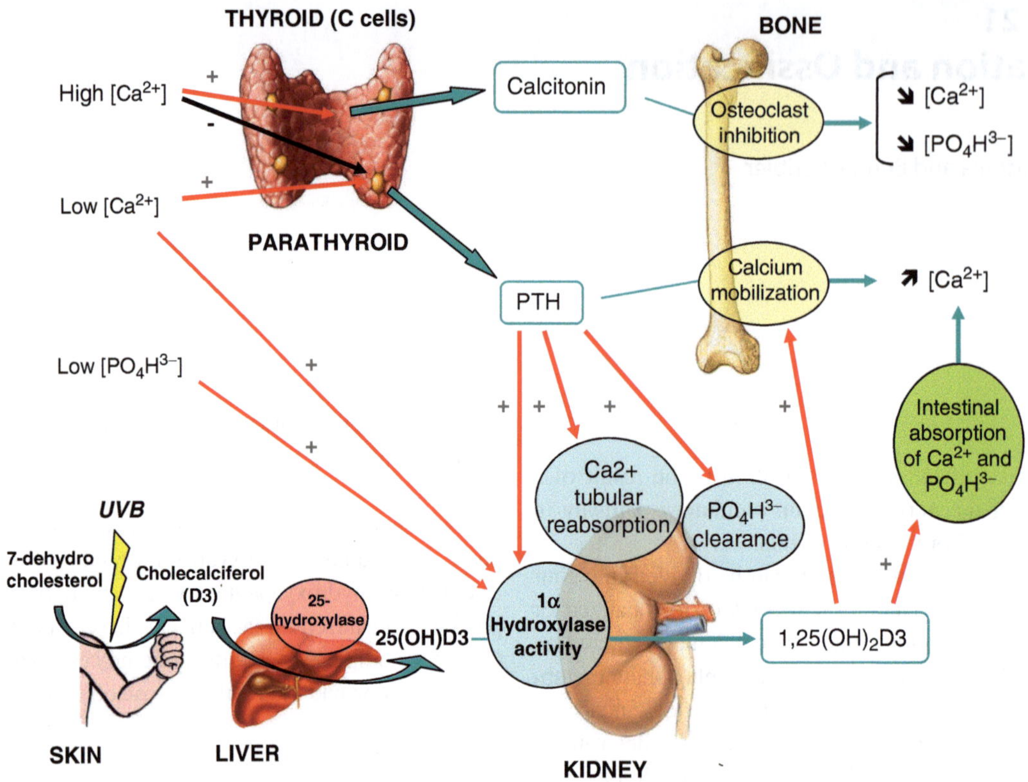

Fig. 21.1 Regulation network of calcium and phosphate plasmatic rates

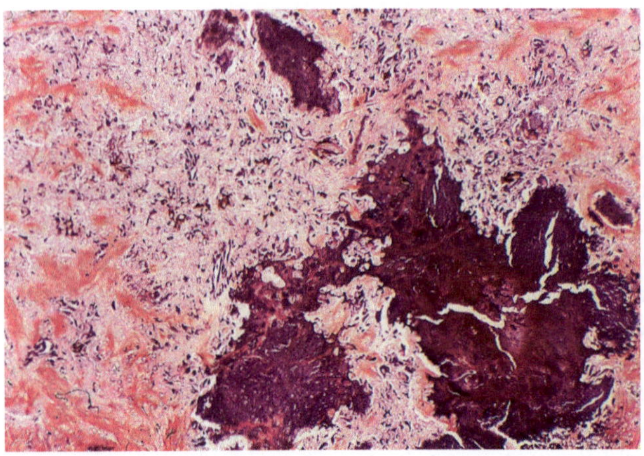

Fig. 21.2 Cutaneous calcinosis (HE stain)

metabolism, including calciphylaxis; (3) idiopathic calcinosis; and (4) iatrogenic calcinosis.

21.2.2 Dystrophic Calcinosis

Dystrophic calcinoses related to localized tissue alterations (1, 2) are summarized in Table 21.1. One of the most frequent causes of localized cutaneous calcification is probably *venous insufficiency* (Fig. 21.3). Calcinosis related to diffuse tissue alterations is seen in the setting of systemic diseases, especially in *connective tissue diseases* (3). It is a frequent feature in systemic sclerosis, especially in the context of CREST syndrome, mainly affecting the pulp of the fingers, but also the periarticular areas, the rachidian axis, and the skin overlying the iliac crests (Fig. 21.4a). Calcification appears in sclerotic skin as well as in uninvolved skin. X-ray examination leads to the discovery of cutaneous calcifications in almost 40% of patients with systemic sclerosis (Fig. 21.4b). Calcification is also seen in morphea, both localized, linear and generalized.

Calcifications occurring in dermatomyositis are larger and more diffuse than in systemic sclerosis. They can affect the skin, the muscles, and the tendons leading to limitations in the mobility of the joints (3). Calcinosis is present in two-thirds of cases of juvenile dermatomyositis and in 20% of adult form. The areas typically involved are those around the joints, the thighs, the arms, and the trunk. Calcinosis is often complicated by painful inflammatory reactions, transepidermal elimination, and cutaneous necrosis in the pressure areas. Severe forms are named "calcinosis universalis" (4).

Calcinosis has been reported in every clinical form of LE (3), although its frequency is lower than in systemic sclerosis or dermatomyositis patients. Asymptomatic cutaneous calcifications can be discovered in as many as 40% of patients

Table 21.1 Exogenous calcinosis and calcinosis related to localized tissue alterations

Transepidermal calcium salts absorption	Calcium gluconate or calcium chloride intravenous injection
	Calcium-containing electrode paste
	Professional exposure to calcium salts or saltpetre
Posttraumatic calcinosis	Heel puncture in neonates
	Intramuscular injections
	Traumatic wounds; lichenification
	Burn scars
	Surgical scars (laparotomy)
	Electrical burns
	Post-radiotherapy
Calcinosis related to vascular alterations	Venous insufficiency
	Phleboliths
	Haematomas
Calcifications related to tissue inflammation	Chronic osteomyelitis
	Chronic adenitis
	Frostbites and ear traumatisms
Post-infectious calcifications	Parasites: cysticercosis, dracunculosis, loa loa filariasis, Bancroft's filariasis, onchocercosis, hydatid cyst
	Leprosy
	Herpes, herpes zoster
Calcifications of cysts and tumors	Follicular tumors: trichoepithelioma, pilomatricoma, basal cell carcinoma, trichoblastic carcinoma
	Sweat gland tumors: syringoma, mixed tumor (chondroid syringoma)
	Epidermal and trichilemmal cyst
	Other tumors: lipoma, dermatofibroma, leiomyoma...
	Cutaneous meningeal heterotopia

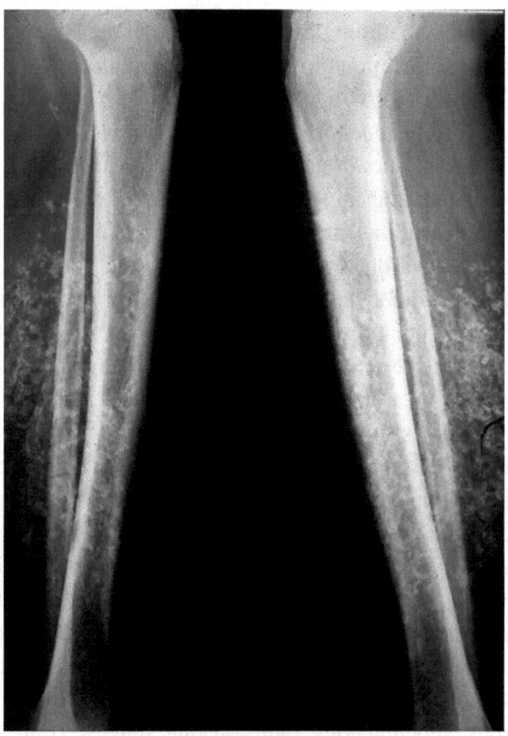

Fig. 21.3 Radiological aspect of cutaneous calcinosis in venous insufficiency

with systemic LE, mainly in the periarticular areas by radiographic examination. Rarely, dermal or subcutaneous calcifications can appear in long-lasting lesions of chronic LE, in subacute LE skin lesions, and lupus panniculitis (5). A form of calcinosis universalis similar to dermatomyositis has been reported in patients suffering from systemic LE (6).

Calcifications have been reported less frequently in many other systemic diseases including porphyria cutanea tarda (7), mixed connective tissue disease (8), nephrogenic systemic fibrosis (9), polyarteritis nodosa and in some inherited diseases such as *pseudoxanthoma elasticum (PXE)* (10), Ehlers–Danlos syndrome, gravis type, Werner syndrome (premature aging with possible soft tissue calcification of the ligaments, tendons, synovial, vasculature, and/or subcutaneous tissue), and Rothmund–Thomson syndrome (small papules on the extremities with dermal calcification; diffuse calcinosis). In PXE, elastic fibers are fragmented, swollen, and clumped in the middle and deep reticular dermis. They appear basophilic because of calcium deposition (Fig. 21.5). Similar calcification is noted in the media and intima of blood vessels.

Anecdotal cutaneous calcinosis has been reported in the context of leukemia (11) and following solid-organ transplantation, bone-marrow transplantation, and especially, liver transplantation (12).

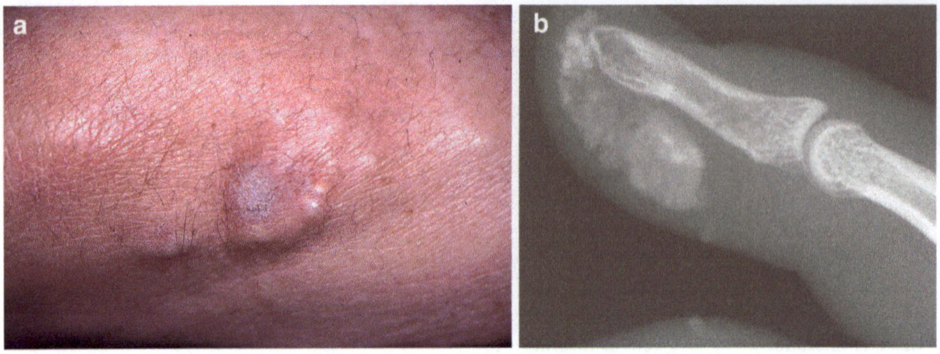

Fig. 21.4 (**a**) Clinical aspect of cutaneous calcification in systemic sclerosis; (**b**) Radiological aspect of calcification of the pulp of the finger in systemic sclerosis

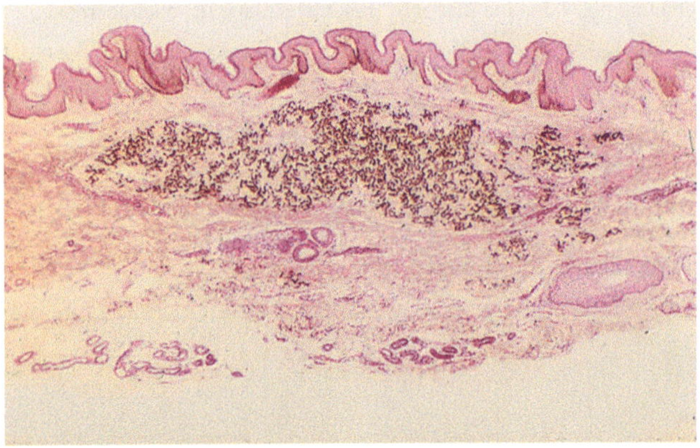

Fig. 21.5 Pseudo-xanthoma elasticum. Histopathological aspect (Orcein stain)

21.2.3 Metastatic Calcinosis

Metastatic calcinoses are related to alterations of calcium-phosphate metabolism. Hyperphosphatemia, indeed, is the major factor implicated in the development of cutaneous calcinosis in the context of hypercalcemia, independently of the blood calcium rate (13).

Cutaneous calcinosis associated with hypercalcemia has been reported in various pathological conditions including sarcoidosis, osteolytic diseases (especially bone metastases), and infectious diseases with granuloma formation (histoplasmosis, tuberculosis). Histiocytes of sarcoidal or infectious granulomas are able to synthesize vitamin D, inducing therefore hypercalcemia. Rarer causes of hypercalcemia with occasional cutaneous calcinosis are seen in vitamin D intoxication and milk alkali syndrome in which calcifications involve the muscles, the eyes, and the visceral organs more often than the skin.

The most frequent clinical manifestations of cutaneous calcinosis develop in the setting of hyperparathyroidism secondary to renal failure. Renal insufficiency leads to a decrease in the 1α hydroxylation of 25(0H)D3 to 1,25$(OH)_2$D3 that is the active form of vitamin D. Its deficiency leads to hypocalcemia and hyperphosphatemia, triggering secondary hyperparathyroidism (13). Bone resorption is increased by the high parathormone (PTH) rate, normalizing calcemia, but worsening hyperphosphatemia. Hydroxyapatite crystallization is triggered locally by various tissue alterations, initiating the cutaneous calcification process. A peculiar clinical manifestation of calcinosis in renal failure patients is *calcific uremic arteriolopathy (calciphylaxis)* (14) characterized by painful necrotic livedo of the limbs with escharotic plaques and mutilating necrosis due to arterial calcifications (Fig. 21.6a). Preexisting protein S or protein C deficiency could favor the development of the lesions. Both imaging study and histopathological examination of the lesions reveal multiple calcifications of the small cutaneous arterioles (Fig. 21.6b).

Calcifying panniculitis results in painful firm nodules, sometimes necrotic, in areas of thick subcutaneous fat tissue (15). Histopathological features show a diffuse calcification of the subcutis without arterial calcification. Calcium deposits decorated with Von Kossa staining underline the cell membranes of the adipocytes, in a way called *en cadre* calcification. Calcifying panniculitis may be triggered by injections and local trauma or may be a complication of infection or gangrene.

A disturbance of the calcium and phosphate metabolism/balance is also seen *in tumoral calcinosis (lipocalcinogranulomatosis, Teutschländer disease)*, a very rare benign condition presenting with massive subcutaneous soft tissue deposits of calcium phosphate near the large joints (16) and in *familial tumoral calcinosis*, which are a heterogeneous group of inherited disorders characterized by the occurrence of cutaneous and subcutaneous calcified masses. Two major forms of the disease are now recognized: hyperphosphatemic and normophosphatemic familial tumoral calcinosis (17). X-rays show enormous subcutaneous radio-opaque masses (Fig. 21.7). Pathological examination reveals irregular subcutaneous round calcifications surrounded by epithelioid histiocytes.

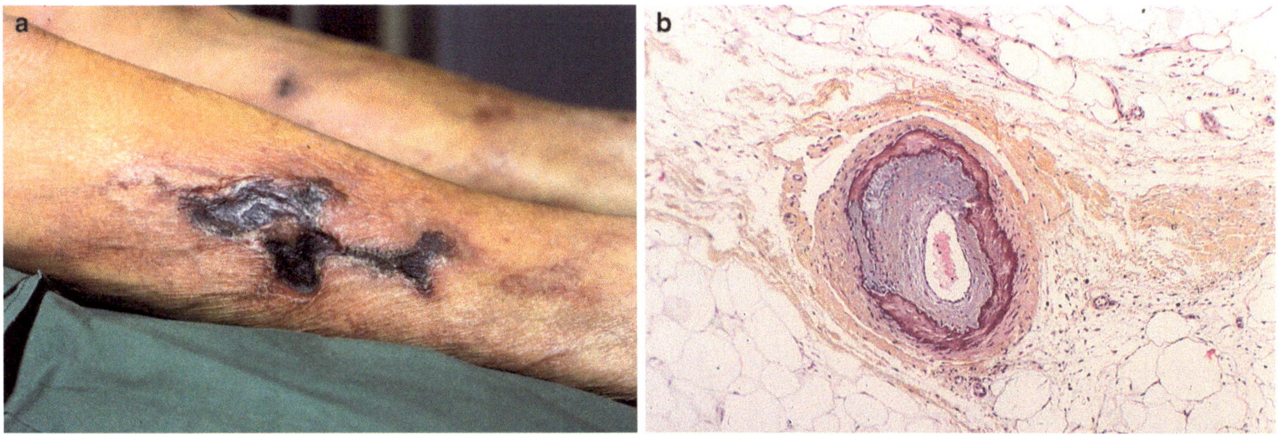

Fig. 21.6 Calciphylaxis in a patient with end-stage renal failure. (**a**) Clinical aspect; (**b**) Calcification of a small cutaneous artery (HE stain)

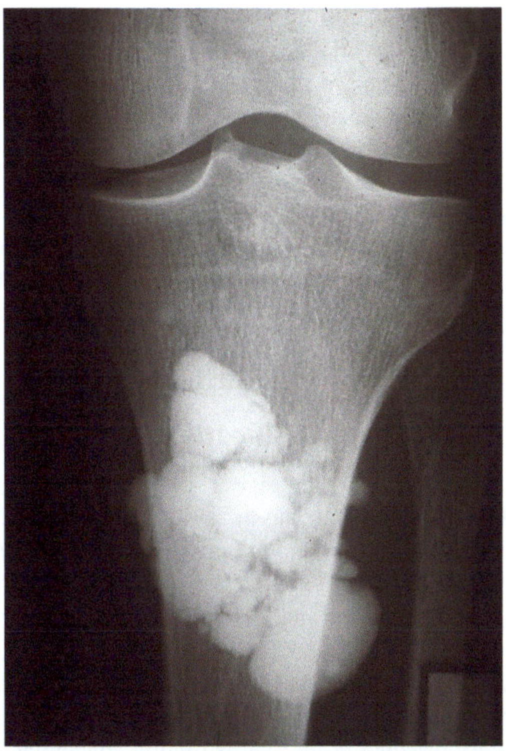

Fig. 21.7 Tumoral calcinosis (Teutschländer disease). Bulky subcutaneous calcified masses in the periarticular area of the knee

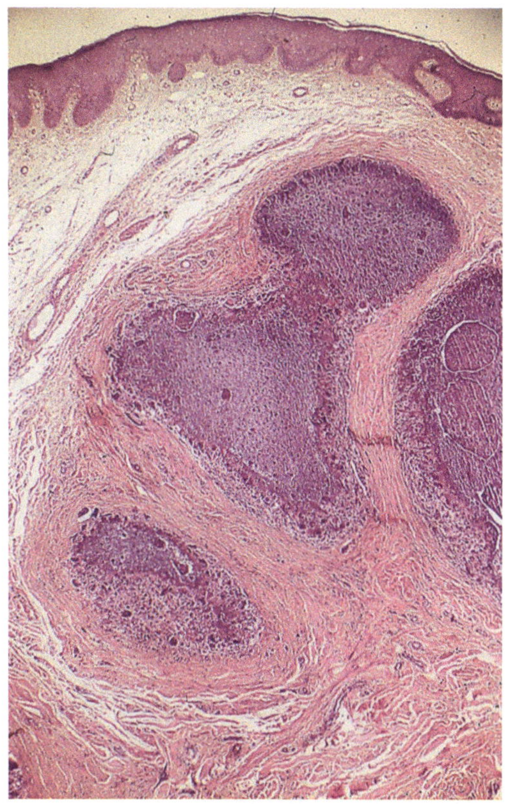

Fig. 21.8 Scrotal calcinosis. Histopathological aspect (HE stain)

21.2.4 Idiopathic Calcinosis

Idiopathic calcinosis is characterized by isolated or multiple papular to nodular lesions, arising in the absence of previous alteration of the skin and of metabolic disorders, including *genital and mammary calcinoses, Winer's solitary calcified nodule, idiopathic calcinosis of the extremities, and extensive idiopathic calcinosis.*

The most frequent condition is *scrotal calcinosis* (18). Vulvar and penile calcinoses have also been described. The lesions are firm and yellow nodules of the skin of the scrotum, the labia majora or the penile shaft, and are often asymptomatic. They display a peculiar histopathologic aspect, showing large dermal calcified masses surrounded by a large granulomatous area containing macrophages and foreign body giant cells (Fig. 21.8). The clinical differential diagnosis is with scrotal or vulvar epidermal cyst.

Mammary calcinosis is often deeply localized in the breast tissue and rarely presents as a dermatological lesion. Idiopathic calcinosis of the areola has exceptionally been reported (19).

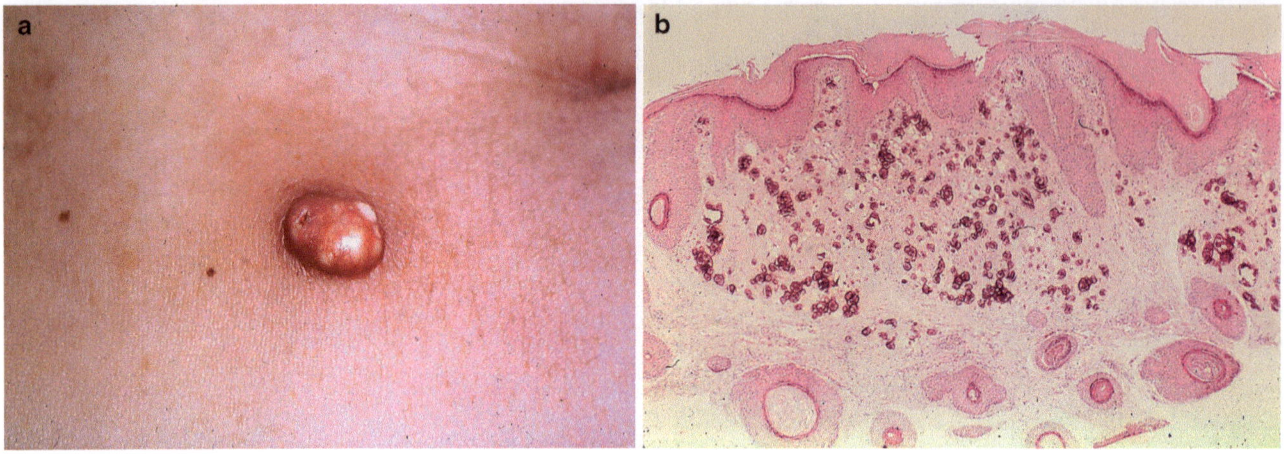

Fig. 21.9 Winer's solitary calcified nodule. (**a**) Clinical aspect. (**b**) Histopathological aspect (HE stain)

Winer's solitary calcified nodule is a solitary small, hard, yellow lesion on the head and neck area, presenting at birth or occurring in early childhood (Fig. 21.9a) (20). Histopathology shows multiple small calcified masses in the upper dermis, surrounded by fibrosis, with absent or very mild inflammatory infiltrate (Fig. 21.9b).

Idiopathic calcinosis of the extremities also named calcinosis circumscripta or subepidermal calcified nodules is characterized by multiple small white papules predominating on the volar aspect of the hands and feet. It has been reported in patients suffering from Down's syndrome (trisomy 21) (21).

Extensive idiopathic calcinosis has often been reported as calcinosis universalis, a term that should be restricted to diffuse calcinosis in dermatomyositis patients. Patients exhibit a diffuse calcification of the skin, the tendons, and the aponeuroses, in the absence of systemic sclerosis or dermatomyositis. The clinical picture and the functional prognosis are close to those of myositis ossificans in children.

21.2.5 Iatrogenic Calcinosis

The cutaneous lesions of iatrogenic calcinosis cutis are typically described as white-yellow papules, plaques, and nodules. They are often multiple and may be associated with erythema, necrosis, or ulceration. *Cutaneous calcinosis secondary to subcutaneous injection of calcium-containing heparin* occurs in patients with renal failure (22). The clinical lesions are characterized by erythematous firm nodules in the areas of subcutaneous injections of low-molecular-weight-calcium-containing heparin in patients with end-stage renal failure and high calcium-phosphate product. Calcified material is transepidermally eliminated. Skin lesions always heal gradually after a few weeks of cessation of the treatment. The biopsy typically shows important calcium deposits in the whole dermis and subcutis, around collagen and elastic fibers, in vessel walls and decorating lipocytes.

Iatrogenic calcinosis cutis has been reported after the *extravasation of calcium-containing intravenous solutions* and following electroencephalographic and electromyographic examinations with electrodes containing calcium chloride paste (23).

21.2.6 Cutaneous Ossification

Cutaneous ossifications have traditionally been divided into primary ossifications (osteoma cutis) and secondary ossifications (2, 24). The latter are related to localized or diffuse tissue alteration and to impaired calcium-phosphate metabolism.

Primary osteomas of the skin (osteoma cutis) may be solitary or multiple.

Solitary osteoma of the skin is often a congenital lesion on the scalp, presenting as a hard radio-opaque nodule of variable size that can ulcerate. Histopathologic examination reveals a well-limited dermal ossified structure, without any associated inflammation (Fig. 21.10). Plaque-like variants, usually on the forehead, have been described in infants (25).

Multiple osteomas cutis are acquired lesions of small size. *Multiple miliary osteomas on the face* (26), or Arzt's disease, consist in multiple tiny, firm yellowish papules on the face of elderly women without any previous history of acne (Fig. 21.11). Another presentation includes disseminated miliary osteomatosis, in which the lesions can be distributed on the whole integument without any relationship with Albright hereditary osteodystrophy.

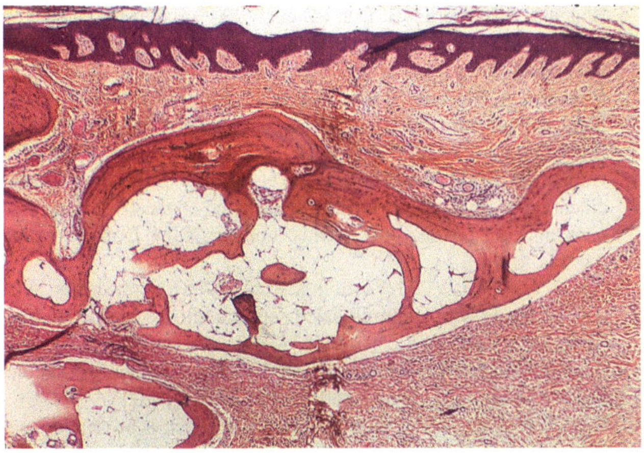

Fig. 21.10 Solitary osteoma cutis. Histopathological aspect (HE stain)

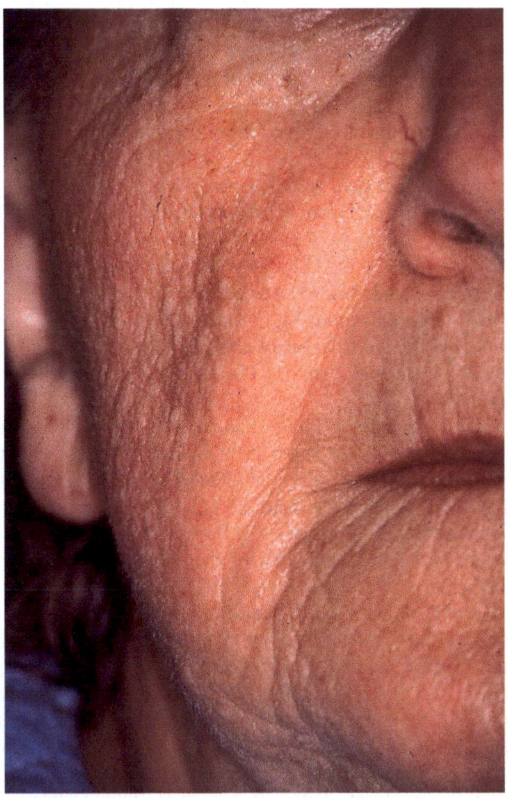

Fig. 21.11 Multiple miliary osteomas on the face

Secondary cutaneous ossifications include ossifications due to tissue alterations and ossifications related to *GNAS* gene alterations.

The former condition is seen in many cutaneous tumors such as benign melanocytic nevus (27), the so-called *osteonevus of Nanta* (1–2% of total melanocytic nevi) whose histopathology shows a small focus of ossification, often situated along a hair follicle among the dermal melanocytic proliferation. Osteomas have also been reported in blue nevus and Spitz nevus and rarely in melanoma. Other tumors exhibiting ossification include follicular tumors (pilomatricoma, basal cell carcinoma, trichoepithelioma), chondroid syringoma (mixed tumor) epidermoid cyst, trichilemmal cyst, dermatofibroma, atypical fibroxanthoma, and hemangioma. *Pilomatricoma* is the most frequent ossifying tumor (10–20% of cases).

Secondary ossification is also found in inflammatory lesions such as postacne facial osteomas that should be distinguished from idiopathic multiple miliary osteomas on the face (28). They appear in the scarring process of acne lesions and may assume a bluish color after prolonged minocyclin treatment. Secondary cutaneous ossification may be encountered in chronic venous insufficiency, surgical scars, intravenous injection sites and in systemic diseases such as diffuse scleroderma, systemic sclerosis, chronic discoid LE, nephrogenic systemic fibrosis, and dermatomyositis.

Ossifications related to GNAS gene alterations include rare inherited ossifying diseases such as progressive osseous heteroplasia (POH), Albright hereditary osteodystrophy (AHO), pseudohypoparathyroidism 1a and 1c (PHP1a/c), and pseudopseudo-hypoparathyroidism (PPHP) (29).

21.3 Treatment and Prognosis

The treatment of primary or secondary localized calcinosis is based on surgical excision of the lesions (30). There is no specific complication due to localized calcinosis, except for transepidermal elimination, which can be painful, but which rarely shows secondary infection.

In diffuse cutaneous calcinosis associated with systemic diseases (scleroderma, dermatomyositis, etc.) and in idiopathic diffuse cutaneous calcinosis, the prognosis relies mainly on possible functional disabilities. Pressure ulcers and secondary infections may arise, portending a worse prognosis. The treatment is quite disappointing. Aluminum hydroxide, biphosphonates, systemic steroids, warfarin, diltiazem hydrochloride, and probenecid have been tried with variable results (31, 32). Sodium etidronate seems more efficient in calcinosis associated with systemic sclerosis than in other diffuse calcinoses. Recently, intravenous immunoglobulin (IVIG) therapy has been offered to patients with diffuse calcifications in systemic sclerosis and dermatomyositis (33). Electric shock wave lithotripsy has seldom been employed to treat calcinosis in dermatomyositis and CREST syndrome (34).

The control of blood phosphate rate is a major objective in the management of patients with renal failure. It allows diminishing the frequency of periarticular and conjunctival hydroxyapatite deposits, but not of vascular deposits.

Calcific uremic arteriolopathy (calciphylaxis) in the context of renal failure carries a poor prognosis. Cutaneous lesions never regress spontaneously. They frequently lead to the death of the patient, through secondary infection and sepsis. The treatment of choice is early parathyroidectomy. Low-calcium dialysis may be of some help, as well as sodium thiosulfate treatment (35). Hyperbaric oxygen therapy has also been proposed in association with other treatments (36).

The other forms of calcinosis in the context of renal failure can be treated with aluminum hydroxide (2 g per day) and low-phosphate diet regimen.

Surgical resection may be the sole treatment option when calcinosis is complicated by infection, nerve compression, or nonhealing ulcer. It is often employed in dermatomyositis patients and in tumoral calcinosis. In the latter condition, recurrence after surgery is observed in as much as 90% of cases.

The treatment of cutaneous ossification relies on surgical excision, if the lesions are esthetically or functionally annoying. Disseminated osteomatosis and miliary osteomas of the face are benign conditions, but they can be disfigurating. Miliary osteomas on the face may be improved by topical 0.05% tretinoin. Physical treatments (37) are the most effective ones including needle microincisions followed by mechanical extirpation of the bony formation, dermabrasion, erbium:YAG laser, or curettage followed by carbon dioxide laser.

Among ossifications related to GNAS mutations, progressive osseous heteroplasia (POH) and rarer progressive forms of PPHP or PHP portend poor functional prognosis, due to progressive ossification of tendons and deep connective tissue. Surgical resection of diffuse lesions tends to lead to recurrence or complications (38). Treatment with pamidronate (biphosphonate) does not resolve preexisting bony formation, but may decrease the occurrence of new ossification, and therefore slow the rate of progressive disability.

References

1. Cribier B, Grosshans E (1992) Cutaneous calcinosis. Ann Dermatol Venereol 119:151–168
2. Rongioletti F, Barnhill RL (2010) Deposition disorders. In: Barnhill RL, Crowson AN, Magro CM, Piepkorn MW (eds) Dermatopathology, 3rd edn. McGraw-Hill, New York, pp 362–386
3. Boulman N, Slobodin G, Rozenbaum M et al (2005) Calcinosis in rheumatic diseases. Semin Arthritis Rheum 34:805–812
4. Yun SJ, Lee JB, Kim SJ et al (2006) Calcinosis cutis universalis with joint contractures complicating juvenile dermatomyositis. Dermatology 212:401–403
5. Morgan KW, Callen JP (2001) Calcifying lupus panniculitis in a patient with subacute cutaneous lupus erythematosus: response to diltiazem and chloroquine. J Rheumatol 28:2129–2132
6. Bhatia S, Silverberg NB, Don PC et al (2001) Extensive calcinosis cutis in association with systemic lupus erythematosus. Acta Derm Venereol 81:446–447
7. Nogueira A, Moreira E, Santos P et al (2009) Calcinosis cutis in porphyria cutanea tarda – not always a marker of disease activity. Eur J Dermatol 19:280–281
8. Goolamali SI, Gordon P, Salisbury J et al (2009) Subcutaneous calcification presenting in a patient with mixed connective tissue disease and cutaneous polyarteritis nodosa. Clin Exp Dermatol 34:e141–e144
9. Nagai Y, Hasegawa M, Shinmi K et al (2008) Nephrogenic systemic fibrosis with multiple calcification and osseous metaplasia. Acta Derm Venereol 88:597–600
10. Buka R, Wei H, Sapadin A et al (2000) Pseudoxanthoma elasticum and calcinosis cutis. J Am Acad Dermatol 43:312–315
11. Satter EK, Maari CH, Morel KD et al (2004) Disseminated linear calcinosis cutis associated with the Koebner phenomenon in an infant with congenital acute monocytic leukaemia. Br J Dermatol 150:753–756
12. Lateo S, Charlton F, Hudson M et al (2005) Cutaneous calcification following liver transplantation. Clin Exp Dermatol 30:484–486
13. Alfrey AC (2004) The role of abnormal phosphorus metabolism in the progression of chronic kidney disease and metastatic calcification. Kidney Int Suppl 90:S13–S17
14. Kalisiak M, Courtney M, Lin A, Brassard A (2009) Calcific uremic arteriolopathy (calciphylaxis): successful treatment with sodium thiosulfate in spite of elevated serum phosphate. J Cutan Med Surg 13(Suppl 1):S29–S34
15. Elamin EM, McDonald AB (1996) Calcifying panniculitis with renal failure: a new management approach. Dermatology 192:156–159
16. Pakasa NM, Kalengayi RM (1997) Tumoral calcinosis: a clinicopathological study of 111 cases with emphasis on the earliest changes. Histopathology 31:18–24
17. Garringer HJ, Malekpour M, Esteghamat F et al (2008) Molecular genetic and biochemical analyses of FGF23 mutations in familial tumoral calcinosis. Am J Physiol Endocrinol Metab 295: E929–E937
18. Yahya H, Rafindadi AH (2005) Idiopathic scrotal calcinosis: a report of four cases and review of the literature. Int J Dermatol 44:206–209
19. Oh CK, Kwon KS, Cho SH et al (2000) Idiopathic calcinosis of the areola of the nipple. J Dermatol 27:121–122
20. Nico MM (2001) Bergonse FN.Subepidermal calcified nodule: report of two cases and review of the literature. Pediatr Dermatol 18:227–229
21. Delaporte E, Gosselin P, Catteau B et al (1997) Perforating milia-like idiopathic calcinosis of the extremities in Down syndrome. Ann Dermatol Venereol 124:159–161
22. Boccara O, Prost-Squarcioni C, Battistella M, Brousse N, Rongioletti F, Fraitag S (2010) Calcinosis cutis: a rare reaction to subcutaneous injections of calcium-containing heparin in patients with renal failure. Am J Dermatopathol 32:52–55
23. Moss J, Syrengelas A, Antaya R, Lazova R (2006) Calcinosis cutis: a complication of intravenous administration of calcium gluconate. J Cutan Pathol 33(Suppl 2):60–62
24. Cribier B, Lipsker D, Grosshans E (1994) Ossification and cutaneous osteoma. Ann Dermatol Venereol 121:918–930
25. Haro R, Revelles JM, Angulo J et al (2009) Plaque-like osteoma cutis with transepidermal elimination. J Cutan Pathol 36:591–593
26. Novak C, Siller G, Wood D (1998) Idiopathic multiple miliary osteomas of the face. Australas J Dermatol 39:109–111
27. Al-Daraji W (2007) Osteo-nevus of Nanta (osseous metaplasia in a benign intradermal melanocytic nevus): an uncommon phenomenon. Dermatol Online J 13(4):16
28. Thielen AM, Stucki L, Braun RP et al (2006) Multiple cutaneous osteomas of the face associated with chronic inflammatory acne. J Eur Acad Dermatol Venereol 20:321–326

29. Adegbite NS, Xu M, Kaplan FS et al (2008) Diagnostic and mutational spectrum of progressive osseous heteroplasia (POH) and other forms of GNAS-based heterotopic ossification. Am J Med Genet A 146A:1788–1796
30. Saddic N, Miller JJ, Miller OF 3rd et al (2009) Surgical debridement of painful fingertip calcinosis cutis in CREST syndrome. Arch Dermatol 145:212–213
31. Cukierman T, Elinav E, Korem M et al (2004) Low dose warfarin treatment for calcinosis in patients with systemic sclerosis. Ann Rheum Dis 63:1341–1343
32. Abdallah-Lotf M, Grasland A, Vinceneux P et al (2005) Regression of cutis calcinosis with diltiazem in adult dermatomyositis. Eur J Dermatol 15:102–104
33. Schanz S, Ulmer A, Fierlbeck G (2008) Response of dystrophic calcification to intravenous immunoglobulin. Arch Dermatol 144:585–587
34. Chan AY, Li E (2005) Electric shock wave lithotripsy (ESWL) as a pain control measure in dermatomyositis with calcinosis cutis-old method, new discovery. Clin Rheumatol 24:172–173
35. Wang HY, Yu CC, Huang CC (2004) Successful treatment of severe calciphylaxis in a hemodialysis patient using low-calcium dialysate and medical parathyroidectomy: case report and literature review. Ren Fail 26:77–82
36. Arenas MD, Gil MT, Gutierrez MD et al (2008) Management of calcific uremic arteriolopathy (calciphylaxis) with a combination of treatments, including hyperbaric oxygen therapy. Clin Nephrol 70:261–264
37. Baskan EB, Turan H, Tunali S et al (2007) Miliary osteoma cutis of the face: treatment with the needle microincision-extirpation method. J Dermatolog Treat 18:252–254
38. Hou JW (2006) Progressive osseous heteroplasia controlled by intravenous administration of pamidronate. Am J Med Genet A 140:910–913

Chapter 22
Pigmentary Deposition Disorders

Jessica Linder, Maria Miteva, and Paolo Romanelli

Key Points

- Pigmentary deposition skin disorders are characterized by abnormal accumulation of pigmented substances that are of endogenous or exogenous derivation.
- Endogenous pigmentary deposition disorders are due to inherited diseases, mainly alkaptonuria (ochronosis).
- Exogenous pigmentary deposition disorders are due to drugs including antimalarials, phenothiazines, tetracyclines, amiodarone, clofazimine, chemotherapeutic agents, and hydroquinone (exogenous ochronosis) or heavy metals including silver, gold, mercury, arsenic, bismuth, and lead.
- Hyperpigmentation due to drugs is usually reversible with discontinuation of the therapy.

Keywords Endogenous pigmentation • Alkaptonuria • Exogenous pigmentation • Drugs • Heavy metals

22.1 Introduction

Pigmentary deposition skin disorders are characterized by abnormal accumulation of pigmented substances that are of endogenous or exogenous derivation. Endogenous pigmentary deposition disorders are due to inherited diseases, mainly alkaptonuria (ochronosis), while the exogenous ones are due to drugs including antimalarials, phenothiazines, tetracyclines, amiodarone, clofazimine, and chemotherapeutic agents or heavy metals including silver, gold, mercury, arsenic, bismuth, and lead. Ochronosis can also be exogenous when it is caused by several medications including hydroquinone, phenol, and resorcinol. Tattoos are also considered in Chap. 23.

P. Romanelli (✉)
Department of Dermatology and Cutaneous Surgery, University of Miami Miller School of Medicine, 1600 NW 10th Avenue, Rosenstiel Building, Miami, FL 33136, USA
e-mail: promanelli@med.miami.edu

22.2 Clinical and Pathological Aspects of Skin Manifestations

22.2.1 Endogenous Deposition Disorders

22.2.1.1 Alkaptonuria (Ochronosis)

Alkaptonuria, or ochronosis, is an autosomal recessive disorder of homogentisic acid (HGA) metabolism, caused by a defect in HGA oxidase. This enzyme is needed for the breakdown of phenylalanine and tyrosine. A defect or deficiency of this enzyme causes buildup of homogentisic acid within cells. Ochronosis can also be exogenous, caused by several medications including hydroquinone, phenol, and resorcinol [1].

The first manifestation of alkaptonuria is a brownish discoloration of the urine seen several days after birth [2]. High amounts of HGA are secreted by the kidneys and, when oxidized, demonstrate a yellow-brown coloration. HGA is also secreted out of sweat glands; the axillary sweat of adolescents can be tinted greenish-blue.

The cutaneous pigmentation seen in alkaptonuria occurs after many years and progressively worsens as more and more pigment is deposited within tissues. The skin appears blue due to the Tyndall effect. Blue discoloration develops at sites where cartilage and tendons are close to the surface of the skin, such as the ear, nose, costochondral junctions, and extensor tendons of the hands. The sclera develops a bluish discoloration known as Osler's sign. Microscopically, the ochronotic pigment of alkaptonuria is yellow-brown (Fig. 22.1a). Pigment is seen in the dermis within the endothelial cells, macrophages, secretory cells of sweat glands, and along the basement membrane. Ocher-colored fibers appear in the dermis and may be crescentic, vermiform, or banana-shaped (Fig. 22.1b) [2]. The changes in exogenous ochronosis are identical to those of the endogenous form.

F. Rongioletti and B.R. Smoller (eds.), *Clinical and Pathological Aspects of Skin Diseases in Endocrine, Metabolic, Nutritional and Deposition Disease*, DOI 10.1007/978-1-60761-181-3_22,

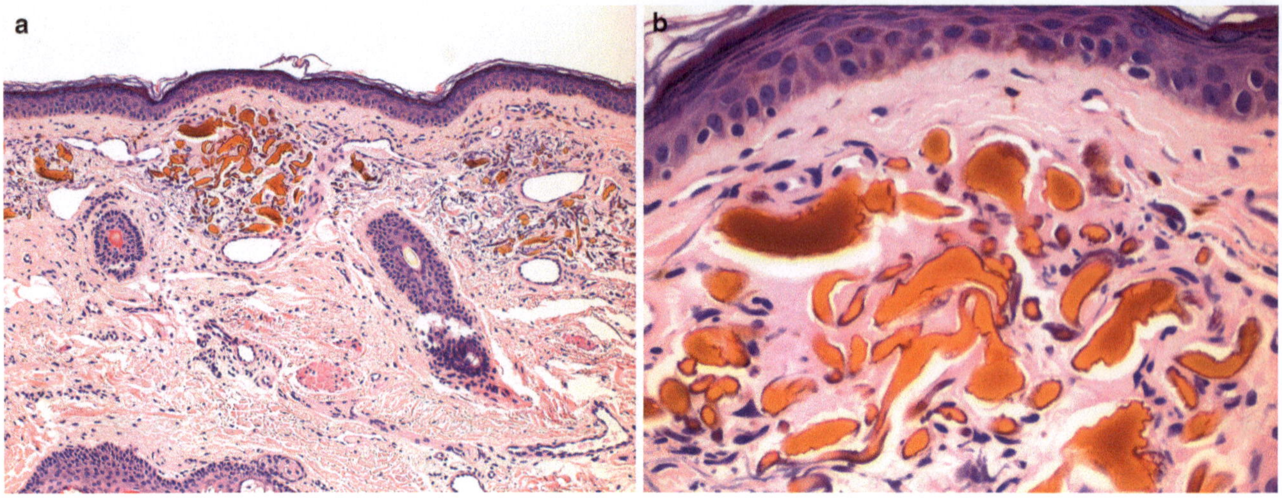

Fig. 22.1 (**a**) Endogenous ochronosis. Banana bodies (HE stain). (**b**) Close-up of banana bodies (HE stain)

22.2.2 Exogenous Deposition Disorders

22.2.2.1 Hyperpigmentation Due to Drugs

Drugs can affect the skin in a variety of ways. Hyperpigmentation can occur by deposition of drug metabolite or drug–melanin complex in the dermis. Drugs can also cause stimulation of melanocytes to produce more melanin. Additionally, drugs can result in postinflammatory pigmentation. There are many drugs that cause increased cutaneous pigmentation, including antimalarials, phenothiazines, tetracyclines, amiodarone, clofazimine, and chemotherapeutic agents [3].

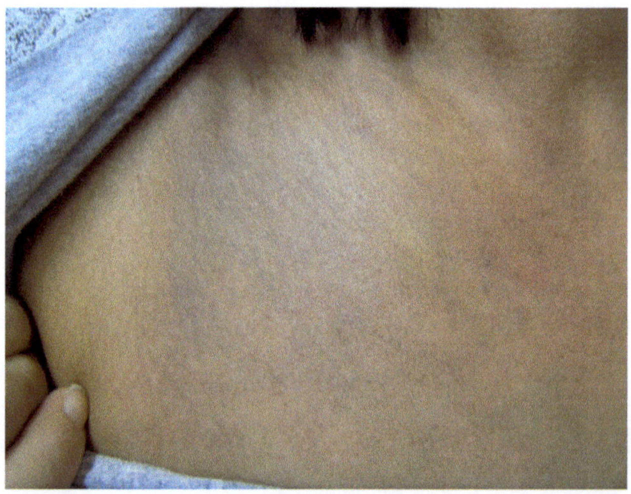

Fig. 22.2 Gray-blue hyperpigmentation after long-term use of antimalarials

Antimalarials

It is estimated that 25% of patients taking antimalarials for longer than 4 months will develop dyspigmentation [4]. The most commonly implicated antimalarial drugs to cause changes in skin pigmentation are chloroquine, hydroxychloroquine, amodiaquine, and quinacrine, which are mostly used in dermatology for the treatment of connective tissue diseases.

These antimalarials produce an irregular, patchy, bluish-gray pigmentation (Fig. 22.2). Color change is more prominent over the tibias and face. The nails and oral mucosa may also be involved. Initially, lesions present as discrete macules resembling ecchymoses, which eventually coalesce. Quinacrine, unlike the other antimalarials, can produce a generalized lemon-yellow coloration of the skin that mimics jaundice. Unlike jaundice, however, it tends to spare the sclera. The blue-gray hyperpigmentation seen with antimalarial use is most likely due to a combination of hemosiderin deposition and drug–melanin complexes [2]. Histologically, yellow to dark brown pigmented granules are seen within the dermis (Fig. 22.3a). Pigment granules stain for melanin and hemosiderin (Fig. 22.3b, c). There is increased melanin within the epidermis [5].

Phenothiazines

Phenothiazines are neuroleptic, antipsychotic drugs. Chronic administration of phenothiazines can lead to hyperpigmentation, particularly in sun-exposed areas of the face, hands, and upper extremities. Chlorpromazine is the most commonly implicated drug of this class [6]. The hyperpigmentation has an additive effect and begins as a tan color, progresses to slate-gray and later purple. The eyes can be affected and

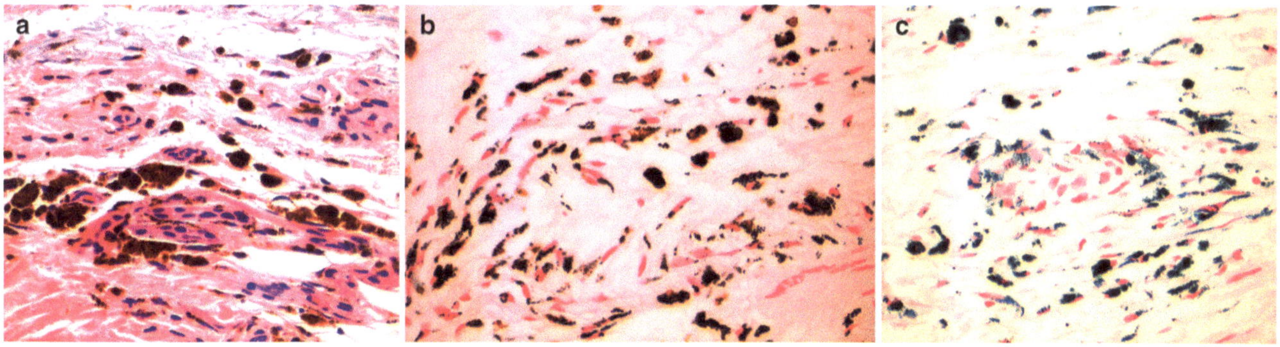

Fig. 22.3 Hyperpigmentation due to antimalarials. (**a**) (HE, stain). (**b**) (Fontana Masson stain for melanin). (**c**) (Perl stain for iron)

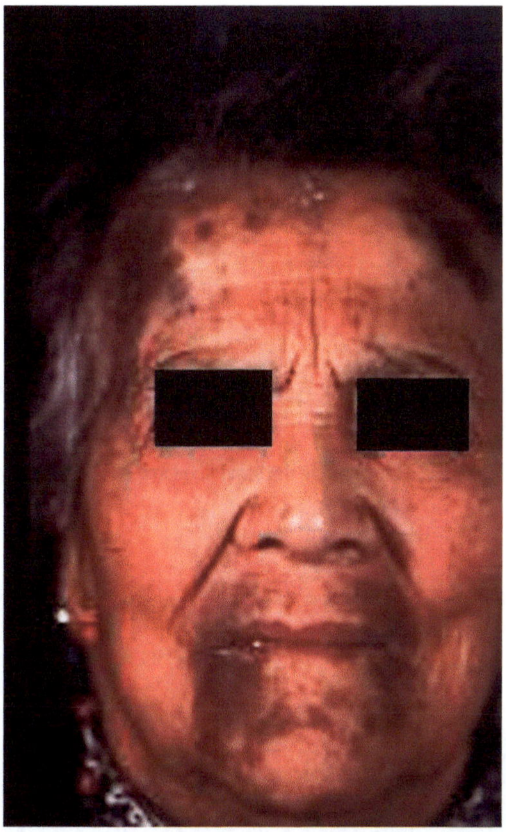

Fig. 22.4 Brownish dyscoloration of the face due to imipramine

demonstrate brown discoloration [6]. Similar pigmentation has been described in patients taking the tricyclic antidepressants, imipramine [7] (Fig. 22.4), and desipramine [8]. They are not commonly used today but are sometimes used to treat major depression as a second-line therapy.

Histologically, yellow-brown pigment granules are seen within dermal macrophages around the superficial capillaries (Fig. 22.5a). Granules have the staining properties of melanin (Fig. 22.5b). Iron stain with Perl is negative (Fig. 22.5c). Electron microscopy demonstrates membrane-bound inclusions within macrophages, endothelial cells, and Schwann cells. Melanin and drug–melanin complexes are present within macrophages in the dermis, and these complexes may be the cause of hyperpigmentation [9].

Tetracyclines

Minocycline is a derivative of tetracycline and is frequently used in the treatment of acne and other inflammatory conditions. When oxidized, minocycline turns black and may lead to dyspigmentation of the skin. There are three clinical types of dyspigmentation seen with minocycline use. Type I hyperpigmentation produces a localized blue-black discoloration in areas of inflammation or previous scarring. Type II hyperpigmentation produces a blue-gray discoloration over the extremities. Type III hyperpigmentation produces diffuse, muddy-brown discoloration of sun-exposed areas (Fig. 22.6a). The nails, sclera, teeth, and mucous membranes may also be affected [10].

Histology varies depending on the type of hyperpigmentation [11]. Type I hyperpigmentation demonstrates intra- and extracellular iron-staining granules within the dermis. Type II pigmentation produces predominantly intracellular, iron-containing pigment granules within the dermis and subcutis. Finally, Type III specimens reveal increased melanin within the dermis and epidermis (Fig. 22.6b, c).

Amiodarone

Amiodarone is used in the treatment of arrhythmias. Approximately 30–76% of patients taking amiodarone experience photosensitivity, and 1–10% will develop hyperpigmentation after taking the drug for more than 4 months [1]. The skin develops a slate-gray discoloration, which is most prominent over sun-exposed areas (Fig. 22.7a). Hyperpigmentation is caused by lipofuscin accumulation within the skin [12].

Histologically, yellow-brown lipofuscin granules are seen within macrophages, especially surrounding blood vessels at the junction of the papillary and reticular dermis (Fig. 22.7b). Electron microscopy reveals electron-dense, membrane-bound bodies within the cytoplasm of macrophages.

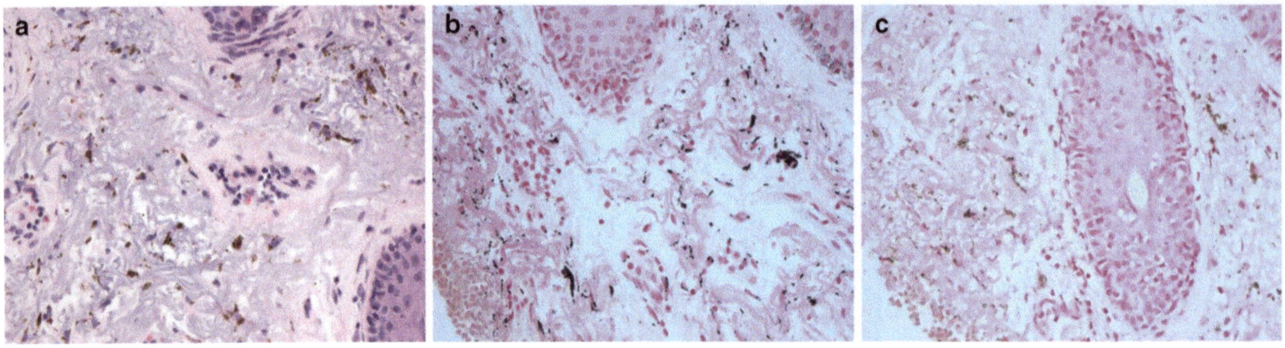

Fig. 22.5 Chlorpromazine pigmentation. (**a**) (HE stain). (**b**) (Fontana stain). (**c**) Negative iron stain with Perl (Courtesy of J.W. Patterson, Charlottesville, VA, USA)

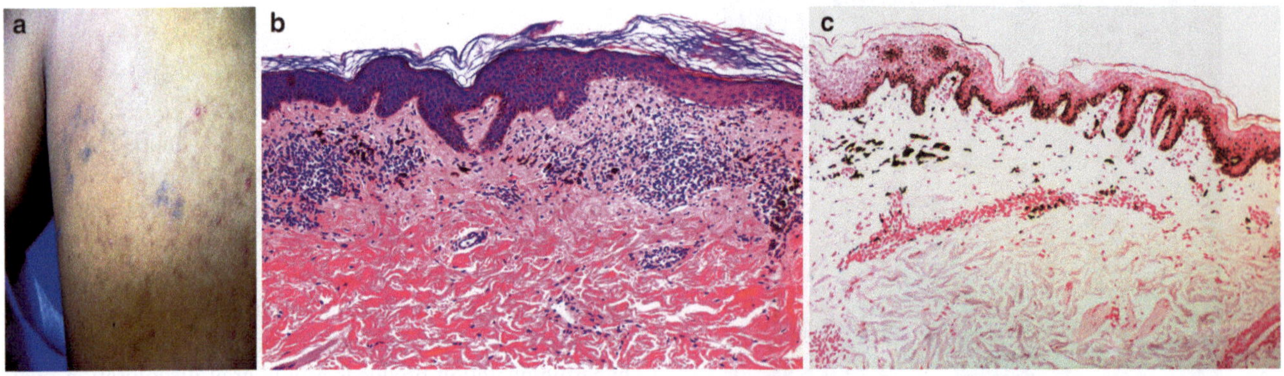

Fig. 22.6 (**a**) Minocyclin hyperpigmentation. (**b**) Minocyclin hyperpigmentation with increased melanin in the basal layer and dermal melanophages (HE stain). (**c**) (Fontana Masson stain for melanin)

Fig. 22.7 Hyperpigmentation due to amiodarone. (**a**) Clinical aspects. (**b**) Amiodarone hyperpigmentation with yellowish-brownish granules in the dermis

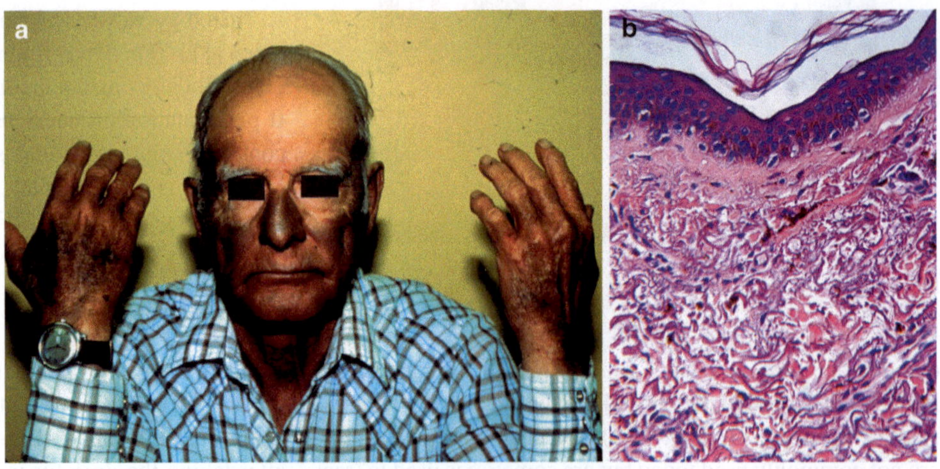

Clofazimine

Clofazimine is used in the treatment of leprosy, rhinoscleroma, discoid lupus, and other mycobacterial infections. Dyspigmentation is caused by deposition of clofazimine in the skin, which causes a reddish hue [1]. Sites of active inflammation will display a deep reddish-blue discoloration. Chronic exposure results in generalized pink-brown discoloration that is more prominent over sun-exposed surfaces.

Histologically, clofazimine pigment will not be evident by routine hematoxylin and eosin stain because the crystals dissolve during preparation. Fresh frozen section, however, will demonstrate vividly red crystals around dermal blood vessels, representing clofazimine crystals.

Chemotherapeutic Agents

Many chemotherapeutic agents can cause hyperpigmentation of the skin including busulfan, bleomycin, doxorubicin, daunorubicin, fluorouracil, cyclophosphamide, dactinomycin, azidothymidine, mechlorethamine, carmustine (BCNU), and hydroxyurea [1]. Skin, hair, nails (Fig. 22.8), and mucous membranes may all be affected. Moreover, involvement may be localized or diffuse [13, 14].

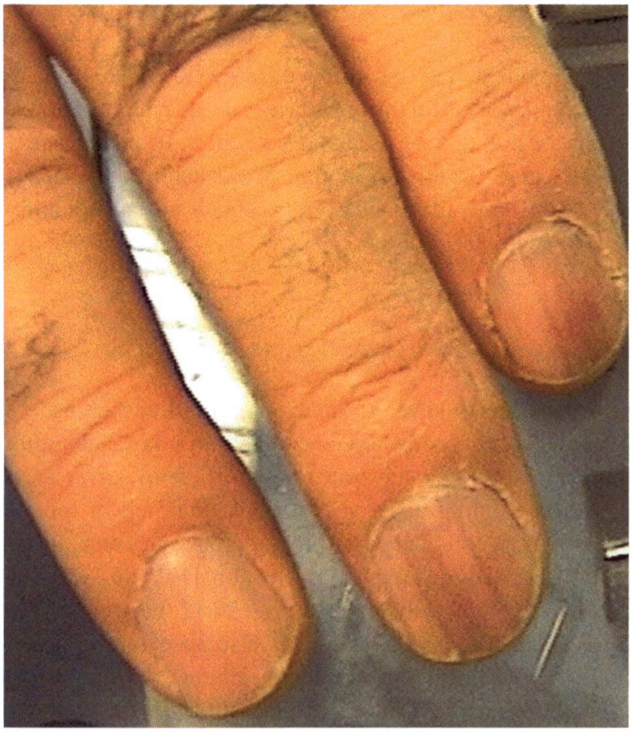

Fig. 22.8 Nail pigmentation due to bleomycin

BCNU and mechlorethamine cause hyperpigmentation when applied topically. Bleomycin causes linear, "flagellate" hyperpigmentation. The exact mechanism of hyperpigmentation caused by chemotherapeutic agents is unknown. Proposed mechanisms include direct stimulation of melanocytes by chemotherapeutic agents and/or postinflammatory change following toxic insult to the keratinocytes.

A case of generalized eruptive lentiginosis induced by chemotherapy has recently been reported, related to intravenous application of CHOP (cyclophosphamide, doxorubicin, vincristine, and oral prednisone) for non-Hodgkin's lymphoma [15]. The lesions occurred after cessation of the chemotherapy and presented as multiple asymptomatic brownish macules distributed over the photo-protected areas of all four extremities, sparing the mucosae, palms, and soles. The pathology examination showed elongated hyperpigmented rete ridges with increased number of S-100 positive cells within the basal layer. The authors concluded that the eruptive lentigines developed secondary to immunosuppression associated with the chemotherapy.

Hydroquinone (Exogenous Ochronosis)

Hydroquinone is used as topical bleaching in treatment of melasma. The principal adverse effects of its chronic use are confetti-like depigmentation and a gray-brown or blue-black hyperpigmentation (Fig. 22.9a, b), as well as pinpoint hyperchromic papules that look like caviar [16]. Histopathology is identical to that of the endogenous form (Fig. 22.9c).

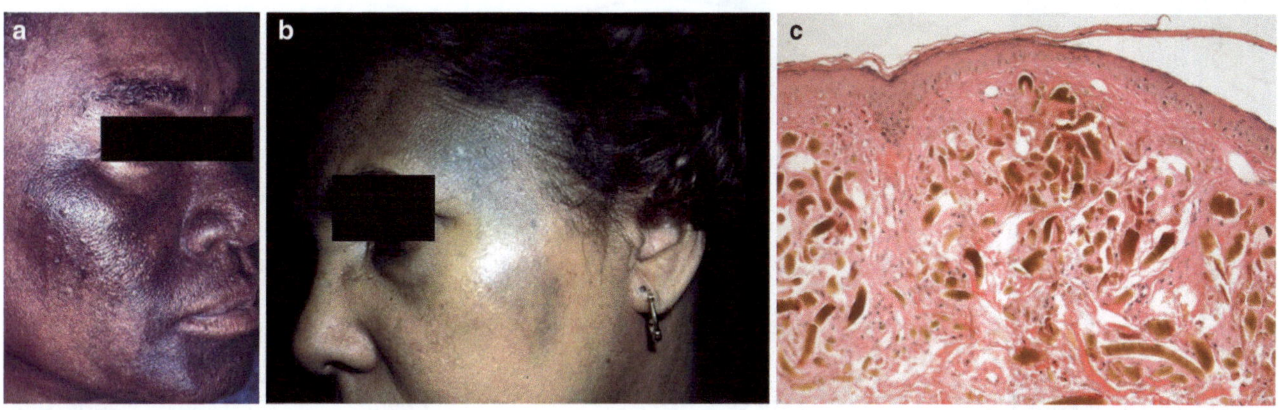

Fig. 22.9 Exogenous ochronosis. (**a**) Blue-black hyperpigmentation after longstanding application of hydroquinone (Courtesy of Kenneth E. Greer, Charlotteville, VA). (**b**) Another case of gray-blue pigmentation of the face (Courtesy of Kenneth E. Greer, Charlotteville, VA, USA). (**c**) Ocher-colored, irregularly shaped fibers in the dermis, similar to endogenous ochronosis (Courtesy of James W. Patterson, Charlottesville, VA, USA)

Iron

Localized brown to black pigmentation after intramuscular injection (mostly gluteal) may develop days or weeks after the treatment for the injected solution (Fig. 22.10). The pigmentation may spread to the neighboring areas and persists 6–8 months up to several years [17].

Acquired Brachial Cutaneous Dyschromatosis

This condition affects primarily middle-aged women and causes asymptomatic, gray-brown patches with geographic borders to erupt over the dorsum of forearms. This pattern is usually bilateral and spares the face (Fig. 22.11a). These lesions are interspersed with hypopigmented macules [18]. Many of the affected individuals have also features of Civatte's poikiloderma. 65% of the patients have hypertension and have been taking antihypertensive drugs, especially angiotensin-converting enzyme inhibitors, before the pigmentation occurred.

In the histopathologic examination of the pigmented lesion, there is epidermal atrophy, increased basal layer pigmentation (Fig. 22.11b, c), actinic elastosis, and superficial teleangiectasias. Characteristically, no pigmentary incontinence is seen. No macrophages are noted in the papillary dermis.

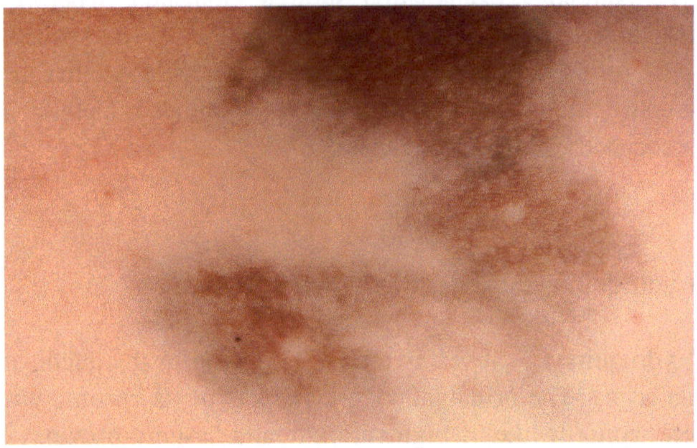

Fig. 22.10 Iron gluteal hyperpigmentation due to intramuscular injections

22.2.2.2 Hyperpigmentation Due to Heavy Metals

Before modern medicine, heavy metals were often utilized as therapeutic agents for many diseases such as syphilis, asthma, psoriasis, rhus dermatitis, and many others. In excess, heavy metals cause hyperpigmentation of the skin. Today, heavy metals are rarely used, and overexposure is a relatively infrequent occurrence.

Silver

Overexposure to silver is known as argyria, which can be generalized or localized. Generalized argyria occurs after exposure to silver substrate or ingestion of silver salts (silver-containing nose or eye drops, ingested or topical silver nitrate, colloidal silver protein drinks, etc) resulting in a diffuse slate-gray hyperpigmentation [19]. Sun-exposed areas are more heavily affected (Fig. 22.12a) and skin folds are spared. Hyperpigmentation is also seen in the sclera, nails (Fig. 22.12b), and mucous membranes. Discoloration typically appears 2–3 years after exposure. In contrast,

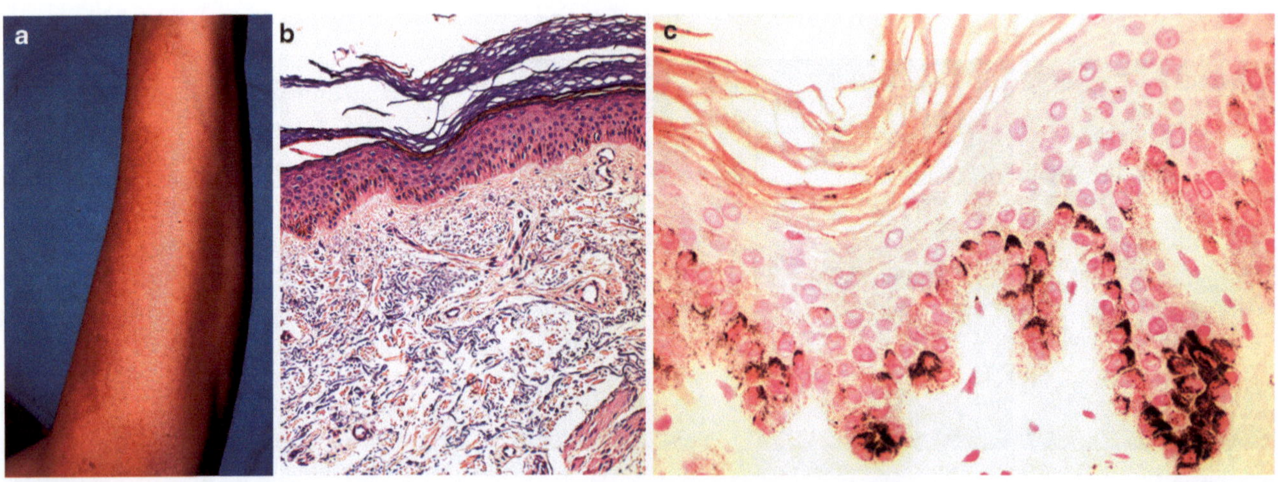

Fig. 22.11 Acquired brachial cutaneous dyschromatosis (ABCD). (**a**) Clinical aspects characterized by a brown patch with geographic borders over the dorsum of forearm. (**b**) Atrophic epidermis, basilar hyperpigmentation (HE stain). (**c**) Basilar hyperpigmentation (Fontana Masson stain for melanin)

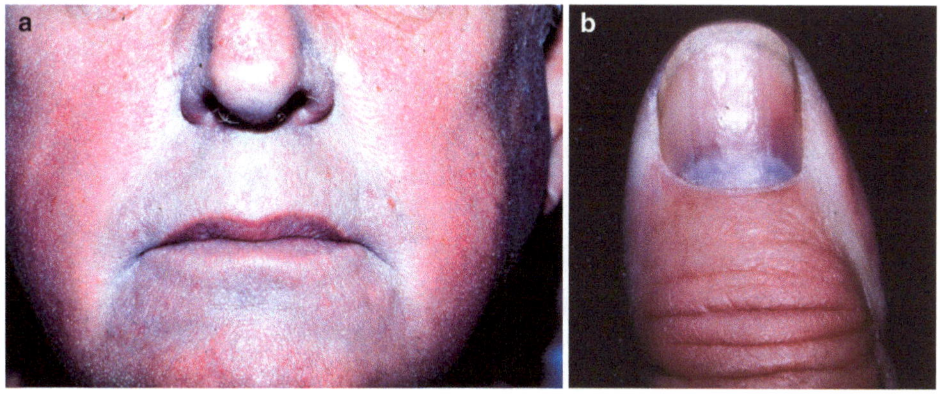

Fig. 22.12 (**a**) Slate-blue-gray hyperpigmentation due to argyria. (**b**) Nail pigmentation in argyria

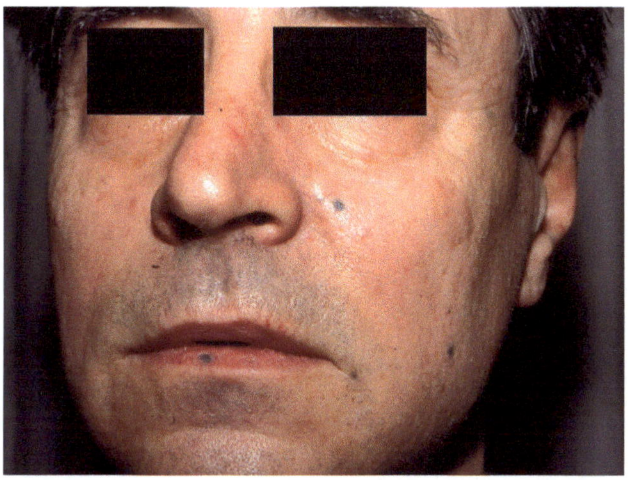

Fig. 22.13 Blue nevi-like occupational argyria

localized cutaneous argyria presents with an asymptomatic blue-gray macule due to diverse etiologies including occupational exposures in workers dealing with metal manufacturing [20], topical medications, alternative medical therapies, body jewelry, and dental procedures (amalgam tattoos). The lesions may mimic blue nevi and even malignant melanoma (Fig. 22.13).

Histologically, brown-black granules are present singly or in clusters within the basement membrane of sweat glands (Fig. 22.14a). Granules are also seen within the connective tissue, where they have a predilection for elastic fibers (Fig. 22.14b) and within the basal lamina of the epidermis (Fig. 22.14c), hair follicles, sebaceous glands, and blood vessels. Silver granules are brilliantly refractile under dark-field microscopy. Ellipsoid black globules within an area of degenerated collagen are reported in blue nevi-like argyria (Fig. 22.14d). There is also an increase in melanin. Electron microscopy reveals electron-dense deposits within macrophages and fibroblasts (Fig. 22.15).

Gold

Today, gold is still sometimes used as an alternative treatment for disease, most notably in the treatment of refractory rheumatoid arthritis. Excess gold exposure, or chrysiasis, causes a blue-gray pigmentation that is limited to sun-exposed areas of the body (Fig. 22.16a). It is more pronounced around the eyes; the nails and mucous membranes are spared. Chrysiasis causes a permanent hyperpigmentation that occurs months to years following exposure. Localized chrysiasis was induced in patients receiving parenteral gold therapy who underwent treatment with a Q-switched ruby laser. This form of chrysiasis resulted from a structural alteration in dermal gold deposits [21].

Histologically, small, round to oval, black granules are seen around blood vessels and within phagolysosomes of dermal macrophages (Fig. 22.16b). The dyspigmentation of chrysiasis is due to deposition of the metal in addition to altered reflection of melanin.

Mercury

Historically, mercury was commonly found in many skin bleaching creams, and long-term use was found to cause a slate-gray discoloration of the skin [22]. The skin folds are affected most prominently, especially at the eyelids, nasolabial folds, and neck folds. Systemically, mercury overexposure can lead to neuropsychiatric toxicity. Dyspigmentation is a result of direct deposition of mercury and an increase in melanin production.

Histologically, mercury granules are brown-black and seen within the upper dermis within macrophages and surrounding capillaries, elastic fibers, and collagen. Granules are brilliantly refractile under dark-field microscopy. The basal epidermis and dermal melanophages demonstrate increased melanin.

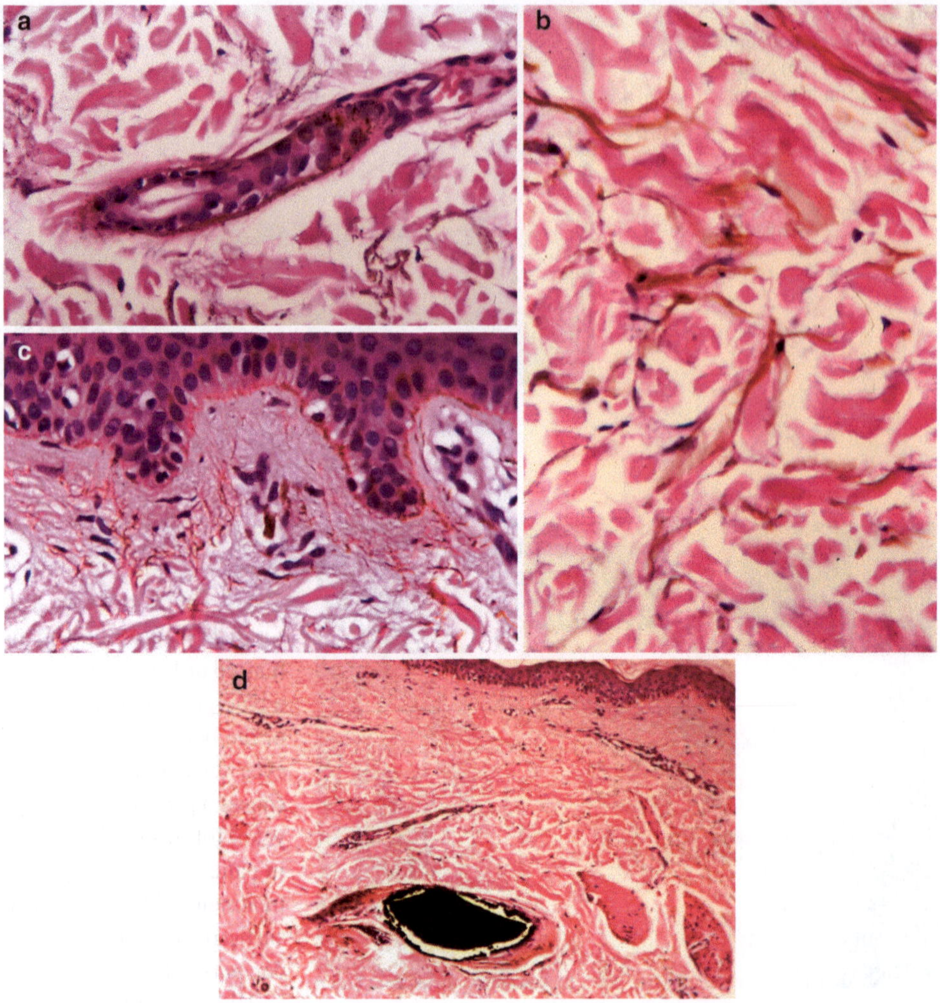

Fig. 22.14 Argyria. (**a**) Deposition of granules in clusters with in the basement membrane of sweat glands. (**b**) Deposition of granules in cluster on the elastic fibers. (**c**) Deposition of silver along the basal lamina of the epidermis and the elastic fibers of papillary dermis. (**d**) Ellipsoid black globule within an area of degenerated collagen in blue-nevi like argyria

Arsenic

Arsenic exposure to humans mainly occurs from the ingestion of arsenic-contaminated water and food [23]. The skin seems to be quite susceptible to the effects of this agent and arsenic-induced skin lesions seem to be the most common and initial symptoms of arsenicosis. Prolonged exposure to arsenic results in a diffuse bronze pigmentation of the skin, which is more prominent in the trunk. It produces a characteristic "raindrop" appearance, where small areas of normal to hypopigmented skin are scattered over a diffuse hyperpigmented background. There is also hyperkeratosis of the palms and soles. The nails demonstrate transverse leukonychia, known as Mees lines. Dyspigmentation occurs 1–20 years following exposure and is due to both deposition of metal and increased production of melanin.

Bismuth

Bismuth-containing compounds have been used in the past to treat many diseases such as venereal disease, psoriasis, and lichen planus. Systemic symptoms of toxicity include nephropathy, stomatitis, vomiting, diarrhea, and neurotoxicity. Bismuth toxicity produces a blue-gray hyperpigmentation of the skin that is generalized and most prominent over the face, neck, and hands [24]. Oral mucosa may also be affected, producing a blue-black gingival line.

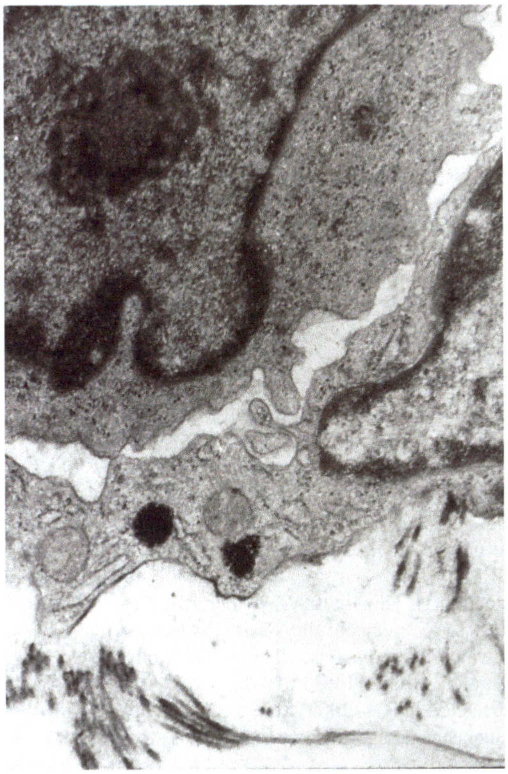

Fig. 22.15 Electron-dense deposits of silver within macrophages in argyria

Histology reveals small granulations in the papillary and reticular dermis.

Lead

Lead toxicity, also known as plumbism, leads to lethargy, gastrointestinal disturbances, peripheral neuritis, and encephalopathy. Eighty percent of patients show a characteristic blue-gray line over the marginal gingivae, known as Burton's line [25].

22.3 Treatment and Prognosis

Over time, alkaptonuria leads to a severe, debilitating arthropathy. Destruction of the joints is due to accumulation of ochronotic pigment. No specific treatment exists either for cutaneous or extracutaneous symptoms of endogenous ochronosis. High-dose ascorbic acid may give some improvement [2]. Exogenous ochronosis induced by topical hydroquinones may be treated with carbon dioxide or Q-switched Nd:YAG lasers.

Hyperpigmentation due to drugs is usually reversible with discontinuation of the therapy. Q-switched lasers have shown benefit when resolution is incomplete or in patients whose pigmentation persists [26]

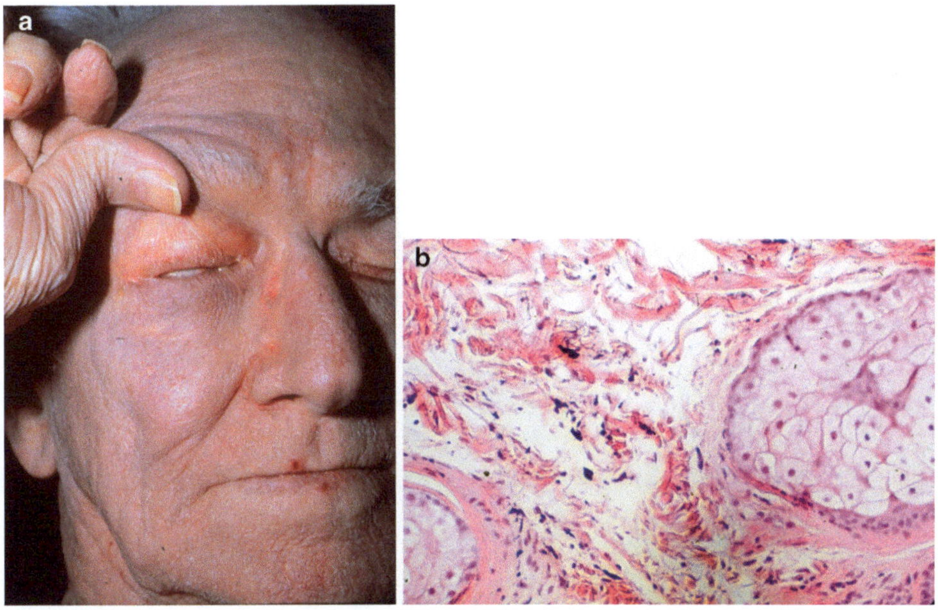

Fig. 22.16 Chrysiasis. (**a**) Slate-gray pigmentation due to chrysiasis. (**b**) Fine blue-black granules within macrophages surrounding vessels in the reticular dermis (H-E stain)

References

1. Lio PA, Sober AJ (2006) Drug-induced or -related pigment. In: Nordlund JJ (ed) The pigmentary system: physiology and pathophysiology. Blackwell, Malden, MA, pp 1026–1054
2. Turgay E, Canat D, Gurel MS, Yuksel T, Baran MF, Demirkesen C (2009) Endogenous ochronosis. Clin Exp Dermatol 34:865–868
3. Dereure O (2001) Drug-induced skin pigmentation: epidemiology, diagnosis and treatment. Am J Clin Derm 2:253
4. Reynaert S, Setterfield J, Black MM (2006) Hydroxychloroquine-induced pigmentation in two patients with systemic lupus erythematosus. J Eur Acad Dermatol Venereol 20:487–488
5. Amichai B, Gat A, Grunwald MH (2007) Cutaneous hyperpigmentation during therapy with hydroxychloroquine. J Clin Rheumatol 13:113
6. Loganathan S (2007) Chlorpromazine-induced skin pigmentation with short-term use in a patient with bipolar disorder: a case report. Prim Care Companion J Clin Psychiatry 9:316–317
7. D'Agostino ML, Risser J, Robinson-Bostom L (2009) Imipramine-induced hyperpigmentation: a case report and review of the literature. J Cutan Pathol 36:799–803
8. Narurkar V, Smoller BR, Hu CH, Bauer EA (1993) Desipramine-induced blue-gray photosensitive pigmentation. Arch Dermatol 129:474–476
9. Sicari MC, Lebwohl M, Baral J, Wexler P, Gordon RE, Phelps RG (1999) Photoinduced dermal pigmentation in patients taking tricyclic antidepressants: histology, electron microscopy, and energy dispersive spectroscopy. J Am Acad Dermatol 40:290–293
10. Youssef S, Langevin KK, Young LC (2009) Minocycline-induced pigmentation mimicking persistent ecchymosis. Cutis 84:22–26
11. Bowen AR, McCalmont THJ (2007) The histopathology of subcutaneous minocycline pigmentation. J Am Acad Dermatol 57:836–839
12. High WA, Weiss SD (2001) Images in clinical medicine. Pigmentation related to amiodarone. N Engl J Med 345:1464
13. Susser WS, Whitaker-Worth DL, Grant-Kels JM (1999) Mucocutaneous reactions to chemotherapy. J Am Acad Dermatol 40: 367–398
14. Sanborn RE, Sauer DA (2008) Cutaneous reactions to chemotherapy: commonly seen, less described, little understood. Dermatol Clin 26:103–119
15. De D, Dogra AL, Kanwar AJ, Saikia UN (2010) Generalized eruptive lentigines induced by chemotherapy. Clin Exp Dermatol 35(4):e113–e115
16. Charlín R, Barcaui CB, Kac BK, Soares DB, Rabello-Fonseca R, Azulay-Abulafia L (2008) Hydroquinone-induced exogenous ochronosis: a report of four cases and usefulness of dermoscopy. Int J Dermatol 47:19–23
17. Christian Raulin C, Werner S, Greve B (2001) Circumscripted pigmentations after iron injections-treatment with Q-switched laser systems. Lasers Surg Med 28:456–460
18. Rongioletti F, Rebora A (2000) Acquired brachial cutaneous dyschromatosis: a common pigmentary disorder of the arm in middle-aged women. J Am Acad Dermatol 42:680–684
19. Brandt D, Park B, Hoang M, Jacobe HT (2005) Argyria secondary to ingestion of homemade silver solution. J Am Acad Dermatol 53:S105–S107
20. Rongioletti F, Robert E, Buffa P, Bertagno R, Rebora A (1992) Blue nevi-like dotted occupational argyria. J Am Acad Dermatol 27:1015–1016
21. Almoallim H, Klinkhoff AV, Arthur AB, Rivers JK, Chalmers A (2006) Laser induced chrysiasis: disfiguring hyperpigmentation following Q-switched laser therapy in a woman previously treated with gold. J Rheumatol 33:620–621
22. Dadzie OE, Petit A (2009) Skin bleaching: highlighting the misuse of cutaneous depigmenting agents. J Eur Acad Dermatol Venereol 23:741–750
23. Rahman MM, Ng JC, Naidu R (2009) Chronic exposure of arsenic via drinking water and its adverse health impacts on humans. Environ Geochem Health 31(Suppl 1):189–200
24. Granstein RD, Sober AJ (1981) Drug- and heavy metal–induced hyperpigmentation. J Am Acad Dermatol 5:1–18
25. Camuglia JE, Grigoriadis G, Gilfillan CP (2008) Lead poisoning and Burton's line. Med J Aust 189:339
26. Stratigos AJ, Katsambas AD (2004) Optimal management of recalcitrant disorders of hyperpigmentation in dark-skinned patients. Am J Clin Dermatol 5:161–168

Chapter 23
Exogenous Cutaneous Deposits with Special Consideration to Skin Reactions to Soft-Tissue Fillers

Franco Rongioletti

Key Points

- Any nonliving material introduced into the skin and resistant to degradation may trigger an inflammatory response.
- The origin and way of introduction goes from traumatic (accidental or self-induced) to cosmetic and surgical procedures to topical application of drugs and products.
- The increased use of exogenous injectable aesthetic microimplants (soft-tissue fillers) is paralleled by an increase in adverse cutaneous reactions.
- The most common clinical presentation of granulomatous reactions includes papules, nodules and stiff infiltration of the skin with or without ulceration.
- Histopathology is a good means to identify the type of exogenous agent, particularly of filler particles.

Keywords Foreign body granulomas • Soft-tissue fillers • Permanent • Biodegradable

23.1 Introduction

Any nonliving material that comes in direct contact with the skin is perceived as foreign and can induce a granulomatous reaction. The main exogenous causes of foreign body granulomas are: silica, talc, sutures, sea-urchin spine, beryllium, zirconium, graphite, mercury, hemostatic agents such as Monsel's solution and aluminum chloride (Drysol®), vegetable matter (including wood splinters, *Lycopodium clavatum* spores), mineral and vegetable oil, polyvinylpyrrolidone, artificial and true hairs, tattoos and dermal fillers for tissue augmentation [1–3].

F. Rongioletti (✉)
Department of Endocrinological and Medical Sciences (DISEM)
Section of Dermatology and Department of Pathology
University of Genova, Genova, Italy
e-mail: franco.rongioletti@unige.it

23.2 Clinical and Pathological Aspects of Skin Manifestations

23.2.1 Skin Reactions to Soft Tissue Fillers

Given the recent boom of the cosmetic industry and the increasing demand for soft tissue augmentation without surgery, various soft-tissue fillers have been developed and put into the market. However, different local or systemic adverse reactions have been reported with increased frequency, both with permanent (more frequent) and biodegradable or resorbable products [4, 5]. Adverse skin reactions may be divided into (1) immediate occurring within days of the injection, and (2) delayed, occurring after weeks or years. The main immediate or early reactions include bruising generally limited to around the injection site, transient swelling, tenderness, hematoma, and infections due to herpes simplex or common skin pathogens such as *Staphylococcus aureus*. Delayed reactions include substantially true granulomas, which are characterized by progressively developing papules, nodules, plaques, or stiff infiltration at the site of injections (Figs. 23.1 and 23.2a–c) that may lead to retracted, disfiguring scars (Fig. 23.2d). They have a variable incidence ranging from 0.01 to 14%. The pathogenesis of these granulomatous reactions includes at least four possibilities: (1) Improper substances injected fraudulently, (2) Hypersensitivity reactions, (3) Impurity of microimplants, (4) Bad technique. Histopathology is very useful to make a diagnosis, as the particular configuration of the vacuoles and cystic structures inside the granulomas reflects the shape of the injected implants particles (Table 23.1). Interferon and other immunostimulatory medications have been described to exacerbate such inflammatory reactions [6].

Permanent fillers carry a higher risk of granulomatous reactions. The major permanent fillers include silicone, microspheres of polymethylmethacrylate suspended in collagen (Artecoll® and Artefill®), ethylmethacrylate microspheres suspended in hyaluronic acid (Dermalive® DermaDeep®), polyvinylpyrrolidone-silicone suspension (Bioplastique), and polyacrylamide (Aquamid). The granulomata induced by silicone show a peculiar pattern of extracellular round or oval

F. Rongioletti and B.R. Smoller (eds.), *Clinical and Pathological Aspects of Skin Diseases in Endocrine, Metabolic, Nutritional and Deposition Disease*, DOI 10.1007/978-1-60761-181-3_23, © Springer Science+Business Media, LLC 2010

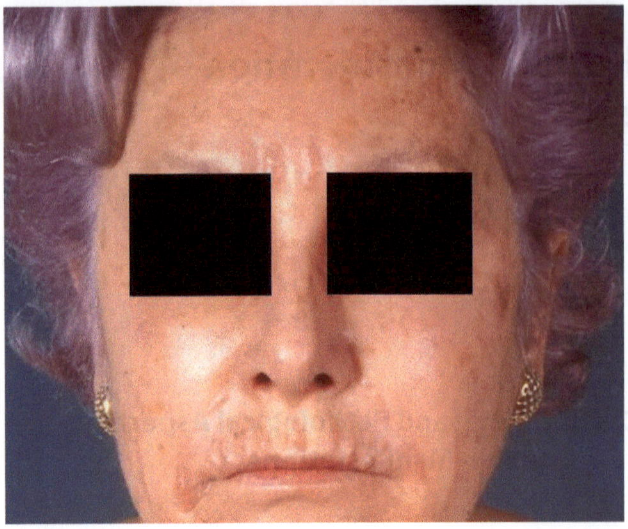

Fig. 23.1 Linear papules and nodules with stiff infiltration on the glabella, nasolabial folds, and around the lips after injection with hyaluronic acid

vacuoles of different size, sometimes confluent, giving the reaction the appearance of Swiss cheese (Fig. 23.3). The vacuoles are surrounded by epithelioid histiocytes with their cytoplasm replete with tiny vacuoles giving them a foamy appearance. These vacuolated histiocytes may mimic lipoblasts (Fig. 23.4), and in the absence of adequate clinical information, a misdiagnosis of liposarcoma can be made [7]. The granulomata induced by microspheres of polymethylmethacrylate suspended in collagen (Artecoll® and Artefill®) are characterized by multiple small, round cystic spaces of approximately the same size and shape, mimicking normal adipocytes (Fig. 23.5), surrounded by epithelioid cells with a few multinucleate giant cells. The granulomas induced by ethylmethacrylate microspheres suspended in hyaluronic acid (Dermalive® DermaDeep®) are characterized by multiple small, translucent pinkish particles of slightly different sizes, polygonal or irregularly shaped, nonbirefringent, unevenly distributed on a background of finely fibrillar collagen with a giant-cell granulomatous reaction (Fig. 23.6).

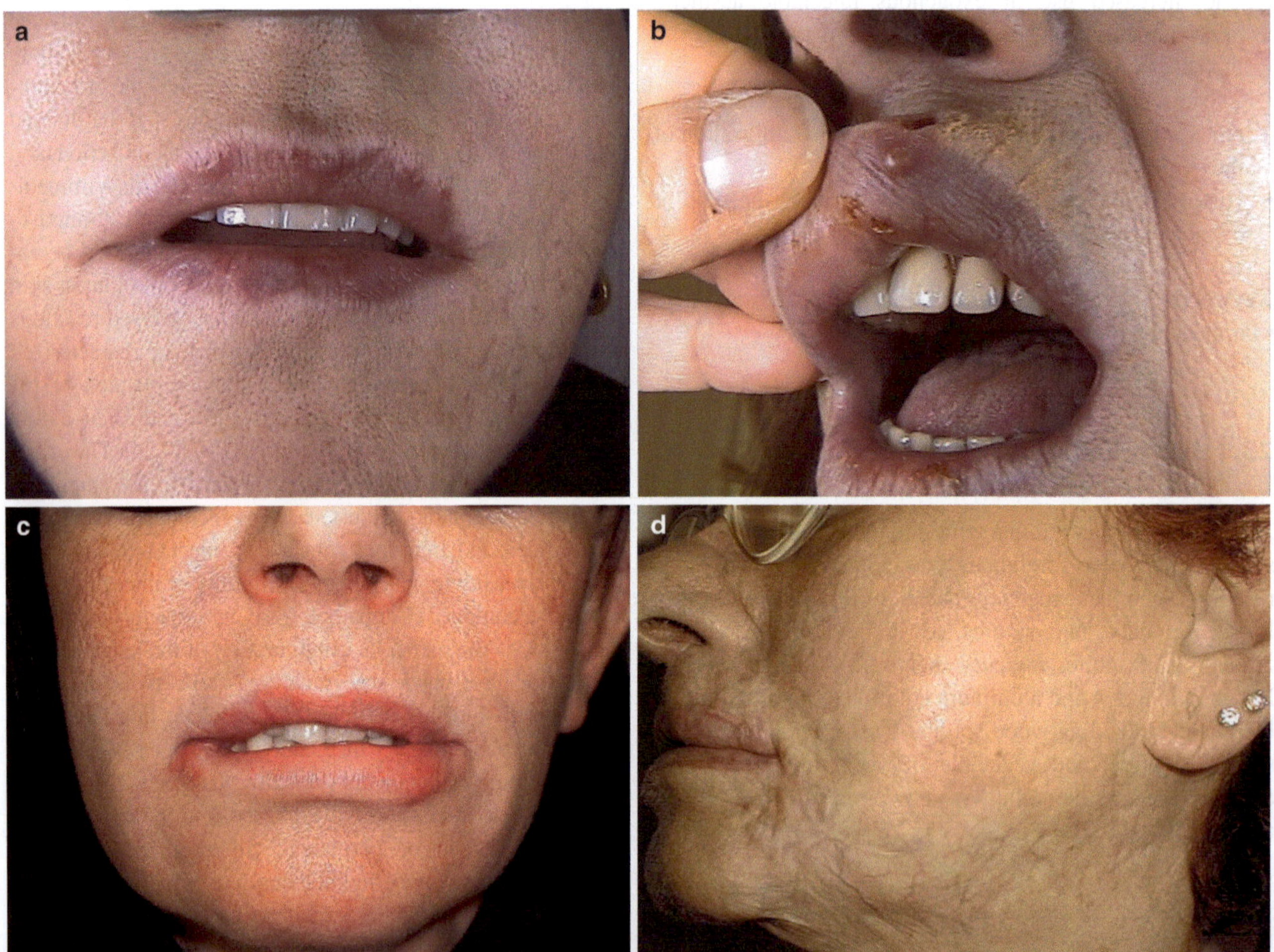

Fig. 23.2 (**a**) Lip granuloma induced by silicone. (**b**) Lip granuloma induced by silicone (Courtesy of M. De Padova, Bologna). (**c**) Lip granuloma due to hyaluronic acid. (**d**) Disfiguring retractional scars due to silicone injection (Courtesy of M. Romagnoli, Genoa, Italy)

Table 23.1 Histologic features of granulomas induced by commonly used cosmetic fillers

Commercial names	Zyderm Zyplast	Restylane® Hylaform®	Sculptra™ New Fill	Silikon 1000 Silskin	Artecoll	Dermalive	Bioplastique
Composition	Purified bovine collagen	Hyaluronic acid	Poly-lactic acid microspheres in mannitol and carbomethoxycellulose	Liquid silicone (polydimethylsiloxane)	Polymethylmethacrylate microspheres in collagen	Acrylic hydrogel particles in hyaluronic acid	Solid silicone particles in polyvinylpyrrolidone
Category	Resorbable	Resorbable	Biodegradable	Permanent	Permanent	Permanent	Permanent
Histologic pattern of granulomas	Thick, brightly eosinophilic, non birefringent collagen lacking the fibrillar nature of native collagen surrounded by histiocytes, foreign giant cells, neutrophils, eosinophils	Irregularly shaped drops of amorphous basophilic material similar to mucin (Alcian blue+) surrounded by giant cells and histiocytes	Translucent particles, birefringent in polarized light with a fusiform or spiky shape surrounded by giant cells and lymphocytes	Extracellular vacuoles of different size (Swiss-cheese pattern). Foamy histiocytes mimicking lipoblasts	Small round vacuoles of the same size and shape mimicking normal adipocytes surrounded by giant cells, vacuolated histiocytes, lymphocytes and eosinophils in a loose sclerotic stroma	Irregularly shaped cystic structures containing translucent pinkish non-birefringent particles of different sizes with a giant cells reaction	Irregularly shaped cystic structures containing "pop-corn-shaped" translucent, non birefringent particles. Giant cells surrounding the spaces and occasionally protruding into them

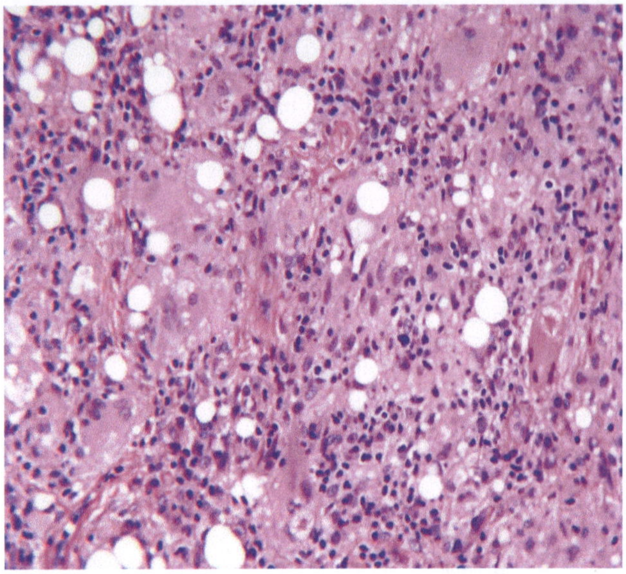

Fig. 23.3 Swiss-cheese granuloma due to silicone (HE stain)

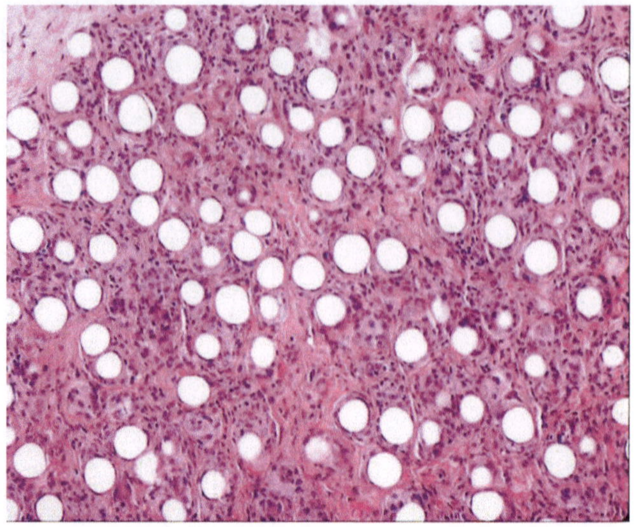

Fig. 23.5 Small *round* vacuoles of the same size and shape mimicking normal adipocytes surrounded by a granulomatous reaction, induced by Artecoll (HE stain)

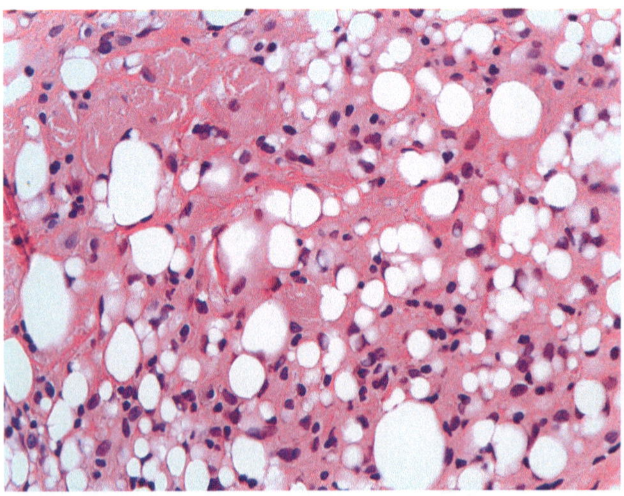

Fig. 23.4 Vacuolated histiocytes mimicking lipoblasts in granuloma induced by silicone (HE stain)

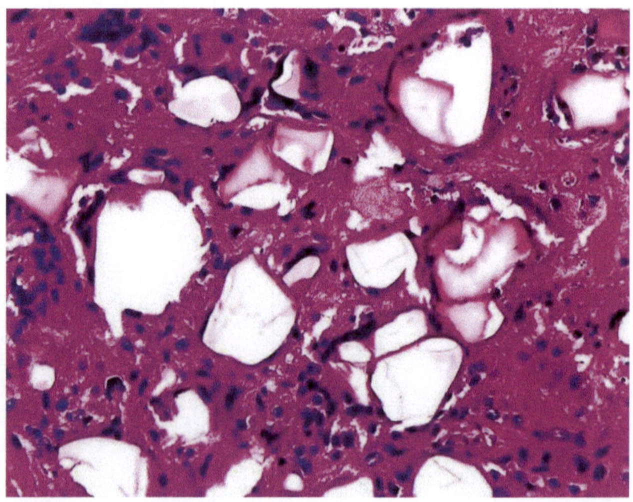

Fig. 23.6 Irregularly shaped cystic structures containing translucent *pinkish* particles of slightly different sizes surrounded by a granulomatous reaction, induced by Dermalive (HE stain)

The granulomata induced by Bioplastique are characterized by numerous irregularly shaped cystic structures that contain many "popcorn-shaped", translucent, nonbirefringent particles of silicone. Multinucleated giant cells surround the cystic spaces, occasionally protruding into them, forming "arabesque" projections, and exhibiting asteroid bodies. Polyacrylamide gel (Aquamid, Outline, Evolution, Bio-Alcamid) may induce a granulomatous reaction surrounding amorphous basophilic material, positive by Alcian blue stain and similar in appearance to hyaluronic acid. The basophilic debris is found in the cytoplasm of the giant cells (Fig. 23.7) [4, 5, 8].

Although not commonly, biodegradable fillers are also capable of inducing granulomatous reactions. The main biodegradable fillers include: *polylactic acid* consisting of microspheres in mannitol and carbomethoxycellulose, approved by the European Union (as New Fill®) and the Food and Drug Administration in the USA (as Sculptra™), for HIV facial lipoatrophy; *hyaluronic acid derivatives* which are at present the treatment of choice in Europe for wrinkles, lip augmentation, and scars; bovine (Zyderm I and II, Zyplast, Resoplast) and human *collagen* and *calcium hydroxylapatite*. The granulomas induced by polylactic acid exhibit multiple translucent particles of different sizes (between 10 and 125 μm) with a fusiform or spiky shape surrounded by numerous giant cells with a mild lymphocytic infiltrate (Fig. 23.8a) [4, 9]. Particles are birefringent in polarized light (Fig. 23.8b), and giant cells occasionally contain asteroid bodies. Hyaluronic acid derivatives, both of bacterial origin

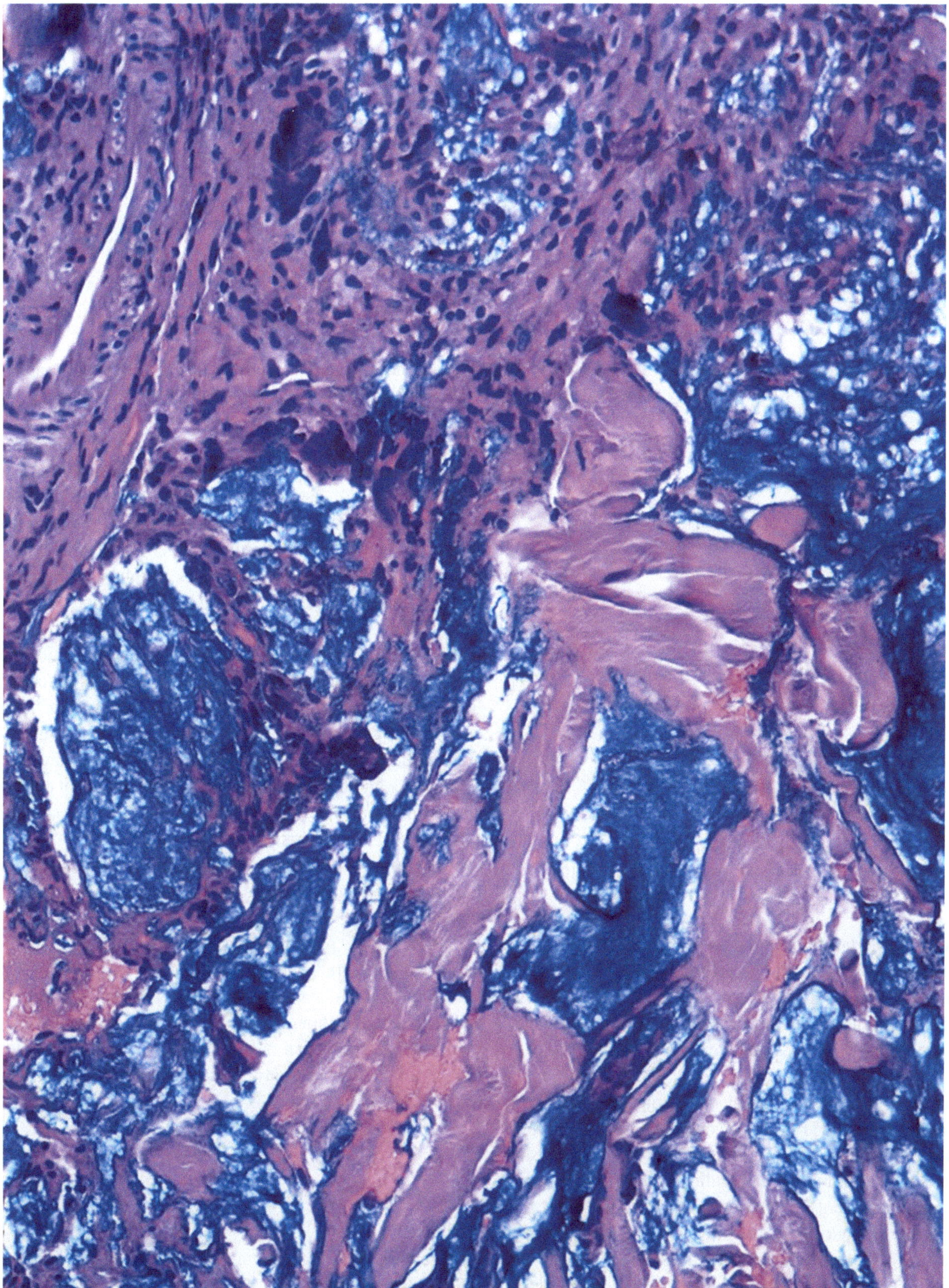

Fig. 23.7 Amorphous basophilic material, composed by polyacrylamide with basophilic debris in the cytoplasm of the giant cells (HE stain)

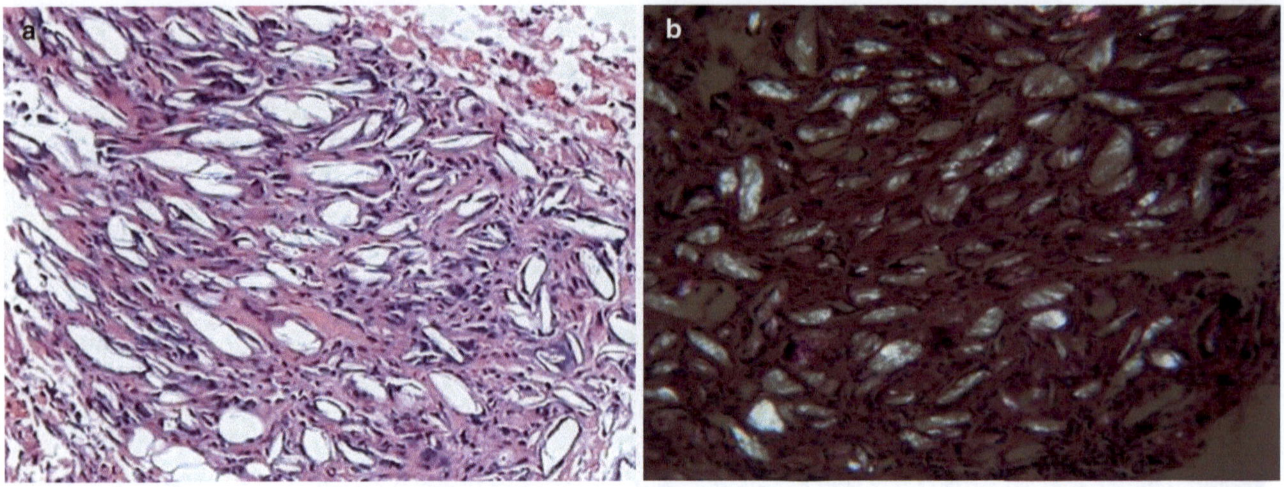

Fig. 23.8 (**a**) Translucent particles with a fusiform or spiky shape surrounded by a giant cells granulomatous reaction, induced by polylactic acid (HE stain). (**b**) The spiky particles of polylactic acid are birefringent with polarized light

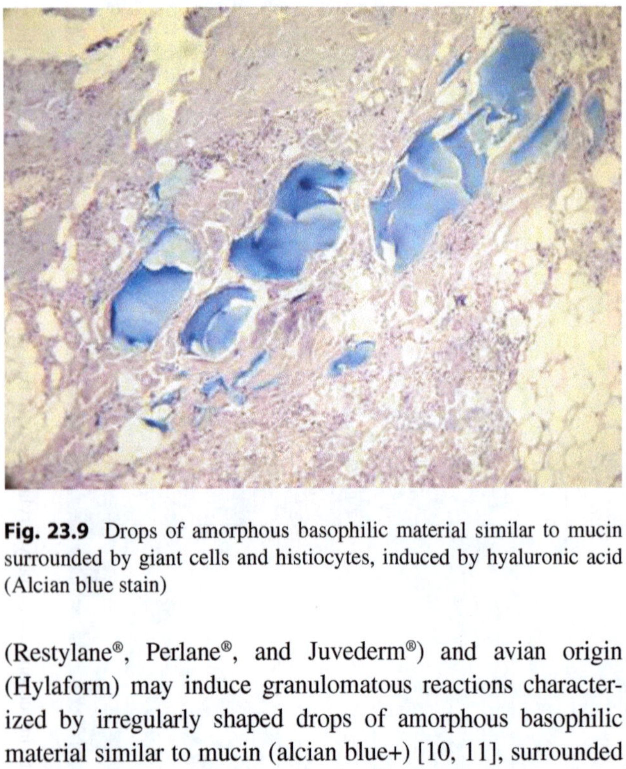

Fig. 23.9 Drops of amorphous basophilic material similar to mucin surrounded by giant cells and histiocytes, induced by hyaluronic acid (Alcian blue stain)

(Restylane®, Perlane®, and Juvederm®) and avian origin (Hylaform) may induce granulomatous reactions characterized by irregularly shaped drops of amorphous basophilic material similar to mucin (alcian blue+) [10, 11], surrounded by multinucleated giant cells and epithelioid histiocytes in the dermis and subcutaneous fat (Fig. 23.9). The development of scleromyxedema after hyaluronic acid injections has been anecdotally described [12]. Bovine collagen (Zyderm) is composed mainly of type I collagen that can be recognized in skin biopsies as it is lightly eosinophilic in hematoxylin–eosin preparations; it is not birefringent under polarized light and stains a pale gray-violet color with Masson's trichrome stain. The human collagen is divided into allogeneic (Dermalogen, AlloDerm, Fascian, Cymetra, Cosmoderm) and autologous (Autologen). The latter preparations are derived from the patient's own tissues. Homologous collagen dispersion (Dermalogen®) and bovine cross-linked collagen (Zyplast®) have been largely used in augmenting human dermis. Three to five percent of patients treated with injectable collagen implants have adverse local reactions, but Dermalogen® proved to be more immunogenic than Zyplast®. Histological analysis reveals the presence of thick, brightly eosinophilic, nonbirefringent bundles of collagen lacking the fibrillar nature of native collagen in the dermis or the subcutis, surrounded by a polymorphic inflammatory reaction with signs of fibroplasias [5, 13]. In addition to the classic features of a foreign-body granuloma, different forms of granulomatous reaction to collagen have been reported at the site of injection including a necrobiotic granuloma resembling granuloma annulare and a sarcoid-like granulomatous panniculitis involving not only the site of injection but also distant sites associated with systemic symptoms [14, 15]. Granulomatous reactions, although rare, occur also with calcium hydroxylapatite (Radiesse), and the presence of blue-gray calcific microspheres are the histologic markers [5].

Migration of "permanent" implants such as silicone and expanded polytetrafluorethylene has been well documented. This occurs much less frequently with temporary fillers that are reabsorbed, although calcium hydroxylapatite has been involved. Migration can occur several years after the injection. An infection or delayed granulomatous reaction may trigger migration [6, 16].

23.2.2 Miscellanea

Most common exogenous agents capable of inducing an inflammatory foreign-body reaction with a clinicopathological correlation are summarized in Table 23.2 (Figs. 23.10 and 23.11a, b).

Table 23.2 Main features of exogenous reactions

Material	Way of entry/source	Clinical features	Histopathology	Other distinctive findings	Other diagnostic methods
Tattoo	Cosmetic Traumatic, accidental Medical purposes	Erythematous papules, nodules Lichenoid papules Eczematous dermatitis Photosensitive reaction	Pigment granules interspersed between the granulomatous infiltrate (extra or intracellular) Lichenoid dermatitis Spongiotic dermatitis Pseudolymphoma	Red dyes containing mercuric sulfide, chrome green, cobalt blue	
Silica	Injuries Wound contamination from soil or glass	Papules and nodules within scars	Crystalline polarizable particles Sarcoidal granulomas	Delayed time of appearance	Spectrographic analysis
Talc	Surgical procedures, i.v. injections, topical treatment of wound	Erythematous papules, Nodules, hard plaques Pyogenic granuloma-like	Polarizable 10–20 μm, round or needle-shaped crystals Sarcoidal or foreign body granulomas		X-ray diffraction
Suture	Surgical procedures	Erythemato-edematous wound with infiltration and fistolisation	Polarizable yellow fibers Foreign body granulomas	Often histological finding in the absence of clinical symptoms	
Zirconium	Deodorant sticks	Brownish papules (axillary skin)	Sarcoidal granulomas		Non polarizable; Spectrographic analysis or X-ray microanalysis
Beryllium	Fluorescent light bulbs	Papules, nodules, ulceration	Sarcoidal granulomas Caseating granulomas		Non polarizable; Spectrographic analysis only
Aluminium	Adjuvant in vaccines	Nodules at injection sites	Granulomas with basophilic granular material		X-ray microanalysis
Starch	Surgical glove powder I.V drug abuse	Papules, nodules	Basophilic ovoid, polarizable, 10–20 μm particles Maltese cross birefringence	PAS positive	
Mercury	Thermometer accident Topical mercurial preparations	Papules, nodules	Round black globules surrounded by necrosis with foreign body reaction		X-ray microanalysis
Injectable steroid	Intralesional steroids	Skin-colored papules and nodules at injection site	Amorphous, pale bluish material surrounded by foreign-body granuloma	Weakly PAS positive	
Sea urchin spines	Traumatic/accidental	Pink, brownish papules, nodules, sometimes pain and umbilication	Sarcoidal or foreign-body granuloma Sometimes necrobiotic granuloma and perforation	Calcium carbonate crystals	
Vegetable matter (including wood splinter, cactus spine)	Traumatic/accidental Occupational	Papules with a central black dot	Uniform smaller spaces with cell walls and internal structures Sarcoidal or foreign-body granuloma	PAS positive (cactus)	
Hair	Traumatic Occupational (barbers, dog groomers)	Barbers' sinus		Diagnosis based on history and clinical features	
Paraffin	Tissue augmentation, elimination of wrinkles, and treatment of male pattern baldness		Sclerosing lipogranuloma with "Swiss-cheese" appearance	Diagnosis based on history and clinical features	

23.3 Treatment and Prognosis

Minor complications of filler injections, such as bruising, can be managed with simple observation and reassurance. For lumpiness, mild asymmetry, or mild overcorrection, gentle massage or additional injection may be effective. Delayed granulomas are the most challenging of the long-term adverse affects to treat [17]. Prognosis is usually good for granulomas induced by biodegradable fillers, while permanent microimplants may lead to undesirable sequelae and permanent disfiguring of the face. Topical, intralesional, or oral corticosteroids are usually considered the treatment of choice. However, this treatment bears the risk of disfiguration by skin atrophy with telangiectasis and scarring. Antimicrobial agents, especially minocycline, are often used successfully as "first-line agents" for the treatment of silicone granulomas. Their effectiveness is likely related not only to their ability to inhibit bacterial growth but also to their direct immunosuppressive activity against granulomas. Persistent hyaluronic acid derivate nodules can be treated with hyaluronidase (18). Other anecdotal treatments include topical imiquimod, topical tacrolimus, intralesional 5-fluorouracil, and systemic isotretinoin. Very recently, agents that bind and inhibit TNF-a, either infliximab or etanercept, may hold particular promise as an effective intervention for extensive silicone granulomas that do not respond to first-line treatment with short-term corticosteroids and antibiotics. However, other systemic immunomodulating medications, including thalidomide, cyclosporine, and mycophenolate mofetil, which offer more targeted immunosuppressive activity, are of potential therapeutic interest. Severe granulomas occasionally require surgical excision (17, 18).

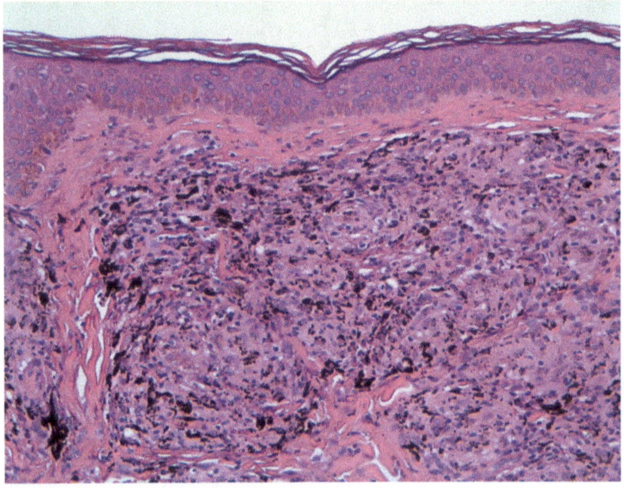

Fig. 23.10 Tattoo reaction (HE stain)

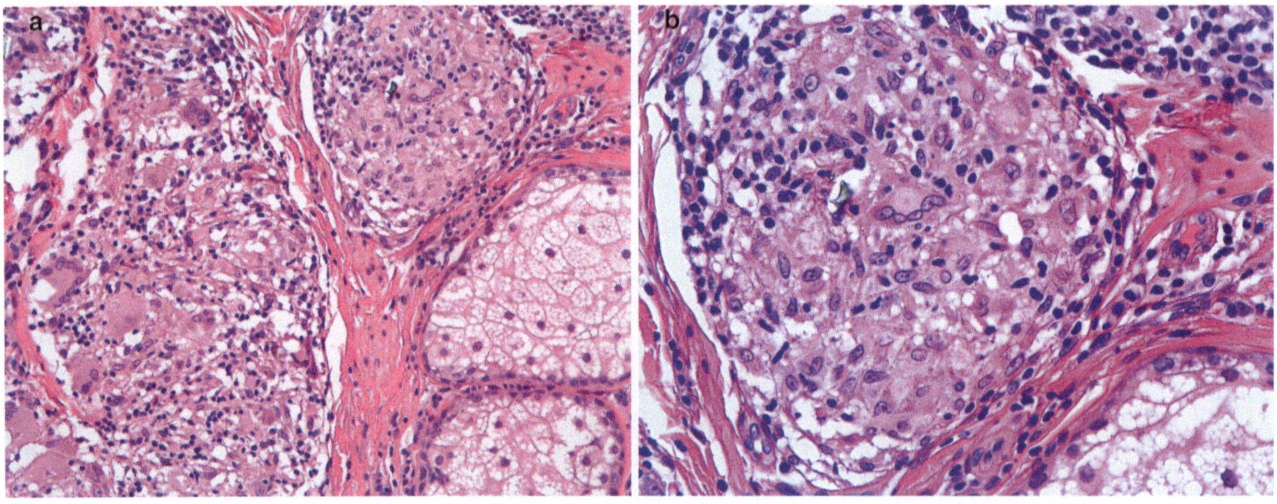

Fig. 23.11 (**a**) Sarcoidal reaction to silica. (**b**) Note the silica particle inside the granuloma (HE stain)

References

1. Abdallah M (2008) Foreign body reactions. In: Bolognia J, Jorizzo JL, Rapini R (eds) Dermatology, 2nd edn. Mosby, Elsevier, St Louis, MO, pp 1437–1446
2. Del Rosario RN, Barr RJ, Graham BS, Kaneshiro S (2005) Exogenous and endogenous cutaneous anomalies and curiosities. Am J Dermatopathol 27:259–267
3. Boztepe G, Rakhshanfar M, Erkin G, Ozkaya O, Sahin S (2005) Cutaneous silica granuloma: a lesion that might be clinically underdiagnosed. Eur J Dermatol 15:194–195
4. Rongioletti F (2008) Granulomatous reactions from aesthetic dermal micro-implants. Ann Dermatol Venereol 135:1S59–1S65
5. Dadzie OE, Mahalingam M, Parada M, El Helou T, Philips T, Bhawan J (2008) Adverse cutaneous reactions to soft tissue fillers- a review of the histological features. J Cutan Pathol 35: 536–548
6. Fischer J, Metzler G, Schaller M (2007) Cosmetic permanent fillers for soft tissue augmentation: a new contraindication for interferon therapies. Arch Dermatol 143:507–510
7. Mustacchio V, Cabibi D, Minervini MI, Barresi E, Amato S (2007) A diagnostic trap for the dermatopathologist: granulomatous reactions from cutaneous microimplants for cosmetic purposes. J Cutan Pathol 34:281–283
8. Vargas-Machuca I, Gonzalez-Guerra E, Angulo J, del Carmen Farina M, Martin L, Requena L (2006) Facial granulomas secondary to Dermalive microimplants: report of a case with histopathologic differential diagnosis among the granulomas secondary to different injectable permanent filler materials. Am J Dermatopathol 28: 173–177
9. Apikian M, Roberts S, Goodman GJ (2007) Adverse reactions to polylactic acid injections in the periorbital area. J Cosmet Dermatol 6:95–101
10. Sidwell RU, Dhillon AP, Butler PE, Rustin MH (2004) Localized granulomatous reaction to a semi-permanent hyaluronic acid and acrylic hydrogel cosmetic filler. Clin Exp Dermatol 29: 630–632
11. Ghislanzoni M, Bianchi F, Barbareschi M, Alessi E (2006) Cutaneous granulomatous reaction to injectable hyaluronic acid gel. Br J Dermatol 154:755–758
12. Rongioletti F, Cattarini G, Sottofattori E, Rebora A (2003) Granulomatous reaction after intradermal injections of hyaluronic acid gel. Arch Dermatol 139:815–816
13. Sclafani AP, Romo T, Parker A, McCormick SA, Cocker R, Jacono A (2002) Homologous collagen dispersion (Dermalogen) as a dermal filler: persistence and histology compared with bovine collagen. Ann Plast Surg 49(2):181–188
14. Barr RJ, King DF, McDonald RM, Bartlow GA (1982) Necrobiotic granulomas associated with bovine collagen test site injections. J Am Acad Dermatol 6:867–869
15. García-Domingo MI, Alijotas-Reig J, Cisteró-Bahima A, Tresserra F, Enrique E (2000) Disseminated and recurrent sarcoid-like granulomatous panniculitis due to bovine collagen injection. J Investig Allergol Clin Immunol 10:107–109
16. Lowe NJ, Maxwell CA, Patnaik R (2005) Adverse reactions to dermal fillers:review. Dermatol Surg 31:1616–1625
17. Wolfram D, Tzankov A, Piza-Katzer H (2006) Surgery for foreign body reactions due to injectable fillers. Dermatology 213: 300–304
18. Sclafani AP, Fagien S (2009). Treatment of injectable soft tissue filler complications. Dermatol Surg 35:1672–1680

Index

MIX
Papier aus verantwortungsvollen Quellen
Paper from responsible sources
FSC® C105338

If you have any concerns about our products,
you can contact us on
ProductSafety@springernature.com

In case Publisher is established outside the EU,
the EU authorized representative is:
Springer Nature Customer Service Center GmbH
Europaplatz 3, 69115 Heidelberg, Germany

Printed by Libri Plureos GmbH
in Hamburg, Germany